LEUKEMIA

Edited by **Margarita Guenova**
and **Gueorgui Balatzenko**

Leukemia
http://dx.doi.org/10.5772/45914
Edited by Margarita Guenova and Gueorgui Balatzenko

Contributors

Jelena Roganovic, Margarita Guenova, Ota Fuchs, Gamal Abdul Hamid, Gerrit Jan Schuurhuis, Wendelien Zeijlemaker, Jesús-María Hernández, Spiro Konstantinov, Maya Zaharieva, G. Amudov

Published by InTech

Janeza Trdine 9, 51000 Rijeka, Croatia

Publishing Process Manager Ana Pantar
Technical Editor InTech DTP team
Cover InTech Design team

Additional hard copies can be obtained from orders@intechopen.com

Leukemia, Edited by Margarita Guenova and Gueorgui Balatzenko
p. cm.
ISBN 978-953-51-1127-6

For EU product safety concerns :
IN TECH d . o . o . , Prolaz Marije Krucifikse Kozulić 3 , 51000 Rijeka , Croatia ,
info@intechopen . com or visit our website at intechopen . com .

Meet the editors

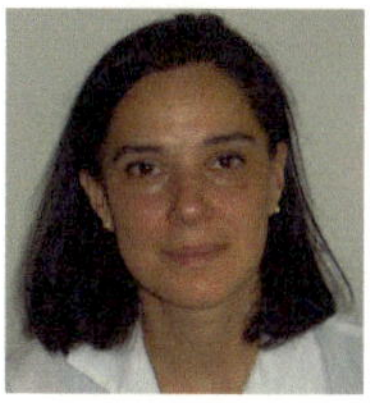

Professor Dr Margarita Guenova received her medical training at the Medical University of Sofia and her PhD degree at the National Center of Haematology in 2000. She is employed as Head of the Laboratory of Haematopathology and Immunology and Professor of Haematology and Blood Transfusion at the National Specialised Hospital for Active Treatment of Haematological Diseases, Sofia, Bulgaria, teaching both undergraduate and graduate studies at the Sofia Medical University. She specializes in the field of leukemia and lymphoma diagnostics. In regard to her scientific interests, she worked on the elucidation of critical mechanisms of leukemia pathogenesis and progression, investigation of clinically relevant biomarkers and potential targets for therapy in leukemias and lymphomas, characterization of leukemic stem cell populations, minimal residual disease and implementation of a multifaceted approach in oncohaematology. Dr Guenova has authored and co-authored many abstracts, articles in peer-reviewed journals and book chapters. She serves on editorial boards and is the President of the Bulgarian Society of Hematology as well as a member of several professional societies such as the Bulgarian Society of Pathology, the Bulgarian Association of Clinical Immunology, the European Hematology Association, the European Association of Haematopathology, the International Society of Haematology.

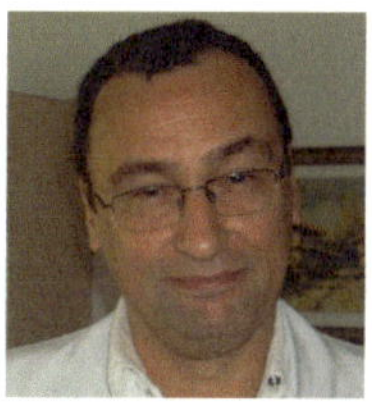

Professor Dr Gueorgui Balatzenko received his medical training at the Medical University of Sofia and his PhD degree at the National Center of Haematology in 2002. He obtained additional qualifications at the Red Cross Blood Bank, Groningen-Drenth, The Netherlands; Institute Paoli-Calmettes Marseille, France; Necker-Enfans Malades, Paris, France. He is Associate Professor of Haematology and Blood Transfusion at the Laboratory of Cytogenetics and Molecular Biology at the National Specialised Hospital for Active Treatment of Haematological Diseases, Sofia, Bulgaria, teaching both undergraduate and graduate studies at the Sofia Medical University. His major interests are in the field of molecular investigations in leukemias. In regard to his scientific achievements, he worked on the elucidation of the incidence and clinical relevance of molecular biomarkers in chronic and acute leukemias, molecular monitoring of treatment response. Dr Balatzenko has authored and co-authored many abstracts, articles in peer-reviewed journals and book chapters. He is a member of several professional societies such as the Bulgarian Society of Hematology, the Bulgarian Society of Genetics, the European Hematology Association, a life member of the UICC, and referee for international journals.

Contents

Preface

Leukemias are a group of heterogeneous neoplastic disorders that differ significantly in terms of morhological, immunophenotypic, cytogenetic and molecular features of malignant cells. These specific features reflect the differences in the spectrum of underlying biological alterations involved in malignant transformation, and/or variations in the level of hematopoietic stem cells hierarchy where the transforming events occur. Classically, leukemias have been classified according to their cellular origin as myeloid or lymphoid, or according to their course as acute or chronic. During the last two decades a broad spectrum of sophisticated equipment and methods were implemented into the routine practice leading to a better understanding of the development of leukemias. This in term resulted in the invasion of new diagnostic criteria, definition of new entities and categories, introduction of novel therapeutic strategies, as well as improved monitoring of theatment effectiveness.

The continuous and rather extensive influx of new information regarding the pathogenesis and treatment of leukemias requires a frequent updating of this topic. The primary objective of this book is to provide the specialists involved in the diagnosis and management of acute and chronic leukemias with comprehensive and concise information on some important theoretical and practical issues of the diagnosis, treatment and follow up of patients with leukemias. An international panel of experts contribute their experience to an update of various aspects of leukemias.

The recent development of the genome wide analysis has provided new and critical knowledge of genetic changes in leukemias. The first chapter concerns recent knowledge of genetic and molecular aberrations in acute lymphoblastic leukemias (ALL), describing risk groups, frequency of cytogenetic abnormalities and their relationship with the prognosis, copy number alterations and somatic mutations. The second chapter reviews the epidemiology, genetics, pathogenesis, classification, clinical presentation, laboratory findings, differential diagnosis, treatment and prognosis in ALL in children.

The third chapter summarizes the major signs, symptoms and laboratory features in acute leukemia. While acute leukemia patients depend on the expert recommendations from their physicians, knowledge of clinical presentation and patient's related prognostic factors can help to improve treatment decision and to identify patients who would benefit most from either intensive or low-intensive treatment or even best supportive care alone. Later in the book, therapy related acute myeloid leukemias are covered, emphasizing, on one side, that these represent the most serious long-term complications to current cancer therapy and the understanding would help to identify patients at risk in order to tailor therapy; while, on the other – that there is clinical and biological overlap between therapy related and high-risk de novo leukaemias suggesting similar mechanisms of leukaemogenesis. Deeper insights into pathogenetic mechanisms will eventually help to establish a more differentiated clinical approach to successfully treat, but hopefully also prevent, these often fatal consequences of cytotoxic therapies.

The advances in basic knowledge on leukemias provide clinicians with important understanding and improved decision making towards the most suitable therapy. Biochemical, structural, and genetic studies may have brought a new era of epigenetic based and immunomodulatory drugs that will form the basis for novel treatment strategies, presented in the fifth chapter of the book. Besides, treatment response is increasingly evaluated with minimal residual disease (MRD) assays. In the past years, there has been growing attention towards understanding the clinical relevance of MRD assessment. The monitoring of MRD levels at various stages of therapy has considerable potential to impact the guidance of treatment for AML patients and improve outcomes. Chapter six presents a comprehensive overview of the methodological approaches for MRD detection, the clinical applications and future directions for improvement of and alternatives for bone marrow MRD detection, including leukemic stem cell targeted therapies. The last chapter covers modern therapies in patients with chronic myeloid leukemia (CML) as one of the best investigated and undoubtedly best understood leukemias today. Current targeted drugs have changed not only the way we treat CML, but it has also changed the approach to developing new cancer drugs.

Each chapter is a separate publication that reflects each author´s views and concepts. However, the book presents a multi-faceted picture of our current understanding of the biology and clinical presentation, the diagnostic and therapeutic challenges in patients with leukemias.

Prof. Dr. Margarita Guenova, MD, PhD
Laboratory of Haemathopathology and Immunology,
National Specialised Hospital for Active Treatment of Haematological Diseases,
Sofia, Bulgaria

Prof. Dr. Gueorgui Balatzenko, MD, PhD
Laboratory of Cytogenetics and Molecular Biology,
National Specialised Hospital for Active Treatment of Haematological Diseases,
Sofia, Bulgaria

Chapter 1

Genetics of Acute Lymphoblastic Leukemia

Ruth Maribel Forero, María Hernández and
Jesús María Hernández-Rivas

Additional information is available at the end of the chapter

http://dx.doi.org/10.5772/55504

1. Introduction

Acute lymphoblastic leukemia (ALL) is mainly a disease of childhood that arises from recurrent genetic alterations that block precursor B- and T-cell differentiation and drive aberrant cell proliferation and survival [1]. Due to the advances in the cytogenetic and molecular characterization of the acute leukemias in the past two decades, genetic alterations can now be identified in more than 80% of cases of ALL [2]. These genetic lesions influence the prognosis and therapeutic approach used for treatment of ALLs [3]. This chapter describe genetic subtypes of ALL according to the hematological malignancies classification (WHO) 2008, risk groups, frequency of cytogenetic abnormalities, and their relationship with the prognosis of ALL, copy number alterations and somatic mutations in ALL.

2. Acute Lymphoblastic Leukemia (ALL) — Genetic subtypes

2.1. Definition and genetic subtypes according to the hematological malignancies classification (WHO) 2008

Acute lymphoblastic leukemia (ALL) is mainly a disease of childhood that arises from recurrent genetic alterations that block precursor B- and T-cell differentiation and drive aberrant cell proliferation and survival [1]. ALL is characterized by the accumulation of malignant, immature lymphoid cells in the bone marrow and, in most cases, also in peripheral blood. The disease is classified broadly as B- and T-lineage ALL [1].

ALL occurs with an incidence of approximately 1 to 1.5 per 100,000 persons. It has a bimodal distribution: an early peak at approximately age 4 to 5 years with an incidence as high as 4 to 5 per 100,000 persons, followed by a second gradual increase at about age 50 years with an incidence of up to 2 per 100,000 persons. ALL, the most common childhood malignancy, represents about 80% of all childhood leukemias; but only about 20% of adult leukemias [4]. The rate of success in the treatment of ALL has increased steadily since the 1960s. The five-year event-free survival rate is nearly 80 percent for children with ALL and approximately 40 percent for adults [5].

Diagnosis of ALL relies on an assessment of morphology, flow cytometry immunophenotyping, and identification of cytogenetic-molecular abnormalities [4]. Conventional and molecular genetics allow the identification of numerical and structural chromosomal abnormalities and the definition of prognostically relevant ALL subgroups with unique clinical features [6, 7]. However, acute lymphoblastic leukemia subtypes show different responses to therapy and prognosis, which are only partially discriminated by current diagnostic tools, may be further determined by genomic and gene expression profiling [4]. More accurate delineation of genetic alterations can also provide information important for prognosis. Minimal residual disease (MRD) detection and quantification have proven important in risk-group stratification for both pediatric and adult ALL [7].

It seems likely that one or several changes in the genome are required for a blast cell to evolve into a leukemic clone, and that all cases probably harbor some form of genetic alteration [7]. Due to the advances in the cytogenetic and molecular characterization of the acute leukemias in the past two decades, genetic alterations can now be identified in greater than 80% of cases of ALL [2]. Improvement in recognizing abnormalities in the blast cells will help in understanding the mechanisms that underlie leukemogenesis.

The cloning and characterization of recurrent chromosomal translocations has allowed the identification of genes critical for understanding of the pathogenesis and prognosis of ALL [5, 8, 9]. These genes are implicated in cell proliferation and/or survival, self-renewal, cell differentiation and, and cell cycle control [10, 11]. The main causes of gene deregulation are: (i) oncogene activation with ensuing ectopic or over-expression, which is mainly due to juxtaposition with T-cell receptor loci; (ii) gain of function mutations; (iii) tumor suppressor gene haploinsufficiency or inactivation, which is usually the result of deletion and/or loss of function mutation; and (iv) chromosomal translocations producing fusion proteins which are associated with specific subgroups of ALL [10].

Efforts to define the genetic lesions that underlie ALL have identified a number of different subtypes of ALL based on their lineage (T- versus B-cell), chromosome number, or the presence or absence of chromosomal translocations. Collectively, these genetic lesions account for approximately 75% of cases, and their presence significantly influences the therapeutic approach used for treatment [3].

B-lineage ALL (B-ALL) shows considerable genetic heterogeneity. Within the category "B lymphoblastic leukemia/lymphoma with recurrent genetic abnormalities", the 2008 World Health Organization classification of hematopoietic neoplasms recognizes seven recurrent genetic abnormalities including t(9;22) (q34;q11.2) *BCR-ABL1*, t(v;11q23) *MLL* rearranged, t(12;21)(p13;q22) *TEL-AML1* (*ETV6-RUNX1*), t(5;14)(q31;q32) *IL3-IGH*, t(1;19) (q23;p13.3) *E2A-PBX1* (*TCF3-PBX1*), hypodiploidy and hyperdiploidy [12].

Burkitt lymphoma/mature B-ALL (BL) was included in the category of mature lymphatic neoplasms in the new WHO classification [12]. BL is characterized by translocation of *MYC* at 8q24.21 with an immunoglobulin gene locus, which in most cases is the immunoglobulin heavy chain locus (*IGH@*, 14q32.33) with rare translocations with the light chain genes for kappa (*IGK@*, 2p11.2) and lambda (*IGL@*, 22q11.2). These translocations result in constitutive expression of the *MYC* gene in peripheral germinal-center B cells, driven by the immunoglobulin gene enhancer [13]. The BL clone must acquire chromosomal aberrations secondary to the *IG-MYC* fusion. The most frequent secondary changes in BL detected by conventional cytogenetics are gains in 1q as well as in chromosomes 7 and 12 [14, 15].

In B-ALL, malignant cells often have additional specific genetic abnormalities, which have a significant impact on the clinical course of the disease. In contrast, although the spectrum of chromosomal abnormalities in T-lineage ALL (T-ALL) has been further widened by the finding of new recurrent but cryptic alterations, no cytogenetically defined prognostic subgroups have been identified [16, 17].

T-ALL is mainly associated with the deregulated expression of normal transcription factor proteins. This is often the result of chromosomal rearrangements juxtaposing promoter and enhancer elements of T-cell receptor genes *TRA@* (14q11), *TRB@* (T-cell receptor b, 7q34-35), *TRG@* (T-cell receptor g, 7p15) and *TRD@* (T-cell receptor d, 14q11) to important transcription factor genes [18]. In most cases, these rearrangements are reciprocal translocations, and lead to a deregulation of transcription of the partner gene by juxtaposition with the regulatory region of one of the TCR loci (e.g. *TCRB/HOXA, TCRA/D-HOX11, TCRA/D-LMO2, TCRA/DLMO1*). These chromosomal aberrations affect a subset of genes with oncogenic properties, such as 1p32(*TAL1*), 1p34(*LCK*), 8q24(*MYC*), 9q34(*TAL2*), 9q34(*TAN1/NOTCH1*), 10q24 (*HOX11*), 11p13 (*RBTN2/LMO2*), 11p15(*RBTN1/LMO1*), 14q32(*TCL1*), 19p13 (*LYL1*), 21q22(*BHLHB1*) and Xq28 (*MTCP1*) [10, 17].

Other type of rearrangement in T-ALL, mostly translocations, results in formation of 'fusion genes' that are associated with specific subgroups of T-ALL (*CALM-AF10*, *NUP98*-t, *MLL*-t and *ABL1*-fusions). In these translocations, parts of both genes located at the chromosomal breakpoints are fused 'in frame' and encode a new chimeric protein with oncogenic properties [10]. Chromosomal translocations producing fusion proteins also are associated with specific subgroups of T-ALL.

In addition, gain of function mutations (*NOTCH1* and *JAK1*) and tumor suppressor gene haploinsufficiency or inactivation, which is usually the result of deletion (*CDKN2A-B*) and/or loss of function mutation (*PTEN*); are frequent in T-ALL. These genetic alterations could be concomitant with other genomic changes [10, 19].

2.2. Risk groups in ALL

During the past three decades, the prognosis of has been improved and the treatment achieved cure rates exceeding 80%. ALL in adults has followed the same trend with long-term survival of about 40%. One main factor behind this improvement is the development of risk-adapted therapy, that permit to stratify the patients in different clinical categories according to risk factors with prognostic influence and to define the intensity and duration of treatment [20].

The prognosis of patients with ALL is influenced by clinical, hematologic and genetic factors, including age, leukocyte count at diagnosis, percentage of blast in peripheral blood, immunophenotype, central nervous system (CNS) involvement, the presence or absence of mediastinal tumor, cytogenetic and molecular alterations and the presence of minimal residual disease (MRD) in different stages of treatment which is currently a defined risk of adapted therapy strategies [20-24].

With respect to age, children less than 24 months and adults more than 50 years old have a worse prognosis, while the better results are achieved for children between 1 and 10 years, followed by adolescents and young adults. The leukocytosis (>30X10^9L in B-ALL and >100X10^9L in T-ALL), the phenotype Pro-B ALL, and T-ALL, are related to a poor outcome and are used to stratify patients as high risk [23].

The study of these prognostic factors allows recognition of three subgroups with outcome clearly differentiated in children: standard risk (40% of cases - 90% survival), intermediate (45-50% - 70-80% survival) and high risk (10-15%-less than 50% survival) [23, 25], and two subgroups in adult, standard-risk (20-25% of cases, 60% survival) and high risk (75-80% - 30% survival) [23, 26].

3. Cytogenetic alterations in ALL

3.1. Cytogenetic alterations in B-cell precursor ALL (BCP-ALL)

A correlation between prognosis and the karyotype at diagnosis in ALL was firstly demonstrated by Secker-Walker (1978) [24]. Subsequently, during the third International Workshop on Chromosomes in Leukemia (IWCL, 1983), the first large series of newly diagnosed ALL were analyzed to establish cytogenetic and prognostic correlations. Sixty-six percent of the patients analyzed showed clonal aberrations, which were identified both high-risk and low-risk ALL patients [27]. Since then it has been considered that the cytogenetic alterations have prognostic value of first order in the ALL.

Development of methods in cytogenetics has contributed to the understanding that ALL is not a homogeneous disease. Chromosome abnormalities have been detected by conventional G-banding in approximately 60–70% of all cases [7, 28]. Abnormal karyotypes have been reported in up to 80% of children and 70% of adults with ALL [29, 30]. There had been considerable developments in fluorescence in situ hybridization (FISH) for the detection of significant chromosomal abnormalities in leukemia in the 1990s [31]. The development of 24-color fluorescence in situ hybridization (FISH), interphase FISH with specific probes, and polymerase chain reaction (PCR) methods has improved the ability to find smaller changes and decreased the proportion of apparently normal karyotype to less than 20% in ALL [7].

In cases with B-ALL (excluding mature B-ALL), the most important subgroups for modal number are hypodiploidy, pseudodiploidy, and hyperdiploidy with a chromosome number greater than 50 [32]. The most structural rearrangements include translocations that generate fusion transcripts with oncogenic potential. The most important of the translocations are t(1;19)(q23;p13)(*TCF3-PBX1* fusion gene; alias *E2A-PBX1*), t(4;11)(q21;q23)(*MLL-AFF1* fusion gene; alias *MLL-AF4*), t(9;22)(q34;q11)(*BCR-ABL1*),and t(12;21)(p13;q22)(*ETV6-RUNX1* fusion gene; previously *TEL-AML1*) [32]. These cytogenetic subgroups have distinctive immunophenotypic characteristic as well as age and prognostic associations [24].

3.1.1. Ploidy alterations

The presence of hypodiploidy (less than 45 chromosomes) is found in only 2% of ALL, and is associated with a very poor outcome [33]. The high hyperdiploidy (with more than 50 chromosomes) is the most common cytogenetic subgroup in childhood BCP-ALL, and associated to a long survival. Hyperdiploidy is more frequent in children (15%) than in adults (6%) [34].

The gain of chromosomes is nonrandom, the eight chromosomes that account for 80% of all gains are: +4(78%), +6 (85%), +10 (63%), +14 (84%), +17 (68%), +18 (76%), +21 (99%), and +X (89%) [24]. Trisomy 4, 10, and 17 are associated to favorable outcome in children [33]. Unlike hypodiploidy ALL patients, hyperdiploid ALL cases have an extremely good prognosis with event-free survival rates near 90% [21]. These patients seem to particularly benefit from high dose methotrexate [33].

Approximately 20% of hyperdiploid ALL have activating mutations in the receptor tyrosine kinase *FLT3*. These mutations are interesting because not only they trigger the activation of the tyrosine kinases as potential oncogenes in hyperdiploid ALL, but also in that it suggests that tyrosine kinase inhibitors could be of benefit to patients with this leukemia. [9].

3.1.2. E2A-PBX1 fusion t(1;19) (q23;p13)

The t(1;19) (q23;p13) represents 5% of children ALL, and 3% in adults ALL, this translocation is frequently associated with the pre-B immunophenotype, in approximately 25% of cases [5, 34, 35]. The t(1;19) (q23;p13) forms a fusion gene that encodes a chimeric transcription factor, *E2A-PBX1* (*TCF3-PBX1* fusion). It disrupts the expression the expression of *HOX* genes and the targets of the *E2A* transcription factor [5]. The t(1;19) has good prognosis with high-dose methotrexate treatment; however this translocation is a risk factor for CNS relapse [1, 21]

3.1.3. BCR-ABL fusion t(9;22) (q34;q11)

As a result of the t(9;22) (q34;q11)/Philadelphia chromosome (Ph+), the *BCR* gene at 22q11.2 is joined to the *ABL* protooncogene at 9q34, giving rise to the *BCR-ABL* fusion gene. The fusion gene encodes an oncogenic fusion protein with enhanced tyrosine kinase activity that interacts with *RAS, AKT*, and *JAK/STAT* pathways [1]. This translocation is found in approximately 3% of children and 30% of adults, and is associated with unfavorable prognosis [34]. Imatinib mesylate plus intensive chemotherapy improve early treatment outcome against Philadelphia chromosome–positive (Ph+) in ALL, one of the highest risk pediatric ALL groups, however imatinib resistance develops rapidly [36].

3.1.4. 11q23-MLL rearrangements

Chromosomal rearrangements of the human *MLL* gene are the most common genetic abnormality in the first year of life, but it occurs in only 8% of children and 10% adults with ALL [34]. The 11q23-*MLL* rearrangements are associated with high-risk pediatric, adult and therapy-associated acute leukemias [37].

Some 104 different *MLL* rearrangements of which 64 fused translocation partner genes (TPGs) are now characterized at molecular level [37]. The five most common *MLL* rearrangements, present about 80% of *MLL*-translocated acute leukemia (*MLL*-t AL), are t(4;11)(q21;q23) encoding *MLL-AF4*, t(9;11)(p22;q23) encoding *MLL-AF9*, t(11;19) (q23;p13.3)-ncoding *MLL-ENL*, t(10;11)(p12;q23)encoding *MLL-AF10*, and t(6;11)(q27;q23)encoding *MLL-AF6* [38].

MLL rearrangements are associated with unfavorable prognosis. However, outcomes could be improved with high-dose cytarabine for some rearrangements [1]. *MLL* fusions with *AF4*, *AF9* and *ENL* recruit small serine/proline-rich proteins with nuclear localization signals, which may generate unique chimeric transcriptional transactivators [1]. The t(4;11)(q21;q23) have poor prognosis and predominance in infancy, especially those < 6 months of age. This rearrangement has been associated with overexpression of *FLT3* [21].

3.1.5. ETV6-RUNX1 t(12;21) (p13;q22)

The t(12;21) (p13;q22) leads to a fusion *ETV6-RUNX1* (*TEL-AML1*). It occurs in 22% of children and 2% adults with ALL [34]. This translocation t(12;21)(p13;q22) is the most common translocation in childhood BCP-ALL [39]. Moreover, is associated to an excellent prognosis with intensive chemotherapy, including asparaginase therapy [1, 21]. *TEL-AML1* is a leukemogenic, chimeric transcription factor encoding the amino-terminal basic helix-loop-helix (bHLH) domain of the ETS family member *TEL* fused to the *AML1* DNA-binding Runt and transactivation domains [40]. *TEL-AML1* may generate a pre-leukemia clone by repression of activated *AML1* target genes or by *TEL* inhibition of other ETS family proteins via binding through the TEL's pointed domain [1].

3.2. Cytogenetic alterations in Burkitt lymphoma/mature B-ALL (BL)

3.2.1. *MYC/IG* (t(8;14), t(2;8) and t(8;22))

The t(8;14)(q24;q32) and its variants t(2;8)(p11;q24) and t(8;22)(q24;q11) are associated with BL [13]. The t(8;14) is most common, found in 85%, whereas t(2;8) and t(8;22) are found in around 5 and 10%, respectively [24]. The crucial event in all three reciprocal translocations is the juxtaposing of *C-MYC* (from 8q24) under the control of immunoglobulin (Ig) gene enhancers of the heavy chain (*IGH*-14q32), kappa light chain (*IGK*-2p12), or lambda light chain (*IGL*-22q11), leading to deregulation and increased transcription of *MYC* [13]. The 2008 World Health Organization classification of hematopoietic neoplasms, established that *MYC* translocations are not specific for BL. Most *MYC/IG* breakpoints in endemic BL originate from aberrant somatic hypermutation. On the other hand, in sporadic cases the translocation involves the *IG* change regions of the *IGH* locus at 14q32 [12].

The abnormalities of *C-MYC* are an important step in the development of BL. *MYC* is a transcription factor with both activating and repressing function and is involved in the regulation of roughly 10–15% of all human genes. *MYC* regulates a number of critical biologic processes such as cell cycle control, cell growth, protein synthesis, angiogenesis, and apoptosis [41]. The upregulation of *C-MYC* disrupts many aspects of cell function, such as cell cycle progression, differentiation, metabolism, apoptosis, telomerase activity, and cell adhesion. These effects of *C-MYC* are likely to be of pathogenetic relevance in human tumors [42].

3.2.2. Secondary chromosome changes in BL

Several cytogenetic reports have correlated the presence of cytogenetic abnormalities with the outcome of patients with non-Hodgkin lymphomas, showing that secondary chromosome changes may influence the clinical phenotype of lymphoid tumors [43].

Most of the secondary chromosome changes are unbalanced rearrangements, leading to DNA gains or losses. These changes have been studied in Burkitt's lymphoma-derived cell lines and primary tumors by cytogenetic techniques including karyotype analysis [44-48], fluorescence in situ hybridization (FISH) [49], multiplex FISH (M-FISH) [50], spectral karyotype analysis (SKY), comparative genomic hybridization (CGH)[43, 51-54], and microarray analysis [55].

Additional recurrent chromosomal abnormalities have involved chromosomes 1, 6, 7, 12, 13, 17, and 22. Gains of the long arm of chromosomes 1 (+1q) or 7 (+7q) or 12 (+12q), deletion (del) 17p13 and abnormalities of band 13q34 usually occur in adult BL, without or in the setting of an HIV infection [13, 44-46, 51, 56]. Some secondary abnormalities have been associated with tumor progression, such as abnormalities on 1q, + 7q and del(13q) which have been independently associated with a worse outcome [43-46, 49, 50].

3.3. Cytogenetic alterations in T-ALL

Conventional karyotyping identifies structural chromosomal aberrations in 50% of T-ALL. Numerical changes are rare, except for tetraploidy which is seen in approximately 5% of cases. The presence of chromosomal abnormalities is not associated to the prognosis [19]. Some nonrandom translocations that are specific to T-lineage malignancies have been identified. They involve genes coding for transcriptional regulators transcriptionally deregulated in malignancies [57].

Extensive characterization of specific chromosomal abnormalities for T-ALL led to the identification of several oncogenes whose expression was up-regulated under the influence of the transcriptional regulation elements of genes which are normally expressed during T-cell differentiation [58]. T-cell malignancies are often associated with unfavorable features compared with childhood precursor B-cell ALL. However, the use of more intensive treatments and risk adapted therapy has significantly improved the outcome of patients with T-ALL. Event-free survival rates of 60% to 70% are now reported in children [57].

3.3.1. Rearrangements involving TCR genes

3.3.1.1. Deregulation of homeobox genes

The homeobox (*HOX*) family of transcription factors is divided into two classes. Class I *HOX* genes are organized in four distinct clusters (*HOXA@, HOXB@, HOXC@* and *HOXD@*) at four chromosomal loci (7p15, 17q21, 12q13, and 2q31 whereas class II *HOX* genes are dispersed throughout the whole genome. In the class I *HOX* genes, the *HOXA@* cluster is involved in T-ALL, while that in the class II *HOX* genes, *TLX1* (*HOX11*) and *TLX3* (*HOX11L2*) have been extensively studied in the context of T-ALL [18].

3.3.1.1.1. TLX1 (HOX11) (t(10;14)(q24;q11) and its variant t(7;10)(q35;q24))

The translocation t(10;14)(q24;q11) and its variant t(7;10)(q35;q24) are a nonrandom alteration identified in T-ALL. Either of these is present in 5% of pediatric to 30% of adult T-ALL [1]. Both of them lead to the transcriptional activation of an homeobox gene, *HOX11* gene (*TLX1; TCL3*), that is not expressed in healthy T-cells, by bringing the *HOX11* coding sequence under the transcriptional control of regulatory sequences of the T-cell receptor gene (*TRA@* or *TRB@* genes, respectively). However, the overexpression of *HOX11* in thymocytes has been also demonstrated in the absence of a 10q24 rearrangement, suggesting that other, trans-acting mechanisms could lead to this aberrant gene expression, probably by disrupting gene silencing mechanisms that operate during normal T-cell development [18, 57, 58].

There is some evidence that *HOX11* may play an important role in leukemogenesis. It has been particularly shown that constitutive expression of *HOX11* favors expansion and, in some instances, immortalization of murine hematopoietic progenitors in vitro [59, 60]. However, *HOX11* has better prognosis than other T-ALL molecular subtypes [1].

3.3.1.1.2. TLX3 (HOX11L2) (t(5;14)(q35;q32))

The cryptic translocation, t(5;14)(q35;q32), is restricted to T-ALL, is present in approximately 20% of childhood T-ALL and 13% of adult cases. This translocation is associated with strong ectopic expression of another homeobox gene called *HOX11L2* (*RNX; TLX3*) [17, 58, 61], because of possibly the influence of regulatory elements of *CTIP2* (*BCL11B*), a gene highly expressed during T-lymphoid differentiation [17, 57]. Other variant chromosomal aberrations, each targeting *TLX3*, have been observed as well, including a t(5;7)(q35;q21), in which the *CDK6* gene is involved on 7q21[18].

Although *TLX1* and *TLX3* themselves and the gene expression profiles of *TLX1* and *TLX3* expressing T-ALL samples are very similar [18], the t(5;14) and/or *HOX11L2* ectopic expression has been associated with a very poor outcome in children with T-ALL [57].

However, the exact prognostic meaning of *TLX3* expression alone or in combination with other markers is not clear [18].

3.3.1.1.3. HOXA@ cluster (inv(7)(p15q34))

Other rearrangement involving *TCR* genes that affecting *HOXA@* cluster (7p15) is associated with the inv(7) (p15q34), t(7;7)(p15;q34), and t(7;14)(p15;q11). The chromosomal inversion inv(7)(p15q34) has been observed in approximately 5% of T-ALL cases. This inversion juxtaposes part of the *TRB@* locus (7q34-35) to part of the *HOXA@* cluster (7p15), resulting in elevated *HOXA10* and *HOXA11* expression. In addition, 2% of the cases showed elevated *HOXA10* and *HOXA11* expression in the absence of inv(7), suggesting that other activating mechanisms may exist [18].

In contrast to *TLX1* and *TLX3*, which are normally not expressed in the hematopoietic system, *HOXA10* and *HOXA11* are expressed in developing thymocytes. While *HOXA11* is expressed at different stages of T-cell differentiation, *HOXA10* expression is only detected at the earliest stages of differentiation, suggesting that its downregulation is required for full maturation of T-cells to the CD4 and CD8 single positive stages [18].

3.3.1.2. Deregulation of TAL1-related genes

TAL1-related genes (*TAL1, TAL2* and *LYL1*), encode a distinct subgroup of basic helix-loop-helix (bHLH) proteins that share exceptional homology in their bHLH sequences [62]. The malignant potential of these proteins is likely to reside largely within their HLH domains that potentially mediate sequence-specific DNA recognition [63].

Although expression of *TAL1, TAL2* or *LYL1* has not been observed during normal T-cell development, the rearranged alleles of these genes are readily transcribed in T-ALL cells, and the ectopic expression of these genes in T-lineage cells may be a contributing factor in T-ALL pathogenesis [62].

3.3.1.2.1. TAL1 (SCL,TCL5) (t(1;14)(p32;q11), t(1;14)(p34;q11) and t(1;7)(p32;q34))

Alteration of the *TAL1* (*SCL, TCL5*), a gene located on chromosome 1p32, is considered as the most common nonrandom genetic defect in childhood T-ALL. *TAL1* disruption is associated with a t(1;14)(p32;q11), t(1;14)(p34;q11) and t(1;7)(p32;q34) (*TRA@/TRAD@-TAL1* respectively) in 1% to 3% of childhood T-ALL [1, 57]. In other 9% to 30% of childhood T-ALL, *TAL1* is overexpressed as a consequence of a nonrandom submicroscopic interstitial deletion between a locus called *SIL* and the 5′ untranslated region (UTR) of *TAL1* at 1p32, giving rise to an *SIL-TAL* fusion transcript [19].

As the translocation as interstitial deletion disrupt the coding potential of *TAL1* in a similar manner, leading to its ectopic overexpression in T-cells [57]. Nevertheless, high expression levels of *TAL1* in the absence of detectable *TAL1* rearrangement are observed in about 40% of T-ALL [19].

The deletions aberrantly triggers activated *TAL1* during thymocyte maturation, promoting transformation [1]. *TAL1* alteration leads to silencing of genes target encoding E47 and E12 variants of E2A transcription factors. Several studies have proposed that the reactivation of silenced genes by administering histone deacetylase (HDAC) inhibitors may prove efficacious in T-ALL patients expressing *TAL1* [18, 57].

3.3.1.2.2. TAL2 (t(7;9)(q34;q32))

As a consequence of t(7;9) (q34;q32), the *TAL2* gene is juxtaposed to the *TRB@* locus. The *TAL2* gene is activated as a result of this translocation. The activation of the *TAL2* or *LYL1* genes is less common, affecting <2% of T-ALL patients [18, 62]. The properties of *TAL2* broadly resemble those described previously for *TAL1*. Therefore, this support the idea that both proteins promote T-ALL by a common mechanism [64].

3.3.1.2.3. LYL1 (t(7;19)(q34;p13))

In the t(7;19)(q35;p13), the *LYL1* coding sequences are juxtaposed to the *TRB@* locus. This gene is constitutively expressed in T-ALL, whereas its expression is absent in normal T-cells. The ectopic *LYL1* expression is found in some human T-cell leukemias, suggesting that it may participate in T-cell leukemogenesis. Similar to *TLX1*, *TLX3*, and *TAL1*, the ectopic expression of *LYL1* is mutually exclusive, although rare exceptions to this rule have been described [18].

LYL1 encodes another class II basic helix-loop-helix (bHLH) transcription factor that forms heterodimers with class I bHLH proteins, including E2A (E47 and E12) and HEB. *LYL1*-transgenic mice developed CD4+CD8+ precursor T-cell ALL (pre-T-LBL), probably by dimerization with E2A, inhibition of CD4 promoter activity, and downregulation of a subset of *E2A/HEB* target genes, suggesting a block in cell differentiation [1, 65]

3.3.1.3. Deregulation of LIM-domain only genes LMO1 and LMO2

3.3.1.3.1. LMO1 (t(11;14)(p15;q11) and LMO2 (t(11;14)(p13;q11))

The genes encoding the LIM-domain only proteins *LMO1* (*RBTN1* or *TTG1*, 11p15) and *LMO2* (*RBTN2* or *TTG2*, 11p13) are frequently rearranged with the T-cell receptor loci in T-ALL, resulting in overexpression of *LMO1/LMO2* [1, 66]. The most common alterations are t(11;14)(p15;q11) and t(11;14)(p13;q11) juxtaposing *LMO1* or *LMO2* to the *TRA@* or *TRAD@* loci [1], nevertheless other genetic alterations have also been reported like t(7;11)(q34;p15) and t(7;11)(q34;p13) translocations, involving *TCRB* and *LMO1* or *LMO2* loci [17].

Generally the ectopic expression of *LMO1* and *LMO2* are not mutually exclusive, because abnormal expression of *LMO1/2* has been found in 45% of T-ALL, even in the absence of typical chromosomal changes, but often in association with deregulation of *LYL1* (*LMO2*) or *TAL1* (*LMO1* and 2) [19]. Studies in transgenic mice have showed that *TAL1* expression in itself is not sufficient to induce T-cell malignancies and that co-expression of *LMO1* or *LMO2* is strictly required [18].

3.3.1.4. Deregulation of family of tyrosine kinases — LCK gene (t(1;7)(p34;q34))

The lymphocyte-specific protein tyrosine kinase (*LCK*), a member of the SRC family of tyrosine kinases, is highly expressed in T-cells and plays a critical role in proximal TCR-based signaling pathways [67]. The *LCK* gene is activated due to the t(1;7)(p34;q34) that juxtaposing *LCK* with *TRB@* loci [18]. *ABL1* is located downstream of *LCK* in the TCR signaling pathway. Based on these results, *SRC* kinase inhibitors and the dual *SRC/ABL* kinase inhibitors could be used for treating T-ALL patients with hyperactive LCK [18].

3.3.1.5. Deregulation of MYB gene — Duplication and t(6;7)(q23;q34)

MYB is the cellular homolog of the *V-MYB* oncogene of the avian myeloblastosis virus. A t(6;7)(q23;q34), juxtaposing *MYB* to *TCRβ* regulatory elements, and a submicroscopic amplification of the long arm of chromosome 6 at 6q23.3 caused by ALU-mediated homologous recombination, has been detected in 8–15% of T-ALL. It leads to upregulation of *MYB* expression and a blockade in T-cell differentiation that could be reversed with *MYB* knockdown [1, 68]. The upregulation of *MYB* has raised expectations that *MYB* may be used as a molecular target for therapy in these patients [66].

Finally, other rearrangements involving TCR genes affect genes like *BCL11B* (inv(14)(q11q32); and t(14;14)(q11;q32)), *TCL1* (inv(14)(q11q32), and t(14;14)(q11;q32)), *CCND2* (t(7;12)(q34;p13.3), and t(12;14)(p13;q11)), *NOTCH1* (t(7;9)(q34;q34.3)), and *OLIG2* gene (t(14;21)(q11;q22)) [19, 24].

3.3.2. Fusion genes rearrangements

3.3.2.1. PICALM-MLLT10 (CALM-AF10) — t(10;11)(p13;q14)

The *PICALM-MLLT10* (*CALM-AF10*) fusion gene is caused by a recurrent translocation, t(10;11)(p13;q14). It is detected in about 10% of childhood T-ALL. and it has been associated with a poor prognosis [11]. This translocation has also been observed in other leukemias, including acute myeloid leukemia [18].

The precise mechanism for *CALM-AF10* mediated transformation is not known, although *CALM-AF10* T-ALL are characterized by overexpression of *HOXA* cluster genes, including *HOXA5, HOXA9*, and *HOXA10*. *CALM-AF10*+ T-ALL has also showed overexpression of several *AF10* downstream genes (*DNAJC1, COMMD3, BMI1* and *SPAG6*) located close to the *AF10* gene breakpoint. From these four *AF10* downstream genes, *BMI1* is the only one known to be associated with an increase of self-renewal of hematopoietic stem cells and oncogenesis [69].

3.3.2.2. MLL-fusions

Translocations implicating *MLL* with various partners represent about 4% of T-ALL cases [18]. The t(11;19)(q23;p13) *MLL-MLLT1* (ENL) gene fusion is the most common *MLL* translocation partner in T-ALL. Nevertheless, other *MLL* translocations also occur in T-ALL [11].

CALM-AF10+ T-ALL and *MLL-t* AL share a specific *HOXA* overexpression, triggering activate common oncogenic pathways [69]. *MLL* fusion proteins enhance transcriptional activity, resulting in increased expression of *HOXA9, HOXA10, HOXC6*, and overexpression of the *MEIS1 HOX* coregulator [18].

MLL controls skeletal patterning, regulates the establishment of functional hematopoietic stem cells, and early hematopoietic progenitor cell development [1, 70]. T-ALL cells with *MLL* fusions are characterized by differentiation arrest at an early stage of thymocyte differentiation, after commitment to the TCR gammadelta lineage [11].

3.3.2.3. ABL1-fusions

Translocations of *ABL1* are rare, except for *NUP214-ABL1* fusion (t(9;9)(q34;q34)) identified in up to 6% of T-ALL as a result of episomal formation with amplification. Recurrent translocations involving *NUP98*, such as the t(4;11)(q21;p15) with the *NUP98/ RAP1GDS1* gene fusion), another protein of the nucleopore complex, are reported very rarely [19]. The t(9;12)(p24;p13) encoding *ETV6-JAK2* fusion gene, with an important leukemogenic role, results in constitutive tyrosine kinase activity in positive T-ALL patients [71].

4. Copy number alterations in acute lymphoblastic leukemia

In spite of continually improving event-free (EFS) and overall survival (OS) for ALL, particularly in children, a number of patients on current therapies will relapse. Therefore it is important to know the group of patients with high risk of relapse [72, 73]. As the risk-stratification of ALL is partly based on genetic analysis, different genomic technologies designed to detect poor-risk additional genetic changes are being expanded substantially. Analyses of somatic DNA copy number variations in ALL aided by advances in microarray technology (array comparative genomic hybridization and high density single nucleotide polymorphism arrays) have allowed the identification of copy gains, deletions, and losses of heterozygosity at ever-increasing resolution [74].

Several microarray platforms have been used for the analysis of DNA copy number abnormalities (CNAs) in ALL, such as array-based comparative genomic hybridization (array-CGH), bacterial artificial chromosome (array-BAC) array CGH and oligonucleotide array CGH (oaCGH), single nucleotide polymorphism array (aSNP) and single molecule sequencing [75]. These microarray platforms vary in resolution, technical performance, and the ability to detect DNA deletions, DNA gains, and copy neutral loss of heterozygosity. These techniques have improved the detection of novel genomic changes in ALL blast cells [76]. The aCGH also detects the majority of karyotypic findings other than balanced translocations, and may provide prognostic information in cases with uninformative cytogenetics [77, 78]. In addition, the use of these methods documented multiple regions of common genetic cryptic alterations. These analyses provide information about multiple submicroscopic recurring genetic alterations including target key cellular pathways. However, many aberrations are still undetected in most cases, and their associations with established cytogenetic subgroups remain unclear [28, 79].

4.1. CNA in BCP-ALL

Most of ALL (79-86%) showed alterations in the number of copies (CNA) by aCGH techniques. The CNA frequently involved chromosomes 1, 6, 8, 9, 12, 15, 17 and 21; and rarely chromosomes 2, 3, 14 and 19. The losses have been more frequent than gains [6, 7, 28, 35, 77, 78, 80-85].

In precursor B-cell ALLs, most of the abnormalities have been gains of 1q (multiple loci), 9q, 17q, amplification of chromosome 21 (predominantly tetrasomy 21), and loss of 1p and 12p. Other recurrent chromosomal rearrangements have been found in both B-and T ALLs, such as loss of 6q (heterogeneous in size), 9p (9p21.3), 11q, and 16q, as well as gain of 6q and 16p. Other recurrent findings have included dim (13q), dim (16q) and enh (17q) [6, 7, 28, 35, 77, 78, 80-85] (Figure 1).

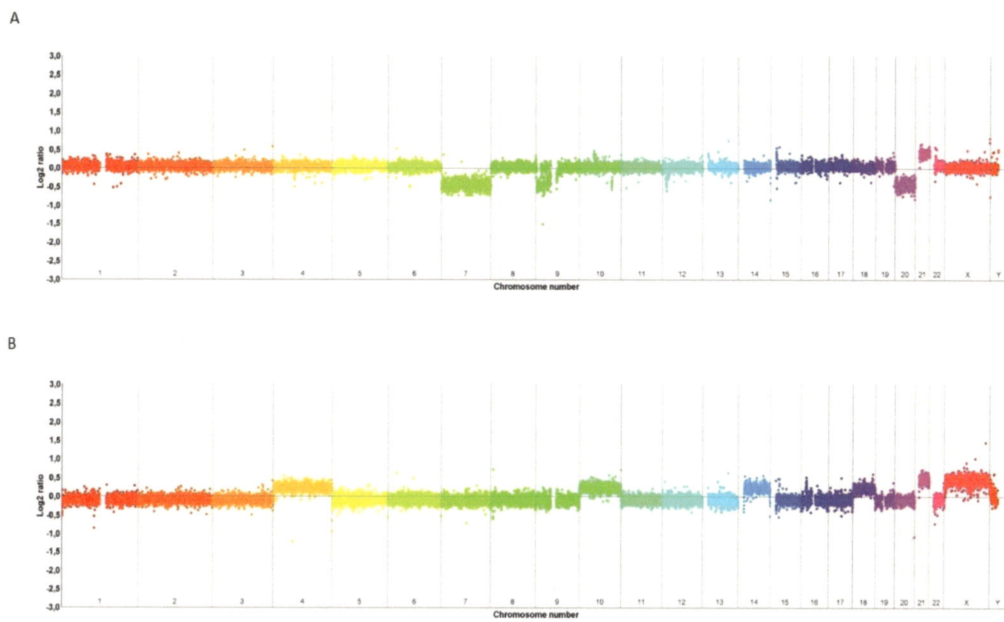

Figure 1. Copy number alterations in two newly diagnosed BCP-ALL patients. A. Male patient with losses of 7, 9p24-q21 and 20 chromosome and gain of 21q chromosome. B. Male patient with whole gains of 4, 10, 14,18, 21, and X chromosome.

Several observations suggest that the CNAs are biologically important. The identification of these recurrent chromosomal rearrangements in ALL has defined Minimal Critical Regions (MCR), which are target small regions of the genome, that are often small enough to pinpoint the few candidate genes that present in these chromosomal regions [75].

Many of these MCR contain genes with known roles in leukemogenesis of ALL. These lesions include deletions of lymphoid transcription factors and transcriptional coactivators (e.g. *PAX5, EBF1, E2-2, IKZF1*-Ikaros, *ETV6* (*TEL*), *ERG, TBL1XR1*, and *LEF1*), tumor suppressor and cell cycle regulatory genes (e.g. *CDKN2A/B, NF1, PTEN, RB1*, and *ATM*), as well as genes with other established roles in B-cell development, such as *RAG1* and *RAG2, FYN, PBEF1* or *CBP/*

PAG. Moreover putative regulators of apoptosis (e.g. *BTG1*), lymphoid signaling molecules (e.g. *BTLA/CD200, TOX*), micro-RNAs (e.g. mir-15a/16-1), steroid receptors (e.g. *NR3C1, NR3C2*), genes at fragile sites (e.g. *FHIT, DMD*), and genes with unknown roles in leukemogenesis of ALL (e.g. *C20orf94/MKKS, ADD3,* and *DMD*) have been located in these regions. It is notable that about 40% of B-progenitor ALL cases present genomic alterations in genes that regulate B-lymphocyte differentiation [6, 7, 28, 35, 77, 78, 80-86] (Table 1).

Loss/gain	Chromosome	Cytoband	Size (Mb)	Start position (Mb)*	End position (Mb)*	Candidate genes	Reference
loss	1	p33	0.039	47.728	47.767	*TAL1*	[75, 85]
loss	1	q44	1.74	245.113	246.853	*LOC440742 Adjacent to gen ZNF528*	[80, 110]
loss	2	p21	0.287	43.425	43.712	*THADA*	[75, 85]
loss	3	p22.3	0.306	35.364	35.670	*No annotated gene ARPP-21*	[85, 110]
loss	3	p14.2	0.254	60.089	60.343	*FHIT*	[75, 83, 85, 110]
loss	3	q13.2	0.148	112.055	112.203	*CD200, BTLA*	[75, 85, 110]
loss	3	q26.32		Various		*TBL1XR1*	[75, 83, 85, 110]
loss	4	q25	0.049	109.035	109.084	*LEF1*	[75, 85, 110]
loss	4	q31.23	0.145	149.697	149.842	*None; telomeric to NR3C2*	[75, 85, 110]
loss	5	q31.3	0.087	142.780	142.867	*NR3C1, LOC389335*	[75, 85]
loss	5	q33.3	0.553	157.946	158.499	*EBF1*	[75, 80, 83, 85, 110]
loss	6	p22.22	0.023	26.237	26.260	*Histone cluster, HIST1H4F, HIST1H4G, HIST1H3F, HIST1H2BH*	[75, 85, 110]
loss	6	q21	0.088	109.240	109.328	*ARMC2, SESN1*	[75, 85, 110]
loss	7	7p		Whole p-arm	Whole p-arm		[35, 85]
loss	7	q21.2	0.209	92.255	92.464	*LOC645862, GATAD1, ERVWE1, PEX1, DKFZP564O0523, LOC442710, MGC40405, CDK6*	[85, 110]
loss	7	p12.2	0.048	50.419	50.467	*IKZF1 (ZNFN1A1, Ikaros),*	[75, 83, 85]
loss	8	q12.1	0.094	60.032	60.126	*Immediately 5' (telomeric) of TOX*	[75, 85, 110]
loss	9	p21.3	0.237	21.894	22.131	*CDKN2A/CDKNA2B, MTAP, MLLT3 (AF9)*	[6, 35, 75, 80, 83, 85, 110]
loss	9	p13.2	0.088	36.932	37.020	*PAX5 CNA or sequence mutation*	[75, 80, 83, 85, 110]
loss	10	q23.31	0.062	89.676	89.738	*PTEN*	[75, 85, 110]
loss	10	q24.1	0.178	97.889	98.067	*BLNK*	[75, 85, 110]
loss	10	q25.1	0.078	111.782	111.860	*ADD3*	[75, 85, 110]
loss	11	p13	0.155	33.917	34.072	*No gene; immediately 5' of LMO2*	[75, 85]
loss	11	p12	0.008	36.618	36.626	*RAG1/2, LOC119710*	[75, 85, 110]
loss	11	q22.3	0.034	36.600	36.634	*ATM*	[80, 110]
loss	11	q23.3	0.274	118.369	118.643	*16 genes distal to MLL breakpoint, including 3' MLL*	[80, 85]
loss	12	p12.1	4.5	19.309	23.809	*KRAS*	[35, 110]

Loss/gain	Chromosome	Cytoband	Size (Mb)	Start position (Mb)*	End position (Mb)*	Candidate genes	Reference
loss	12	p13.2	0.086	11.813	11.899	*ETV6, KLRA-D family*	[6, 35, 75, 80, 83, 85, 110]
loss	12	q21.33	0.218	92.291	92.509	*BTG1*	[75, 80, 85, 110]
loss	13	q14.11	0.031	41.555	41.586	*ELF1 , C13orf21, LOC400128*	[75, 85, 110]
loss	13	q14.2	0.149	49.016	49.165	*RB1*	[6, 75, 80, 83, 85, 110]
loss	13	q14.2-3	0.889	50.573	51.462	*DLEU2, RFP2, KCNRG, MIRN16-1, MIRN15A, DLEU1, FAM10A4, LOC647154, LOC730194, DLEU7*	[75, 85]
loss	15	q12	0.038	26.036	26.074	*ATP10A*	[80, 110]
loss	15	q14	–	–	–	*SPRED1 (5')*	[75, 110]
loss	15	q15.1	0.792	41.258	42.050	*18 genes including LTK and MIRN626*	[85, 110]
loss	17	17p		Whole p-arm	Whole p-arm	*TP53*	[83]
loss	17	q11.2	0.169	29.066	29.235	*LOC729690, SUZ12P, CRLF3, LOC646013, C17orf41, C17orf42, [NF1]¶*	[75, 83, 85, 110]
loss	17	q21.1	0.045	37.931	37.976	*IKZF3 (ZNFN1A3, Aiolos)*	[75, 85, 110]
loss	19	p13.3	0.229	1.351	1.580	*63 genes telomeric to TCF3; region may include TCF3*	[75, 85, 110]
loss	20	20p12.1	0.035	10.422	10.457	*C20orf94*	[75, 85]
loss	20	q11.22	1.426	32.304	33.730	*Several genes , VPREB1*	[6, 110]
loss	21	q22.12	0.004	36.428	36.432	*No gene, but immediately distal to RUNX1*	[75, 85]
loss	21	q22.2	0.023	39.784	39.807	*ERG*	[75, 85, 110]
gain	1	q23.3-q44	81.326	164.759	qtel	*719 genes telomeric of PBX1, including 3' region of PBX1*	[75, 85]
Gain	6	q23.3	0.182	135.492	135.674	*MYB, MIRN548A2, AHI1*	[75, 80, 85]
Gain	9	9q		Whole q-arm	Whole q-arm	*ABL*	[83, 85]
Gain	9	q34.12-q34.3	7.676	133.657	qtel	*155 genes telomeric of ABL1, including 3' region of ABL1*	[75, 85, 110]
Gain	10	10p		Whole p-arm	Whole p-arm	–	[83, 85]
Gain	21	21	46.8	Whole chromosome	Whole chromosome	*Several genes*	[6, 83]
Gain	21	21q		Whole q-arm	Whole q-arm	*AML1, BACH, ERG*	[35, 83]
Ampl	21	iAMP21**	11.713	–	–	*Several genes*	[6]
Gain	21	q22.3	0.589	42.775	43.364	*7 genes*	[80]
Gain	21	q22.11-12	4.022	32.322	36.344	*34 genes*	[80]
Gain	21	q22.11-q22.12	2.303	33.974	36.277	*33 genes including RUNX1*	[75, 85]

Loss/gain	Chromosome	Cytoband	Size (Mb)	Start position (Mb)*	End position (Mb)*	Candidate genes	Reference
Gain	22	q11.1-q11.23	21.888	ptel	23.563	*277 genes telomeric (5') of BCR, including 5' region of BCR*	[75, 85]

* Assembly GRCh37/hg19 from Genome Reference Consortium

Table 1. Recurring regions of copy number alteration reported in ALL and involved genes with known or putative roles on leukemogenesis and cancer.

The average number of CNAs per ALL case is usually low, suggesting that this disease is not characterized by inherent genomic instability. This has been shown in a large SNP arrays study performed on pediatric ALL cases (B-progenitor and T-lineage). It allowed to identify a relatively low number of CNAs in ALL -a mean of 6.5 lesions per case- indicating that gross genomic instability is not a feature of most ALL cases [75, 85], although it is higher that the number of genomic changes in myeloid malignancies. Furthermore, similar studies have found 4.2 lesions per case in the precursor B-cell childhood ALLs (3.1 losses and 1.1 gains), and 2.6 lesions per case in the T-ALLs (1.7 losses and 0.9 gains) [80].

In spite of the large number of novel alterations, most of them have been focal deletions (less than a megabase) that involve only one or a few genes in the minimal region of genetic alteration. Apart from high hyperdiploid ALL, gains of DNA have been specifically uncommon and a few of them were focal gains [75, 85].

The pattern and number of CNAs is similar in the genetic ALL subtypes. Notably, less than one deletion per case was observed in *MLL*-rearranged ALL, typically presenting early in infancy. Therefore it has been suggested that a few additional genetic lesions are required for inducing leukemia. In contrast, other ALL subtypes such as *ETV6-RUNX1* and *BCR-ABL1,* typically presenting later than childhood, had over 6 copy number alterations per case, and some cases had over 20 lesions. These results are consistent with the concept that the initiating translocations are developed early in childhood, previous to clinically manifest leukemia (particularly for *ETV6-RUNX1* leukemia). Additional lesions are subsequently required for establishment of the leukemic clone. The deletion of *IKZF1* is also a lesion in *BCR-ABL1* ALL, but it is exceptionally uncommon in *ETV6-RUNX1* ALL [75, 76, 85-87].

High-resolution genomic profiling studies in childhood ALL also reveals recurrent genetic lesions, affecting genes with an established and critical role in leukemogenesis such as *CDKN2A, ETV6* (*TEL*), *RUNX1* (*AML1*) and other genes, such as *MLL,* that are used to stratify the patients [80]. Furthermore, many of these recurrent CNA were different between B-ALL and T-ALL subtypes. For example, deletions involving *ADD3, C20orf94, ERG, ETV6,* the fragile histidine triad gene *FHIT, TBL1XR1,* and a histone cluster at 6p22 were common in B-ALL but rare in T-ALL, whereas deletion of *CDKN2A/B* (9p21), are more frequent in T-ALL (72%-90%) than B-ALL (34%) [11, 76, 85].

4.2. CNA in T-ALL

Genome-wide profiling in T-ALL has been used to identify copy number alterations accompanying novel structural abnormalities, such as the *NUP214-ABL1* and *SET-NUP214* fusion genes. The amplification on extrachromosomal episomes of *ABL1* has been associated with the cryptic fusion of *NUP214* to *ABL1* gene, in around 6% of individuals with T-ALL. This fusion gene triggers the constitutive expression of the chimeric protein tyrosine kinase *NUP214-ABL1* and it is sensitive to the tyrosine kinase inhibitor imatinib. This amplification could improve outcome or decrease treatment-related morbidity of T-ALL cases, but large studies are needed to confirm these results [88]. Moreover, the cryptic and recurrent deletion, del(9)(q34.11q34.13), in pediatric T-ALL cases, results in a conserved *SET-NUP214* fusion product, that contribute to T-ALL pathogenesis by inhibition of T-cell maturation by the transcriptional activation of the *HOXA* genes [89].

Using SNP, BAC, or oligo-array CGH platforms, focal deletions have also identified in T-ALL, leading to deregulated expression of *TAL1* [85] and *LMO2* [90]; deletions of the *RB1* [85]; deletion and mutation of *PTEN* [85, 91]; deletion or mutation of the U3 ubiquitin ligase *FBXW7* [92]; and duplications of the protooncogene *MYB*, present in about 8% of T-ALL cases, that occur in combination with other genetic rearrangements contributing to T-cell differentiation arrest (*TAL/LMO, TLX1, TLX3, HOXA*) [68, 75, 93].

4.3. CNA in BL

High rates of CNAs have been reported in BL. CNAs have been observed in 65% [53] and 76% [43] of BL cases by conventional CGH. CNAs have been reported in 54% and 100% of BL patients by oaCGH and aSNP respectively [14, 55]. In addition, high-resolution molecular inversion probe (MIP) SNP assay have been reported 64% of CNAs in BL [94].

CGH and aCGH studies on cases of BL have shown that the increased number of gains and losses are significantly associated with shorter survival [43]. Gains are more frequent than losses in a range from 52% to 65% [14, 53, 94]. These studies have reported gains on chromosomes 1q, 7, 8q, 12, 13, 22 and Xq and losses in 6q, 13q, 14q, 17p, and Xp [14, 15, 43, 51, 53-55, 94, 95]. Some studies have also identified cases with gains on 2p [43, 55], 3q27.3 [14], 4p [43], 15q [51, 55], and 20p12-q13 [51].

It has been demonstrated that chromosomal gains or losses in the most frequently altered regions in BL, such as 1cen-q22, 1q31-q32, 7q22-qter, 8q24-qter, 13q31-q32, and 17p13-pter, influence changes in locus-specific gene expression levels of many genes that probably are associated with pathogenesis of BL. For example, the chromosomal region 1q showed increased gene expression levels in cases with gains, and correlates with the expression of germinal center-associated genes. By contrast, genetic losses in the chromosomal region 17p13 lead to a down regulation of genes located in this region, not only *TP53*, but also many other genes such as *AURKB*, that may influence the biological behavior as a consequence of deregulated expression [53].

4.4. CNA analysis of paired diagnostic and relapse ALL samples

Detailed comparative analysis of paired diagnostic and relapse ALL samples, using high resolution genomic profiling, have showed the next findings: i) frequent changes in DNA copy number abnormalities have been observed at relapse, ii) there are loss of copy number lesions present at diagnosis in ALL relapse samples, and acquisition of new additional (secondary) lesions in the relapse samples in nearly all analyzed patients, iii) deletions were more common than gains about newly acquired copy number abnormalities in the relapse samples. These data support the clonal evolution in ALL. The pattern of deletions on the antigen receptor loci was comparable between relapse and diagnosis, suggesting the emergence of a related leukemic clone, rather than the development of a distinct second leukemia. It should be noted that several cases were found in which the diagnosis and relapse samples carrying alternative lesions affecting the same gene(s), including *CDKN2A* and *PAX5*, suggesting that the inactivation of these genes were secondary but essential events required to develop a full-blown leukemia. Additionally, genomic abnormalities distinct from those presented at diagnosis has been identified lately, involved genes such as, *IKZF1, IKZF2, IKZF3, RAG, ADD3, ETV6, BTG1, DMD* and *IL3RA/CSF2RA,* suggesting that they confer a selective advantage and resistance to therapy in ALL [75, 96, 97].

These findings indicate that relapse is frequently the result of the emergence of a leukemic clone that shows significant genetic differences from the diagnostic clone. Whether these represent rare clones at the time of diagnosis or are the emergence of new clones should be further investigated [96].

5. Somatic mutations in acute lymphoblastic leukemia

Genome-wide profiling of DNA copy number alterations (CNA) coupled with focused candidate gene resequencing has identified novel genetic alterations in key signaling pathways in the pathogenesis of both B-progenitor and T-ALL. These findings are associated with leukemogenesis, treatment outcome in ALL, and are being exploited in the development of new therapeutic approaches and in the identification of markers of poor prognosis [72, 98].

5.1. Gene mutations in BCP-ALL

Somatic mutations in several genes are present in BCP-ALL. These mutations have identified in genes which are involved in RAS signaling (48%), B-cell differentiation and development (18%), JAK/STAT signaling (11%), TP53/RB1 tumor suppressor (6%) and noncanonical pathways and in other/unknown genes (17%) [72]. The incidence of the most recurrently mutated genes in ALL is described in the Table 2.

The frequency of alterations in the TP53/RB1, RAS, and JAK signaling pathways is much higher in High Risk B-Precursor Childhood Acute Lymphoblastic Leukemia (HR B-ALL)

http://dx.doi.org/10.5772/55504

BCP-ALL			
Pathway	**Gene**	**Frequency**	**Reference**
RAS signaling	*NRAS*	17%	[72]
	KRAS	16%	
	FLT3	7%	
	PTPN11	5%	
	NF1	3%	
B-cell differentiation and development pathway	*PAX5*	15%	
	IKZF1 (IKAROS)	3%	
JAK/STAT signaling	*JAK1*	2%	
	JAK2	9%	
TP53/RB1 pathway	*TP53*	4%	
	RB1	1%	
	CDKN2A/CDKN2B	1%	
Others	*TBL1XR1*	2%	
	ETV6	4%	
	CREBBP	2%	
	Unknown genes	9%	
T-ALL			
Pathway	**Gene**	**Frequency**	**Reference**
Cell cycle defects	*CDKN2A/CDKN2B*	96%	[18]
	TP53, RB, p27	4%	
Differentiation impairment	*TAL1 plus LMO1/2*	39%	
	LYL plus LMO2	20%	
	TLX1	7%	
	TLX3	20%	
	HOXA10/11	7%	
	PICALM-MLLT10	5-10%	
	MLL-fusions	4%	
	TAL2	<1%	
Proliferation and survival	*ABL1-fusions*	8%	
	NRAS	5%	
	FLT3	5%	
	LCK	<1%	
	ETV6-PBL2	<1%	
	ETV6-JAK2	<1%	
	PTEN	<1%	
	Unknown genes	"/>78%	
Self-renewal capacity	*NOTCH*	56%	
	Unknown genes	"/>44%	

Table 2. Frequency of the different mutations observed in ALL.

cohort than reported for unselected pediatric B-precursor ALL patients. In this subgroup of patients have been recently proposed new targeted therapeutics, such as the RAS/ MAPK signaling pathway [98].

5.1.1. Ras signaling

Deregulation of the *RAS-RAF*-mitogen-activated protein kinase/extracellular signal-regulated kinase (*ERK*) kinase (*MEK*)-*ERK* signaling cascade is often caused by somatic mutations in genes encoding proteins that influence the activity of this pathway, such as *NRAS, KRAS2, FLT3, PTPN11,* and *BRAF* [99]. As observed in myeloid malignancies, up-regulated RAS signaling, due to mutations in RAS genes or in genes coding for proteins controlling *RAS* function, represent a major pathway driving the aberrant growth of malignant B-cell precursors [100].

In BCP-ALL, a number of associations with other genetic changes are already known, such as the link between mutations of genes within the RAS signaling pathway and high hyperdiploidy [79, 99, 101]. These mutations have been found in ~60% of high hyperdiploid childhood cases ALL. They are invariably mutually exclusive, and additional cooperative genetic events in this subgroup of patients [99, 101, 102].

5.1.1.1. NRAS and KRAS

RAS genes are part of the small GTPase family and consist of three separate genes, *NRAS, KRAS2*, and *HRAS*. *HRAS* is rarely mutated in hematologic tumors and is expressed at a low level compared to the other two isoforms in the hematopoietic cells in leukemia [102]. The *RAS* proteins activate several downstream pathways to promote proliferation, differentiation, survival, and apoptosis, depending on cellular conditions [102].

Mutations in *NRAS* and *KRAS* have been recognized as a recurring molecular event in childhood ALL, with a reported incidence of between 15% and 30% [98, 100, 102]. The incidence and spectrum of mutations at diagnosis and relapse are similar, although the presence is not a significant risk factor [99, 101]. Moreover, it has not been found any association of *RAS* mutation with an adverse clinical outcome [103]. The presence or number of mutations in the RAS signaling pathway have not been associated with relapse-free survival [98].

5.1.1.2. FLT3

Activating mutations in the receptor tyrosine kinase *FLT3* have been identified in approximately 20-25% of hyperdiploid and *MLL*-rearranged ALL samples [9, 104]. This observations supports the idea that the activation of tyrosine kinases as potential oncogenes in hyperdiploid ALL, as well as that leukemogenic fusion proteins such as MLL fusions cooperate with activated kinases to promote leukemogenesis [9]

Furthermore, small molecule tyrosine kinase inhibitors have activity against *MLL*-rearranged and hyperdiploid ALL with activating mutations in *FLT3*. Therefore *FLT3* inhibitors are validated as a potential therapeutic target in this leukemia [9]. The presence of *FLT3* mutations in those patients with relapsed ALL harbored these alterations at diagnosis, suggested that *FLT3* inhibition could represent a therapeutic opportunity in at least a subset of patients with relapsed ALL [104].

5.1.1.3. *PTPN11*

PTPN11 encodes SHP2, a protein tyrosine phosphatase that positively controls *RAS* function. Somatic missense mutations in *PTPN11* cause SHP2 constitutive activation and enhance signaling through the mitogen-associated protein (MAP) kinase pathways [5].

PTPN11 mutations occur in approximately 6 to 7.3% of children with B-cell precursor ALL [5, 100]. Although *PTPN11* defects have been negatively associated with most of the gene rearrangements (*TEL-AML1, E2APBX1, BCR-ABL,* and *AF4-MLL*), and other gene lesions (*NRAS* and *KRAS2*), it has been observed higher prevalence of *PTPN11* mutations in children and adolescents with hyperdiploid DNA content [100].

PTPN11 mutations have been observed at disease presentation but are undetectable at remission, supporting the presence of the mutated gene in the leukemic clone and role of *PTPN11* lesions in leukemogenesis. Nevertheless, the prognostic significance of these mutations remains unknown [100].

5.1.1.4. *BRAF*

The *BRAF* gene, a member of RAF family, intermediates downstream in the *RAS/RAF/MAP* kinase pathway. This gene has been described mutated in most of hairy cell leukemias, but is less frequently mutated in acute leukemias, indicating that the *RAS-RAF* kinase pathway in some leukemias may be desregulated by somatic mutations of *BRAF* [105].

Mutations in *BRAF* have been reported with a frequency of 20% in B-cell ALLs cases [105, 106]. *BRAF* is expressed in hematopoietic cells, and the expression of activated *BRAF* could relieve the cytokine dependence and could result in the transformation of hematopoietic cells [105]. The functional significance of the most of the BRAF mutations is unknown, though all mutations are located within the kinase activation domain of *BRAF* [106]. Therapies that target *RAS-RAF-MEK-ERK-MAP* kinase pathway would be very valuable in treating tumors with activating mutations of BRAF [105].

5.1.2. *B-cell differentiation and development pathway*

5.1.2.1. *PAX5*

PAX5 (*paired box 5*) encodes a transcription factor which is known as B-cell specific activator protein. This protein plays a key role in B-cell commitment by activating essential components of B-cell receptor signaling and repressing the transcription of genes that are necessary for T-lymphopoiesis [107]. *PAX5* is the most common transcription factor which is altered in both children and adults B-ALL (32% of cases) [108]. Alterations of *PAX5*, including deletions, focal amplifications, novel translocations, and sequence mutations, have not influence treatment outcome [107].

By SNP arrays, monoallelic deletion of *PAX5* has been observed in about 30% of children and adults with B-ALL, resulting in loss of PAX5 protein expression or in the production of a PAX5 isoform lacking the DNA binding domain and/or transcriptional regulatory domain [107, 109]. It has been demonstrated that the *PAX5* deletions are present in a dominant leukemic clone, consistent with a role in leukemogenesis during the establishing the leukemic clone [85, 110].

By sequencing, inactivating mutations of *PAX5* have been observed between 7–30 % of B-ALL cases [107]. These somatically acquired mutations have different patterns of alterations among some genetic subtypes of pediatric ALL [85]. The most point mutations of *PAX5* are hemizygous reducing or inhibiting normal *PAX5* functional activity [85].

Inactivating point mutations in *PAX5* have more effect on the intracellular transcriptional network within primary leukemic cells. These mutations are clustered in exons encoding the DNA-binding or transcriptional regulatory domains, which leads to lose or to alter DNA-binding or transcriptional regulatory function [85].

Chromosomal translocations *PAX5* are relatively rare, occurring in 2.5% of B-ALL cases; it has been reported at least 12 different fusion partners including transcription factors, structural proteins, and protein kinases (e.g. *ETV6, ENL, FOXP1, ZNF521, PML, C20ORF112, AUTS2, JAK2, POM121, HIPK1, DACH1, LOC392027, SLCO1B3, ASXL1,* and *KIF3B*) [107, 111].

In *PAX5* rearrangements, the DNA binding domain of *PAX5* and/or a variable amount of the C-terminal trans-activating domains are fused to functional domains of the partner genes, resulting in a loss of *PAX5* function rather than in a gain of functional elements [107, 110]. The fusion proteins may also influence the expression of genes which are normally regulated by the partner protein, each of which has been implicated in B-cell development or hematopoietic malignancies [85].

5.1.2.2. IKZF1 (IKAROS)

IKZF1 has been established as one of the most clinically relevant genes in pathogenesis of ALL, because it plays a key role in tumor suppression in pediatric B-cell ALL and in high-risk B-cell ALL [112]. Deletions or mutations of this gene have been described in 15% of all pediatric B-ALL. However the incidence in BCR-ABL ALL is higher (80%) and is associated with a poor outcome. In addition, recent genomic profiling studies (GEP) have produced strong evidence that *IKAROS* plays a key role in tumor suppression in pediatric B-cell ALL and in high-risk B-cell ALL. Thus the GEP of ALL cases with losses in IKZF1 is similar to the observed in BCR-ABL1 positive ALL [112]. Further studies, in larger series of patients, are needed to assess the clinical value of the deletion/mutations in *IKAROS* in the other subtypes of ALL.

5.1.3. JAK/STAT signaling

5.1.3.1. JAK

Activating mutations involving the pseudokinase and kinase domains of Janus kinases (primarily *JAK2*, but also *JAK1* and *JAK3*) have been reported in 10% of *BCR-ABL1*-negative high-risk pediatric ALL cases [86, 98, 113]. The childhood high-risk ALL cases, which harbor activating mutations *JAK*, have a gene-expression profile similar to *BCR-ABL1* pediatric ALL ("*BCR-ABL1*–like" -Ph-like), and are associated to a poor outcome [98].

These mutations are transforming in-vitro, and trigger constitutive *JAK-STAT* activation of the mouse Ba/F3 hematopoietic cell line expressing the erythropoietin receptor transduced with mutant *JAK* alleles [108]. This transformation is abrogated by pharmacologic *JAK1/2* inhibitors, suggesting that these agents may be a useful approach for treating patients harboring these mutations [108, 113].

The presence of *JAK* mutations have been associated with concomitant *IKZF1* and *CDKN2A/B* alterations, suggesting that genetic lesions target multiple cellular pathways, including lymphoid development (*IKZF1*), tumor suppression (*CDKN2A/B*), and activation of tyrosine kinase signaling (*BCR-ABL1, JAK*, or other kinase mutations) that cooperate to induce aggressive lymphoid leukemia in high-risk *BCR-ABL1*-ALL [113].

Particularly, gain-function mutations in *JAK2* are a common molecular event which is present about 18% of ALL Down's syndrome (DS-ALL) cases [114]. These findings suggest that *JAK2* inhibition might be a useful therapeutic approach in *JAK2*-mutated acute ALL associated with Down syndrome, because children with DS-ALL are especially sensitive to toxic effects of conventional chemotherapy [115].

5.1.3.2. Mutations in JAK regulators. CRLF2 and IL7R

CRLF2 encodes cytokine receptor–like factor 2 (also known as TSLPR-thymic stromal lymphopoietin receptor), a lymphoid signaling receptor molecule that forms a heterodimeric complex with interleukin-7 receptor alpha (*IL7R*) and binds TSLP [116]. *CRLF2*-mediated signaling promotes B lymphoid survival and proliferation [117].

Signaling from the TSLP receptor activates signal transducer and activator of transcription (*STAT5*) by phosphorylation of JAK1 and JAK2 through association with *IL-7R* and *CRLF2*, respectively [118]. Genetic alterations dysregulating *CRLF2* expression may contribute to the pathogenesis of ALL [117], by induced activation of STAT proteins, especially STAT5 and STAT1 [119].

CRLF2 rearrangements, such as *IGH@-CRLF2* or *P2RY8-CRLF2* fusion, are present in up to 60% of children with Down Syndrome ALL (DS-ALL) and about 10–15% of high-risk *BCR-ABL1* negative childhood and adult ALL [22]. In both DS-ALL and non-DS-ALL, approximately half of *CRLF2* rearranged cases have concomitant activating *JAK* mutations (the most common in *JAK2* but occasionally in *JAK1*), suggesting that the two alterations cooperate downstream in the signal transduction and transformation [108, 116].

Furthermore, in high-risk ALL, *IKZF1* alterations, *CRLF2* rearrangement and *JAK* mutations are frequently observed together. They are associated with very poor outcome, even with current maximal intensive therapy [108, 117]. These leukemias may be sensitive to *JAK* inhibitors, suggesting the potential for a targeted therapy. Thereby, detection of *IKZF1, CRLF2,* and *JAK* mutations should be considered at diagnosis in childhood ALL [117].

Moreover, somatic mutations of Interleukin-7 receptor (*IL7R*) (the heterodimeric partner of *CRLF2*) have been reported in pediatric B and T ALL. Some *IL7R* mutations have been observed in both diagnosis and relapse, but other mutations have been only present in relapse, whereas *CRLF2* expression have been already described at diagnosis, suggesting that the *IL7R* mutation may be a progression event [120]. Mutations of *IL7R* are gain-of-function mutations that cooperate with *CRLF2* to form a constitutively activated TSLP receptor. *IL7R* activating mutations trigger cytokine-independent growth of progenitor lymphoid cells, and constitutive activation of STAT and mTOR pathways [120].

5.1.4. TP53/RB1 pathway

Mutations of the tumor suppressor gene *TP53* have been associated with resistance to treatment and worse prognosis of patients in several tumors. Alterations of the *TP53* gene are important at relapse in childhood ALL, in which they independently predict high risk of treatment failure in a significant number of patients[121].

The presence of *TP53* mutations is associated with a reduced response rate to reinduction therapy. In addition, *TP53* mutations correlate with a shortened duration of survival (from time of relapse and from time of diagnosis), even after successful reinduction therapy [122].

The clinical significance of exclusive deletions might be explained by *TP53* haploinsufficiency. Moreover, an additional mutation appeared during or after relapse therapy in some relapse patients with exclusive deletion and nonresponse to treatment or second relapse, indicating outgrowth of fully *TP53* altered clones that might contribute to the poor outcome [121].

5.2. Gene mutations in T-ALL

T-ALL has been associated with four different classes of mutations: (i) Affecting the cell cycle (*CDKN2A/CDKN2B*); (ii) Impairing differentiation (*HOX* genes, *MLL, LYL1, TAL1/2* and *LMO1/2*); (iii) Providing a proliferative and survival advantage (*LCK* and *ABL1*); (iv) Providing self-renewal capacity (*NOTCH1*) [10, 11, 18, 123]. The genes most recurrently mutated in T-ALL are described in Table 2.

5.2.1. CDKN2A/CDKN2B

In up to 90% of ALL cases, the *CDKN2A/2B* genes, located in tandem at chromosome 9p21, are inactivated by cryptic deletions, promoter hypermethylation, inactivating mutations or (post)-transcriptional modifications. Homozygous or heterozygous inactivation of the genomic *CDKN2A* and *CDKN2B* loci are the most frequent genetic abnormalities in T-ALL [124].

Inactivation of *CDKN2A* and *CDKN2B* by homozygous deletion has been described in 65% and 23% of T-ALL samples, respectively. Hemizygous *CDKN2A* and *CDKN2B* deletions are observed in approximately 10% and 15% of the samples [18].

The haploinsufficiency or inactivation of these tumor suppressor genes are involved in the development of T-ALL, because they not only promote uncontrolled cell cycle entry, but also disable the p53-controlled cell cycle checkpoint and apoptosis machinery. Thus, *RB1* and *TP53* pathways have been identified as possible targets for therapy of T-ALL [10, 11, 18, 19, 123].

5.2.2. Tp53

The acquisition of mutations in *TP53* has been described in T-cell lines and T-ALL patients [123, 125]. The *TP53* mutations are infrequent at diagnosis (5% of T-ALL cases) and tend to be associated with poor clinical outcome [123]. Copy number and sequence alterations of *TP53* have been observed in 6.4%-24% of patients with T-cell ALL relapse, suggesting the importance of these alterations in the progression of the disease, in which they independently predict high risk of treatment failure in a significant number of patients [121, 123].

5.2.3. NOTCH1

Gain-of-function mutations in *NOTCH1* have been identified in more than 50% of T-ALL samples resulting in constitutive NOTCH signaling [126]. They have been associated with a favorable early treatment response [11, 127]. *NOTCH1* is a transmembrane receptor that plays a role in normal hematopoiesis as an early transcription factor and regulates self-renewal of stem cells and lineage commitment of lymphoid progenitor cells towards T-cell development [11, 128]. The intracellular NOTCH (ICN) released after proteolytic cleavage step of *NOTCH1* mediates in the nucleus the expression of various target genes including *HES1, HEY1, MYC, PTCRA, DTX1* and members of the NFkB pathway. At the protein level, activation of *NOTCH1* mutations could also cause phosphorylation of multiple signaling proteins in the mTOR pathway [11]. *NOTCH1* receptor is a promising target for drugs such as gamma-secretase inhibitors which block a proteolytic cleavage required for *NOTCH1* activation signaling pathway [91].

The presence of subclonal duplications of the chromosomal region 9q34 are present in about 33% of pediatric T-ALL patients; the critical region encloses many genes including *NOTCH1*. Although this duplication appears as an independent genetic event from both the episomal *NUP214-ABL1* amplification and the *NOTCH1* mutations, it could induce subtle changes in *NOTCH1* expression levels and contribute to global *NOTCH1* activation in T-ALL [11, 129].

5.2.4. FBXW7

F-box protein FBXW7 is an E3-ubiquitin ligase that regulates the half-life of other proteins including CyclinE, cMYC and cJUN [11]. Heterozygous *FBXW7* single mutations have been identified in 8–30% of T-ALL patients, and usually are combined with *NOTCH1* mutations affecting the heterodimerization (HD) domain. *FBXW7* mutations render *FBXW7* inactive to prime target proteins like *NOTCH1* for proteosomal degradation, therefore these mutations represent an alternative mechanism for *NOTCH1* activation in T-ALL [11]. The presence of both *FBXW7* and *NOTCH1* mutations has been associated with good treatment response in T-ALL patients [130].

5.2.5. JAK1

Somatic activating *JAK1* mutations occur about 10-20% of adults with T-cell precursors ALL, and have low prevalence in children and adolescents T-ALL [131]. *JAK1* gene defects are associated with a poor response to therapy, frequent relapse, and reduced overall survival, identifying such mutations as a novel informative prognostic marker in adult T-ALL [132].

JAK1 gene encodes a cytoplasmic tyrosine kinase that it is noncovalently associates with a variety of cytokine receptors and plays a nonredundant role in lymphoid cell precursor proliferation, survival, and differentiation. T-cell origin with mutated *JAK1* share a gene expression signature which is characterized by transcriptional up-regulation of genes positively controlled by JAK signaling [132].

Gain-of-function mutations in *JAK1* may be concomitant with other genomic changes, such as *NOTCH1* defects. The activation of *JAK1* and *NOTCH1* transduction pathways might cooperate in T-ALL pathogenesis and/or progression [10, 19, 132].

5.2.6. PTEN

PTEN loss of function mutation and deletions occur in approximately 25% to 35% of cases of T-cell ALL [98]. *PTEN* mutations and loss of PTEN protein could be also found as a secondary event during disease progression, thereby it could represent a progression marker rather than an initiating event in T-ALL [11].

The PTEN phosphatase has been identified as an important regulator of downstream (pre)TCR signaling. It directly opposes the activity of the phosphor-inosital-3 kinase (PI3K) functioning as a negative regulator of the oncogenic PI3K-AKT signaling [11, 133]. Inactivation of *PTEN* has been associated with activation of the PI3K-AKT pathway resulting in enhanced cell size, glucose uptake and proliferation [91]. Furthermore, the detection of abnormalities in the *PTEN, PI3K,* and *AKT* genes in a large subset of primary T-ALL samples have demonstrated a prominent role for oncogenic PI3K-AKT signaling in the pathogenesis of T-ALL [133].

Independent from activation following (pre)TCR stimulation, *PTEN* is negatively regulated by *NOTCH1* [11]. There are some small molecule inhibitors of γ-secretase (GSIs) which block *NOTCH1* activation in T-ALL cell lines with prototypical activating mutations in *NOTCH1*, However some of them are GSI-resistant. This resistance to GSI action is mediated by molecular abnormalities in signaling pathways that promote cell growth downstream of *NOTCH1* [91]. It has been reported that mutational loss of *PTEN* is associated with human T-ALL resistance to pharmacological inhibition of *NOTCH1* performed by GSIs [91]. Therefore *PTEN* deletions appeared to impart a high risk of induction failure with contemporary chemotherapy in T-ALL patients [91]

5.2.7. RAS

In T-ALL, activating *RAS* mutations have been identified only in 4–10% of cases without a prognostic impact [98, 123, 134, 135]. Nevertheless, it has been identified an alternative *RAS* activation mechanism in T-ALL cases with *NF1* microdeletions on chromosome 17 without clinical evidence for neurofibromatosis with mutations on the remaining *NF1* allele. *NF1* is a negative regulator of the RAS signaling pathway. The presence of mutations on the remaining *NF1* allele, confirmed the potential *NF1* inactivation as an alternative *RAS* activation mechanism in these T-ALL cases. Therefore, T-ALL patients with activated *RAS* could potentially benefit from additional treatment with *RAS* inhibitors, such as farnesylthiosalicylic acid [11].

5.2.8. WT1

WT1 mutations is a recurrent genetic alteration in T-ALL. They are present in around 10% of T-ALL both in childhood and adults [136]. These mutations are highly associated with direct or indirect aberrant *HOX* genes expression in T-ALL cases with aberrant rearrangements of the oncogenic *TLX1, TLX3,* and *HOXA* transcription factor oncogenes [137]. Survival analysis have demonstrated that *WT1* mutations do not confer adverse prognosis in either pediatric and adult T-ALL cases [136].

5.2.9. Mutated genes in Early Thymic Progenitors (ETP)-ALL

A new T-ALL subgroup, which is defined by a specific gene expression profile and a characteristic immunophenotype (CD1a-, CD8-, CD5weak with expression of stem cell or myeloid markers), has been recently described in pediatric T-ALL patients with poor outcome. This subgroup likely originates from early thymic progenitors (ETP) and has been called ETP-ALL. Recently, it has been described the high presence of *FLT3* mutations in ETP-ALL [138] while in T-ALL patients with a non-ETP immunophenotype are rare (1-3%). In some patients, these mutations are only present in leukemic subclones [139, 140],, indicating that FLT3 mutations may represent a T-ALL progression marker rather than an initiating event [11].

Moreover a recent study of whole-genome sequencing in ETP-ALL cases, has identified activating mutations in genes regulating cytokine receptor and RAS signaling in 67% of cases (*NRAS, KRAS, FLT3, IL7R, JAK3, JAK1, SH2B3 and BRAF*), inactivating lesions disrupting hematopoietic development involving 58% of patients (*GATA3, ETV6, RUNX1, IKZF1* and *EP300*) and histone-modifying genes in 48% of patients (*EZH2, EED, SUZ12, SETD2* and *EP300*) [141]. The global transcriptional profile of ETP ALL was similar to normal and myeloid leukemia hematopoietic stem cells. These findings could be related to the prognosis of ETP ALL patients [141].

In summary, the recent development of the genome wide analysis has provided new and critical knowledge of genetic changes in ALL. These new chromosomal imbalances and mutations could provide new insights for the management of the disease that is still associated with a dismal prognosis in the adult patients.

Acknowledgements

This work was partially supported by grants from the "Fondo de Investigaciones Sanitarias - FIS" (FIS 02/1041, FIS 09/01543 and FIS 12/0028), grant Paula Estevez 2010 of the "Fundación Sandra Ibarra de Solidaridad contra el Cáncer". "Fundación Samuel Solorzano Barruso", research project 106/A/06 SACYL and by the "Acción Transversal del Cáncer" project, through an agreement between the Instituto de Salud Carlos III (ISCIII), Spanish Ministry of Science and Innovation, and the University of Salamanca's Cancer Research Foundation (Spain) and the Research Network RTIIC (FIS). RMF is fully supported by an agreement of study commission remunerated (No. 223-2011) granted by the "Universidad Pedagógica y Tecnológica de Colombia - Colombia". MHS is supported by a grant from "Spanish Foundation of Hematology and Hemotherapy."

Author details

Ruth Maribel Forero[1,2], María Hernández[1] and Jesús María Hernández-Rivas[1,3*]

*Address all correspondence to: jmhr@usal.es

1 IBSAL,IBMCC, Centro de Investigación del Cáncer, Universidad de Salamanca-CSIC, Spain

2 Universidad Pedagógica Y Tecnológica de Colombia, Colombia

3 Servicio de Hematología, Hospital Clínico Universitario de Salamanca, Spain

References

[1] Teitell, M.A. and P.P. Pandolfi, *Molecular genetics of acute lymphoblastic leukemia.* Annu Rev Pathol, 2009. 4: p. 175-98.

[2] Bacher, U., A. Kohlmann, and T. Haferlach, *Gene expression profiling for diagnosis and therapy in acute leukaemia and other haematologic malignancies.* Cancer Treat Rev, 2010. 36(8): p. 637-46.

[3] Downing, J.R. and C.G. Mullighan, *Tumor-specific genetic lesions and their influence on therapy in pediatric acute lymphoblastic leukemia.* Hematology Am Soc Hematol Educ Program, 2006: p. 118-22, 508.

[4] Jabbour, E.J., S. Faderl, and H.M. Kantarjian, *Adult acute lymphoblastic leukemia.* Mayo Clin Proc, 2005. 80(11): p. 1517-27.

[5] Pui, C.H., M.V. Relling, and J.R. Downing, *Acute lymphoblastic leukemia.* N Engl J Med, 2004. 350(15): p. 1535-48.

[6] Bungaro, S., et al., *Integration of genomic and gene expression data of childhood ALL without known aberrations identifies subgroups with specific genetic hallmarks.* Genes Chromosomes Cancer, 2009. 48(1): p. 22-38.

[7] Usvasalo, A., et al., *Acute lymphoblastic leukemias with normal karyotypes are not without genomic aberrations.* Cancer Genet Cytogenet, 2009. 192(1): p. 10-7.

[8] Rowley, J.D., *The critical role of chromosome translocations in human leukemias.* Annu Rev Genet, 1998. 32: p. 495-519.

[9] Armstrong, S.A. and A.T. Look, *Molecular genetics of acute lymphoblastic leukemia.* J Clin Oncol, 2005. 23(26): p. 6306-15.

[10] Gorello, P., et al., *Combined interphase fluorescence in situ hybridization elucidates the genetic heterogeneity of T-cell acute lymphoblastic leukemia in adults.* Haematologica, 2010. 95(1): p. 79-86.

[11] Van Vlierberghe, P., et al., *Molecular-genetic insights in paediatric T-cell acute lymphoblastic leukaemia.* Br J Haematol, 2008. 143(2): p. 153-68.

[12] Swerdlow, S.H., et al., *WHO classification of tumours of haematopoietic and lymphoid tissues.* 4ª ed. 2008, IARC Lyon: World Health Organization.

[13] Miles, R.R., S. Arnold, and M.S. Cairo, *Risk factors and treatment of childhood and adolescent Burkitt lymphoma/leukaemia.* Br J Haematol, 2012. 156(6): p. 730-43.

[14] Scholtysik, R., et al., *Detection of genomic aberrations in molecularly defined Burkitt's lymphoma by array-based, high resolution, single nucleotide polymorphism analysis.* Haematologica, 2010. 95(12): p. 2047-55.

[15] Boerma, E.G., et al., *Translocations involving 8q24 in Burkitt lymphoma and other malignant lymphomas: a historical review of cytogenetics in the light of todays knowledge.* Leukemia, 2009. 23(2): p. 225-34.

[16] Chiaretti, S., et al., *Gene expression profile of adult T-cell acute lymphocytic leukemia identifies distinct subsets of patients with different response to therapy and survival.* Blood, 2004. 103(7): p. 2771-8.

[17] Cauwelier, B., et al., *Molecular cytogenetic study of 126 unselected T-ALL cases reveals high incidence of TCRbeta locus rearrangements and putative new T-cell oncogenes.* Leukemia, 2006. 20(7): p. 1238-44.

[18] De Keersmaecker, K., P. Marynen, and J. Cools, *Genetic insights in the pathogenesis of T-cell acute lymphoblastic leukemia.* Haematologica, 2005. 90(8): p. 1116-27.

[19] Graux, C., et al., *Cytogenetics and molecular genetics of T-cell acute lymphoblastic leukemia: from thymocyte to lymphoblast.* Leukemia, 2006. 20(9): p. 1496-510.

[20] Usvasalo, A., et al., *Prognostic classification of patients with acute lymphoblastic leukemia by using gene copy number profiles identified from array-based comparative genomic hybridization data.* Leuk Res, 2010. 34(11): p. 1476-82.

[21] Pui, C.H., et al., *Biology, risk stratification, and therapy of pediatric acute leukemias: an update.* J Clin Oncol, 2011. 29(5): p. 551-65.

[22] Izraeli, S., *Application of genomics for risk stratification of childhood acute lymphoblastic leukaemia: from bench to bedside?* Br J Haematol, 2010. 151(2): p. 119-31.

[23] Sancho, J.M.C., *Avances en el diagnóstico y tratamiento, y significado pronóstico de la infiltración neuromeníngea en leucemias agudas y linfomas agresivos,* in *Facultad de Medicina.* 2011, Universidad Autónoma de Barcelona. : Barcelona. p. 36.

[24] Heim, S. and F. Mitelman, *Cancer cytogenetics.* Third ed. Acute Lymphoblastic Leukemia. 2009, New Jersey: John Wiley & Sons, Inc. Hoboken.

[25] Pui, C.H., D. Campana, and W.E. Evans, *Childhood acute lymphoblastic leukaemia--current status and future perspectives.* Lancet Oncol, 2001. 2(10): p. 597-607.

[26] Ribera, J.J.O.y.J.M., *Leucemia Aguda Linfoblástica.* 16 ed. Farreras-Rozman, Medicina Interna., ed. F.C.e. En C Rozman. 2009, Barcelona: Elsevier.

[27] Mittelman, F., *The Third International Workshop on Chromosomes in Leukemia. Lund, Sweden, July 21-25, 1980. Introduction.* Cancer genetics and cytogenetics, 1981. 4(2): p. 96-98.

[28] Kuchinskaya, E., et al., *Array-CGH reveals hidden gene dose changes in children with acute lymphoblastic leukaemia and a normal or failed karyotype by G-banding.* Br J Haematol, 2008. 140(5): p. 572-7.

[29] Kim, J.E., et al., *A rare case of acute lymphoblastic leukemia with t(12;17)(p13;q21).* Korean J Lab Med, 2010. 30(3): p. 239-43.

[30] Harrison, C.J. and L. Foroni, *Cytogenetics and molecular genetics of acute lymphoblastic leukemia.* Rev Clin Exp Hematol, 2002. 6(2): p. 91-113; discussion 200-2.

[31] Harrison, C.J., et al., *Interphase molecular cytogenetic screening for chromosomal abnormalities of prognostic significance in childhood acute lymphoblastic leukaemia: a UK Cancer Cytogenetics Group Study.* Br J Haematol, 2005. 129(4): p. 520-30.

[32] De Braekeleer, E., et al., *Cytogenetics in pre-B and B-cell acute lymphoblastic leukemia: a study of 208 patients diagnosed between 1981 and 2008.* Cancer Genet Cytogenet, 2010. 200(1): p. 8-15.

[33] Graux, C., *Biology of acute lymphoblastic leukemia (ALL): clinical and therapeutic relevance.* Transfus Apher Sci, 2011. 44(2): p. 183-9.

[34] Downing, J.R. and K.M. Shannon, *Acute leukemia: a pediatric perspective.* Cancer Cell, 2002. 2(6): p. 437-45.

[35] Steinemann, D., et al., *Copy number alterations in childhood acute lymphoblastic leukemia and their association with minimal residual disease.* Genes Chromosomes Cancer, 2008. 47(6): p. 471-80.

[36] Schultz, K.R., et al., *Improved early event-free survival with imatinib in Philadelphia chromosome-positive acute lymphoblastic leukemia: a children's oncology group study.* J Clin Oncol, 2009. 27(31): p. 5175-81.

[37] Meyer, C., et al., *New insights to the MLL recombinome of acute leukemias.* Leukemia, 2009. 23(8): p. 1490-9.

[38] Meyer, C., et al., *The MLL recombinome of acute leukemias.* Leukemia, 2006. 20(5): p. 777-84.

[39] Forestier, E., et al., *Outcome of ETV6/RUNX1-positive childhood acute lymphoblastic leukaemia in the NOPHO-ALL-1992 protocol: frequent late relapses but good overall survival.* Br J Haematol, 2008. 140(6): p. 665-72.

[40] Golub, T.R., et al., *Fusion of the TEL gene on 12p13 to the AML1 gene on 21q22 in acute lymphoblastic leukemia.* Proc Natl Acad Sci U S A, 1995. 92(11): p. 4917-21.

[41] Frick, M., B. Dorken, and G. Lenz, *New insights into the biology of molecular subtypes of diffuse large B-cell lymphoma and Burkitt lymphoma.* Best Pract Res Clin Haematol, 2012. 25(1): p. 3-12.

[42] Hecht, J.L. and J.C. Aster, *Molecular biology of Burkitt's lymphoma.* J Clin Oncol, 2000. 18(21): p. 3707-21.

[43] Garcia, J.L., et al., *Abnormalities on 1q and 7q are associated with poor outcome in sporadic Burkitt's lymphoma. A cytogenetic and comparative genomic hybridization study.* Leukemia, 2003. 17(10): p. 2016-24.

[44] Lones, M.A., et al., *Chromosome abnormalities may correlate with prognosis in Burkitt/Burkitt-like lymphomas of children and adolescents: a report from Children's Cancer Group Study CCG-E08.* J Pediatr Hematol Oncol, 2004. 26(3): p. 169-78.

[45] Poirel, H.A., et al., *Specific cytogenetic abnormalities are associated with a significantly inferior outcome in children and adolescents with mature B-cell non-Hodgkin's lymphoma: results of the FAB/LMB 96 international study.* Leukemia, 2009. 23(2): p. 323-31.

[46] Onciu, M., et al., *Secondary chromosomal abnormalities predict outcome in pediatric and adult high-stage Burkitt lymphoma.* Cancer, 2006. 107(5): p. 1084-92.

[47] Xiao, H., et al., *American Burkitt lymphoma stage II with 47,XY,+20,t(8;14)(q24;q32).* Cancer Genet Cytogenet, 1990. 48(2): p. 275-7.

[48] Lai, J.L., et al., *Cytogenetic studies in 30 patients with Burkitt's lymphoma or L3 acute lymphoblastic leukemia with special reference to additional chromosome abnormalities.* Ann Genet, 1989. 32(1): p. 26-32.

[49] Nelson, M., et al., *An increased frequency of 13q deletions detected by fluorescence in situ hybridization and its impact on survival in children and adolescents with Burkitt lymphoma: results from the Children's Oncology Group study CCG-5961.* Br J Haematol, 2010. 148(4): p. 600-10.

[50] de Souza, M.T., et al., *Secondary abnormalities involving 1q or 13q and poor outcome in high stage Burkitt leukemia/lymphoma cases with 8q24 rearrangement at diagnosis.* Int J Hematol, 2011. 93(2): p. 232-6.

[51] Zunino, A., et al., *Chromosomal aberrations evaluated by CGH, FISH and GTG-banding in a case of AIDS-related Burkitt's lymphoma.* Haematologica, 2000. 85(3): p. 250-5.

[52] Zimonjic, D.B., C. Keck-Waggoner, and N.C. Popescu, *Novel genomic imbalances and chromosome translocations involving c-myc gene in Burkitt's lymphoma.* Leukemia, 2001. 15(10): p. 1582-8.

[53] Salaverria, I., et al., *Chromosomal alterations detected by comparative genomic hybridization in subgroups of gene expression-defined Burkitt's lymphoma.* Haematologica, 2008. 93(9): p. 1327-34.

[54] Barth, T.F., et al., *Homogeneous immunophenotype and paucity of secondary genomic aberrations are distinctive features of endemic but not of sporadic Burkitt's lymphoma and diffuse large B-cell lymphoma with MYC rearrangement.* J Pathol, 2004. 203(4): p. 940-5.

[55] Toujani, S., et al., *High resolution genome-wide analysis of chromosomal alterations in Burkitt's lymphoma.* PLoS One, 2009. 4(9): p. e7089.

[56] Berger, R. and A. Bernheim, *Cytogenetics of Burkitt's lymphoma-leukaemia: a review.* IARC Sci Publ, 1985(60): p. 65-80.

[57] Cave, H., et al., *Clinical significance of HOX11L2 expression linked to t(5;14)(q35;q32), of HOX11 expression, and of SIL-TAL fusion in childhood T-cell malignancies: results of EORTC studies 58881 and 58951.* Blood, 2004. 103(2): p. 442-50.

[58] Ballerini, P., et al., *HOX11L2 expression defines a clinical subtype of pediatric T-ALL associated with poor prognosis.* Blood, 2002. 100(3): p. 991-7.

[59] Hawley, R.G., et al., *Transforming function of the HOX11/TCL3 homeobox gene.* Cancer Res, 1997. 57(2): p. 337-45.

[60] Keller, G., et al., *Overexpression of HOX11 leads to the immortalization of embryonic precursors with both primitive and definitive hematopoietic potential.* Blood, 1998. 92(3): p. 877-87.

[61] Bernard, O.A., et al., *A new recurrent and specific cryptic translocation, t(5;14)(q35;q32), is associated with expression of the Hox11L2 gene in T acute lymphoblastic leukemia.* Leukemia, 2001. 15(10): p. 1495-504.

[62] Wadman, I., et al., *Specific in vivo association between the bHLH and LIM proteins implicated in human T cell leukemia.* EMBO J, 1994. 13(20): p. 4831-9.

[63] Xia, Y., et al., *TAL2, a helix-loop-helix gene activated by the (7;9)(q34;q32) translocation in human T-cell leukemia.* Proc Natl Acad Sci U S A, 1991. 88(24): p. 11416-20.

[64] Xia, Y., et al., *Products of the TAL2 oncogene in leukemic T cells: bHLH phosphoproteins with DNA-binding activity.* Oncogene, 1994. 9(5): p. 1437-46.

[65] Zhong, Y., et al., *Overexpression of a transcription factor LYL1 induces T- and B-cell lymphoma in mice.* Oncogene, 2007. 26(48): p. 6937-47.

[66] Harrison, C.J., *Cytogenetics of paediatric and adolescent acute lymphoblastic leukaemia.* Br J Haematol, 2009. 144(2): p. 147-56.

[67] Palacios, E.H. and A. Weiss, *Function of the Src-family kinases, Lck and Fyn, in T-cell development and activation.* Oncogene, 2004. 23(48): p. 7990-8000.

[68] Clappier, E., et al., *The C-MYB locus is involved in chromosomal translocation and genomic duplications in human T-cell acute leukemia (T-ALL), the translocation defining a new T-ALL subtype in very young children.* Blood, 2007. 110(4): p. 1251-61.

[69] Dik, W.A., et al., *CALM-AF10+ T-ALL expression profiles are characterized by overexpression of HOXA and BMI1 oncogenes.* Leukemia, 2005. 19(11): p. 1948-57.

[70] Krivtsov, A.V. and S.A. Armstrong, *MLL translocations, histone modifications and leukaemia stem-cell development.* Nat Rev Cancer, 2007. 7(11): p. 823-33.

[71] Lacronique, V., et al., *A TEL-JAK2 fusion protein with constitutive kinase activity in human leukemia.* Science, 1997. 278(5341): p. 1309-12.

[72] Harrison, C.J., *Key pathways as therapeutic targets.* Blood, 2011. 118(11): p. 2935-6.

[73] Harrison, C.J., et al., *Three distinct subgroups of hypodiploidy in acute lymphoblastic leukaemia.* Br J Haematol, 2004. 125(5): p. 552-9.

[74] Macconaill, L.E. and L.A. Garraway, *Clinical implications of the cancer genome.* J Clin Oncol, 2010. 28(35): p. 5219-28.

[75] Mullighan, C.G. and J.R. Downing, *Global genomic characterization of acute lymphoblastic leukemia.* Semin Hematol, 2009. 46(1): p. 3-15.

[76] Mullighan, C.G., *Genomic analysis of acute leukemia.* Int J Lab Hematol, 2009. 31(4): p. 384-97.

[77] Rabin, K.R., et al., *Clinical utility of array comparative genomic hybridization for detection of chromosomal abnormalities in pediatric acute lymphoblastic leukemia.* Pediatr Blood Cancer, 2008. 51(2): p. 171-7.

[78] Yasar, D., et al., *Array comparative genomic hybridization analysis of adult acute leukemia patients.* Cancer Genet Cytogenet, 2010. 197(2): p. 122-9.

[79] Harrison, C., *New genetics and diagnosis of childhood B-cell precursor acute lymphoblastic leukemia.* Pediatr Rep, 2011. 3 Suppl 2: p. e4.

[80] Kuiper, R.P., et al., *High-resolution genomic profiling of childhood ALL reveals novel recurrent genetic lesions affecting pathways involved in lymphocyte differentiation and cell cycle progression.* Leukemia, 2007. 21(6): p. 1258-66.

[81] Strefford, J.C., et al., *Genome complexity in acute lymphoblastic leukemia is revealed by array-based comparative genomic hybridization.* Oncogene, 2007. 26(29): p. 4306-18.

[82] Paulsson, K., et al., *Microdeletions are a general feature of adult and adolescent acute lymphoblastic leukemia: Unexpected similarities with pediatric disease.* Proc Natl Acad Sci U S A, 2008. 105(18): p. 6708-13.

[83] Okamoto, R., et al., *Genomic profiling of adult acute lymphoblastic leukemia by single nucleotide polymorphism oligonucleotide microarray and comparison to pediatric acute lymphoblastic leukemia.* Haematologica, 2010. 95(9): p. 1481-8.

[84] Dawson, A.J., et al., *Array comparative genomic hybridization and cytogenetic analysis in pediatric acute leukemias.* Curr Oncol, 2011. 18(5): p. e210-7.

[85] Mullighan, C.G., et al., *Genome-wide analysis of genetic alterations in acute lymphoblastic leukaemia.* Nature, 2007. 446(7137): p. 758-64.

[86] Mullighan, C.G., *Genomic profiling of B-progenitor acute lymphoblastic leukemia.* Best Pract Res Clin Haematol, 2011. 24(4): p. 489-503.

[87] Greaves, M.F. and J. Wiemels, *Origins of chromosome translocations in childhood leukaemia.* Nat Rev Cancer, 2003. 3(9): p. 639-49.

[88] Graux, C., et al., *Fusion of NUP214 to ABL1 on amplified episomes in T-cell acute lymphoblastic leukemia.* Nat Genet, 2004. 36(10): p. 1084-9.

[89] Van Vlierberghe, P., et al., *The recurrent SET-NUP214 fusion as a new HOXA activation mechanism in pediatric T-cell acute lymphoblastic leukemia.* Blood, 2008. 111(9): p. 4668-80.

[90] Van Vlierberghe, P., et al., *The cryptic chromosomal deletion del(11)(p12p13) as a new activation mechanism of LMO2 in pediatric T-cell acute lymphoblastic leukemia.* Blood, 2006. 108(10): p. 3520-9.

[91] Palomero, T., et al., *Mutational loss of PTEN induces resistance to NOTCH1 inhibition in T-cell leukemia.* Nat Med, 2007. 13(10): p. 1203-10.

[92] O'Neil, J., et al., *FBW7 mutations in leukemic cells mediate NOTCH pathway activation and resistance to gamma-secretase inhibitors.* J Exp Med, 2007. 204(8): p. 1813-24.

[93] Lahortiga, I., et al., *Duplication of the MYB oncogene in T cell acute lymphoblastic leukemia.* Nat Genet, 2007. 39(5): p. 593-5.

[94] Schiffman, J.D., et al., *Genome wide copy number analysis of paediatric Burkitt lymphoma using formalin-fixed tissues reveals a subset with gain of chromosome 13q and corresponding miRNA over expression.* Br J Haematol, 2011. 155(4): p. 477-86.

[95] Capello, D., et al., *Genome wide DNA-profiling of HIV-related B-cell lymphomas.* Br J Haematol, 2010. 148(2): p. 245-55.

[96] Mullighan, C.G., et al., *High-Resolution SNP Array Profiling of Relapsed Acute Leukemia Identifies Genomic Abnormalities Distinct from Those Present at Diagnosis.* ASH Annual Meeting Abstracts, 2007. 110(11): p. 234-.

[97] Kuiper, R.P., et al., *Detection of Genomic Lesions in Childhood Precursor-B Cell ALL in Diagnosis and Relapse Samples Using High Resolution Genomic Profiling.* ASH Annual Meeting Abstracts, 2007. 110(11): p. 995-.

[98] Zhang, J., et al., *Key pathways are frequently mutated in high-risk childhood acute lymphoblastic leukemia: a report from the Children's Oncology Group.* Blood, 2011. 118(11): p. 3080-7.

[99] Case, M., et al., *Mutation of genes affecting the RAS pathway is common in childhood acute lymphoblastic leukemia.* Cancer Res, 2008. 68(16): p. 6803-9.

[100] Tartaglia, M., et al., *Genetic evidence for lineage-related and differentiation stage-related contribution of somatic PTPN11 mutations to leukemogenesis in childhood acute leukemia.* Blood, 2004. 104(2): p. 307-13.

[101] Paulsson, K., et al., *Mutations of FLT3, NRAS, KRAS, and PTPN11 are frequent and possibly mutually exclusive in high hyperdiploid childhood acute lymphoblastic leukemia.* Genes Chromosomes Cancer, 2008. 47(1): p. 26-33.

[102] Wiemels, J.L., et al., *RAS mutation is associated with hyperdiploidy and parental characteristics in pediatric acute lymphoblastic leukemia.* Leukemia, 2005. 19(3): p. 415-419.

[103] Perentesis, J.P., et al., *RAS oncogene mutations and outcome of therapy for childhood acute lymphoblastic leukemia.* Leukemia, 2004. 18(4): p. 685-92.

[104] Armstrong, S.A., et al., *FLT3 mutations in childhood acute lymphoblastic leukemia.* Blood, 2004. 103(9): p. 3544-6.

[105] Lee, J.W., et al., *BRAF mutations in acute leukemias.* Leukemia, 2003. 18(1): p. 170-172.

[106] Gustafsson, B., et al., *Mutations in the BRAF and N-ras genes in childhood acute lymphoblastic leukaemia.* Leukemia, 2005. 19(2): p. 310-2.

[107] Iacobucci, I., et al., *Cytogenetic and molecular predictors of outcome in acute lymphocytic leukemia: recent developments.* Curr Hematol Malig Rep. 7(2): p. 133-43.

[108] Roberts, K.G. and C.G. Mullighan, *How new advances in genetic analysis are influencing the understanding and treatment of childhood acute leukemia.* Curr Opin Pediatr, 2011. 23(1): p. 34-40.

[109] Iacobucci, I., et al., *The PAX5 gene is frequently rearranged in BCR-ABL1-positive acute lymphoblastic leukemia but is not associated with outcome. A report on behalf of the GIMEMA Acute Leukemia Working Party.* Haematologica, 2010. 95(10): p. 1683-90.

[110] Mullighan, C.G., et al., *Deletion of IKZF1 and prognosis in acute lymphoblastic leukemia.* N Engl J Med, 2009. 360(5): p. 470-80.

[111] Zhou, Y., et al., *Advances in the molecular pathobiology of B-lymphoblastic leukemia.* Hum Pathol, 2012. 43(9): p. 1347-62.

[112] Payne, K.J. and S. Dovat, *Ikaros and tumor suppression in acute lymphoblastic leukemia.* Crit Rev Oncog, 2011. 16(1-2): p. 3-12.

[113] Mullighan, C.G., et al., *JAK mutations in high-risk childhood acute lymphoblastic leukemia.* Proc Natl Acad Sci U S A, 2009. 106(23): p. 9414-8.

[114] Bercovich, D., et al., *Mutations of JAK2 in acute lymphoblastic leukaemias associated with Down's syndrome.* Lancet, 2008. 372(9648): p. 1484-92.

[115] Mullighan, C.G., *JAK2--a new player in acute lymphoblastic leukaemia.* Lancet, 2008. 372(9648): p. 1448-50.

[116] Mullighan, C.G., et al., *Rearrangement of CRLF2 in B-progenitor- and Down syndrome-associated acute lymphoblastic leukemia.* Nat Genet, 2009. 41(11): p. 1243-6.

[117] Harvey, R.C., et al., *Rearrangement of CRLF2 is associated with mutation of JAK kinases, alteration of IKZF1, Hispanic/Latino ethnicity, and a poor outcome in pediatric B-progenitor acute lymphoblastic leukemia.* Blood, 2010. 115(26): p. 5312-21.

[118] Rochman, Y., et al., *Thymic stromal lymphopoietin-mediated STAT5 phosphorylation via kinases JAK1 and JAK2 reveals a key difference from IL-7-induced signaling.* Proc Natl Acad Sci U S A, 2010. 107(45): p. 19455-60.

[119] Buettner, R., L.B. Mora, and R. Jove, *Activated STAT signaling in human tumors provides novel molecular targets for therapeutic intervention.* Clin Cancer Res, 2002. 8(4): p. 945-54.

[120] Shochat, C., et al., *Gain-of-function mutations in interleukin-7 receptor-alpha (IL7R) in childhood acute lymphoblastic leukemias.* J Exp Med, 2011. 208(5): p. 901-8.

[121] Hof, J., et al., *Mutations and deletions of the TP53 gene predict nonresponse to treatment and poor outcome in first relapse of childhood acute lymphoblastic leukemia.* J Clin Oncol, 2011. 29(23): p. 3185-93.

[122] Diccianni, M.B., et al., *Clinical significance of p53 mutations in relapsed T-cell acute lymphoblastic leukemia.* Blood, 1994. 84(9): p. 3105-12.

[123] Kawamura, M., et al., *Alterations of the p53, p21, p16, p15 and RAS genes in childhood T-cell acute lymphoblastic leukemia.* Leuk Res, 1999. 23(2): p. 115-26.

[124] Cayuela, J.M., et al., *Multiple tumor-suppressor gene 1 inactivation is the most frequent genetic alteration in T-cell acute lymphoblastic leukemia.* Blood, 1996. 87(6): p. 2180-6.

[125] Cheng, J. and M. Haas, *Frequent mutations in the p53 tumor suppressor gene in human leukemia T-cell lines.* Mol Cell Biol, 1990. 10(10): p. 5502-9.

[126] Weng, A.P., et al., *Activating mutations of NOTCH1 in human T cell acute lymphoblastic leukemia.* Science, 2004. 306(5694): p. 269-71.

[127] Breit, S., et al., *Activating NOTCH1 mutations predict favorable early treatment response and long-term outcome in childhood precursor T-cell lymphoblastic leukemia.* Blood, 2006. 108(4): p. 1151-7.

[128] Sambandam, A., et al., *Notch signaling controls the generation and differentiation of early T lineage progenitors.* Nat Immunol, 2005. 6(7): p. 663-70.

[129] van Vlierberghe, P., et al., *A new recurrent 9q34 duplication in pediatric T-cell acute lymphoblastic leukemia.* Leukemia, 2006. 20(7): p. 1245-53.

[130] Malyukova, A., et al., *The tumor suppressor gene hCDC4 is frequently mutated in human T-cell acute lymphoblastic leukemia with functional consequences for Notch signaling.* Cancer Res, 2007. 67(12): p. 5611-6.

[131] Vainchenker, W. and S.N. Constantinescu, *JAK/STAT signaling in hematological malignancies.* Oncogene, 2012.

[132] Flex, E., et al., *Somatically acquired JAK1 mutations in adult acute lymphoblastic leukemia.* J Exp Med, 2008. 205(4): p. 751-8.

[133] Gutierrez, A., et al., *High frequency of PTEN, PI3K, and AKT abnormalities in T-cell acute lymphoblastic leukemia.* Blood, 2009. 114(3): p. 647-50.

[134] Yokota, S., et al., *Mutational analysis of the N-ras gene in acute lymphoblastic leukemia: a study of 125 Japanese pediatric cases.* Int J Hematol, 1998. 67(4): p. 379-87.

[135] von Lintig, F.C., et al., *Ras activation in normal white blood cells and childhood acute lymphoblastic leukemia.* Clin Cancer Res, 2000. 6(5): p. 1804-10.

[136] Tosello, V., et al., *WT1 mutations in T-ALL.* Blood, 2009. 114(5): p. 1038-45.

[137] Renneville, A., et al., *Wilms' Tumor 1 (WT1) Gene Mutations in Pediatric T-Acute Lymphoblastic Leukemia.* ASH Annual Meeting Abstracts, 2009. 114(22): p. 3075-.

[138] Neumann, M., et al., *High Rate of FLT3 Mutations In Adult ETP-ALL.* ASH Annual Meeting Abstracts, 2010. 116(21): p. 1031-.

[139] Paietta, E., et al., *Activating FLT3 mutations in CD117/KIT(+) T-cell acute lymphoblastic leukemias.* Blood, 2004. 104(2): p. 558-60.

[140] Van Vlierberghe, P., et al., *Activating FLT3 mutations in CD4+/CD8- pediatric T-cell acute lymphoblastic leukemias.* Blood, 2005. 106(13): p. 4414-5.

[141] Zhang, J., et al., *The genetic basis of early T-cell precursor acute lymphoblastic leukaemia.* Nature, 2012. 481(7380): p. 157-63.

Chapter 2

Acute Lymphoblastic Leukemia in Children

Jelena Roganovic

Additional information is available at the end of the chapter

http://dx.doi.org/10.5772/55655

1. Introduction

Extraordinary advances in the treatment outcome of childhood acute lymphoblastic leukemia (ALL) rank as one of the most successful stories in the history of oncology, with the current rate of approximately 80% of children being cured [1-5]. The improvements made have been mainly due to the development of intensive multiagent chemotherapy, identification of clinical and biologic variables predictive for outcome and their use in stratifying treatment, significant advances in supportive care, and development of large-scale, highly disciplined multi-institutional national and international clinical trials [6,7]. In spite of this success, there remains place for improvement, including the development of better treatment for the minority of patients who relapse, the development of less toxic therapy, and focusing attention on screening and management of late effects that may potentially arise as a result of antileukemic treatment [8,9].

2. Epidemiology

ALL is the most common childhood malignancy, accounting for close to 25% of all cancers in children and 72% of all cases of pediatric leukemia [10,11]. ALL occurs at an annual rate of 3 to 4 cases per 100.000 children less than 15 years of age [12]. Approximately 3,000 children in the United States and 5,000 children in Europe are diagnosed with ALL each year [13]. A sharp peak in incidence is observed among children aged 2 to 5 years. Males are affected more often than females except in infants, the difference being greater among pubertal children. There is a geographic variation in the frequency of ALL. The incidence is lowest in North Africa and the Middle East, and highest in the industrialized Western countries, suggesting that this may reflect more exposure to environmental leukemogens [6]. Numerous investigators have reported the occurrence of leukemic clusters in different geographic areas, thus pointing towards infectious and/or environmental causes of at least some cases of ALL [14-17]. Several studies have suggested a link between maternal reproductive history and the risk of ALL. Fetal loss is associated with a higher risk for ALL in subsequent children [18]. There is evidence that increased in utero growth rates and Insulin Growth Factor (IGF) pathways play a role in the development of ALL [19,20].

3. Pathogenesis

ALL represents the malignant proliferation of lymphoid cells blocked at early stages of differentiation. Although a variety of hypotheses regarding potential pathogenic mechanisms in the development of pediatric ALL have been described, the etiology for the overwhelming majority of children with ALL remains unclear. The favored concept is that leukemogenesis reflects a complex interaction between multiple genetic and environmental factors [21].

Genetic factors play a significant role in the etiology of ALL. Molecular techniques have documented the presence of the same leukemia-specific genetic abnormalities in neonatal blood Guthrie spots and stored cord blood as in diagnostic samples from children with ALL [22]. This is evidence that important initiating events that contribute to leukemogenesis may begin *in utero* [23,24]. Consistent with Knudson's two-hit hypothesis [25], postnatal oncogenic mutations may subsequently lead to clinically detectable leukemia [26]. Recent genome-wide association studies have identified germline single nucleotide polymorphisms that predispose subjects to development of ALL. The affected genes include *ARID5B* and *IKZF*, which are involved in B-cell transcriptional regulation and differentiation [27,28].

The occurrence of familial leukemia has been reported, including aggregates within the same generation or in several generations. Siblings of children with ALL have two- to four-fold greater risk of developing the disease than unrelated children [29]. There is a higher risk for ALL in identical twins. The overall concordance rate of ALL in monozygotic twins is estimated to be as high as 25%, and is thought to be the result of shared *in utero* circulation [30]. Leukemias with the (4,11) translocation and the *MLL-AF4* fusion gene have a very high concordance rate and a brief latency, while others may present with disease after a long latency period [31]. The risk for ALL among both mono- and dizygotic twins is highest in infancy, diminishes with age, and after the age of 7 years the risk to the unaffected twin approaches that for general population [30].

Several constitutional chromosomal abnormalities and specific inherited syndromes have been linked to childhood ALL. Children with Down syndrome (DS) are 10 to 20 times more likely to develop ALL and acute myeloid leukemia (AML) than non-DS children [32]. ALL predominates in all but the neonatal age group, but the high incidence of AML (megakaryocytic) in patients with DS under age 5 causes the overall ratio of ALL: AML to be close to 1:1 [33,34]. Higher risk of ALL is documented in children with Beckwith-Wiedeman syndrome, neurofibromatosis and Schwachman's syndrome. Other underlying disorders may be chromosomal-breakage syndromes such as ataxia-teleangiectasia, Bloom's syndrome, Fanconi anemia, and Nijmegen breakage syndrome [21].

In addition to genetic influences, environmental factors including irradiation and certain chemicals, viral infection and immunodeficiency may also play a role.

Exposure to ionizing radiation is linked to leukemia. The high incidence of leukemia is documented in survivors of the atomic bomb explosions in Japan during World War II, ALL being more frequent in children and AML in adults [35]. There is an increased risk of leukemia in children exposed to diagnostic irradiation *in utero*, particularly during the first trimester [36]. The risk for developing leukemia from postnatal exposure to diagnostic radiography is difficult to determine [37]. One study suggested 0.8% increased risk of leukemia in pediatric orthopedic patients who required repeated diagnostic radiographs [38]. Therapeutic irradiation has been implicated as well. An increased ALL incidence is observed in neonates administered irradiation to treat thymic enlargement and children who received scalp irradiation for treatment of tinea capitis [6]. Conflicting results exist about the risk from exposure to electromagnetic fields [39,40] and routine emissions from nuclear power plants [41,42].

With the exception of chronic postnatal exposure to household paints and paint solvents [43], the role of other toxic chemicals in the development of childhood ALL is controversial. There is strong evidence that chemotherapy, including alkylating agents and epipodophyllotoxins, has leukemogenic potential, mostly causing secondary AML [44]. Other factors that may potentially be involved in the development of childhood ALL include parental chemical exposure. Maternal exposures to DNA-damaging agent dipyrone and baygon, indoor insecticides, and pesticides in the garden have been linked to ALL [45]. The risk appears to be enhanced by the presence of *CYP-1A1m1* and *CYP-1A1m2* polymorphisms [46]. Paternal exposures to pesticides and fungicides, alcohol consumption, and smoking history have been associated with ALL in offspring [47,48].

The role of viral infection in the pathogenesis of childhood leukemia has been studied extensively. The interest has been due mainly to the overlapping age patterns of childhood infection and peak incident ALL, documented viral etiology for some animal and human cancers, and the seasonal variation in ALL incidence rates. Various associations have been described between ALL and influenza, chicken pox, measles and mumps, happening either to the mother during the pregnancy or to the index child [6]. The only common feature of these studies is the lack of consistency. A possible inverse association with hepatitis A virus, as a measure of general hygiene, has been shown [49]. Epstein-Barr virus (EBV) has been associated with B-cell leukemia and endemic Burkitt lymphoma [50,51]. Since both EBV-positive and EBV-negative B-cell leukemia/lymphoma have comparable gene rearrangements and postulated oncogenic mechanisms, it is doubtful that EBV is causative.

Children with various primary immunodeficiencies, including severe combined immunodeficiency, X-linked agammaglobulinemia, and Wiskott-Aldrich syndrome, as well as those receiving chronic treatment with immunosuppressive drugs, have an increased risk of developing lymphoid malignancies predominantly lymphomas. ALL may occur but is uncommon [6]. The development of malignancy in immunocompromised patients frequently correlates with infection, whether it is de novo, reactivated, or chronic.

4. Classification

It has long been recognized that ALL is a biologically heterogeneous disease. The classification depends on characterizing leukemic lymphoblasts to determine the morphology, immunophenotype, and cytogenetic and molecular genetic features. Morphology alone usually is adequate to establish a diagnosis but the other studies have a major influence on the choice of optimal therapy and the prognosis.

4.1. Morphologic classification

A number of classification systems have been proposed to classify lymphoblasts morphologically. Generally accepted is the system proposed by the European French-American-British (FAB) Cooperative Working Group in 1976 [52]. The FAB system defines three categories of lymphoblasts (Figure 1). L1 blasts are typically smaller with scant cytoplasm and inconspicuous nucleoli. L2 blasts are pleomorphic larger cells with more abundant cytoplasm and prominent nucleoli. Lymphoblasts of L3 type, notable for deeply basophilic cytoplasm and cytoplasmic vacuolization, are morphologically identical to Burkitt's lymphoma cells containing *myc* translocations [53]. Approximately 85% of children with ALL have predominant L1 morphology, 14% have L2, and 1% has L3.

With the exception of L3 subtype, these distinctions hold little practical value [54]. The recent World Health Organization (WHO) International panel on ALL recommended that the FAB classification be abandoned and advocated the use of the immunophenotypic classification mentioned below [55]. The 2001 WHO scheme subdivided cases into precursor B-cell, precursor T-cell, and mature B-cell ALL (Table 1). The WHO classification was updated in 2008, and has become worldwide accepted as based on the recognition of distinct diseases using a multidisciplinary approach. It incorporates morphologic, biologic, and genetic information into a working nomenclature that has clinical relevance [56].

4.2. Immunological classification

The development of monoclonal antibodies targeted to specific cell surface and cytoplasmatic antigens has revolutionized biological classification of ALL. It has been recognized that ALL subtypes correspond to distinct stage of lymphocyte maturation, but leukemia cells often demonstrate aberrant antigen expression. Hence, a panel of antibodies is needed to establish the diagnosis and to distinguish among the different immunologic subclasses of blasts [57]. Typical patterns are: CD19/CD22/CD79a (B-lineage), CD7/cytoplasmatic CD3 (T-lineage), and CD13/CD33/CD65/MPO (myeloid) [58]. B-lineage ALL accounts for 80% of childhood ALL. CD10 is commonly expressed on the cell surface, and this leukemic subset is referred to as *CALLA*$^{+}$ or common ALL. B-cell leukemias can be further subclassified as early pre-B, pre-B, transitional pre-B and mature B. Mature B-cell ALL, which accounts for only 1-3% of pediatric ALL is regarded as being synonymous with L3 morphological FAB type, and should be differentiated from other B-lineage ALL. T-lineage ALL cases can be classified according to the stages of normal thymocyte development that they resemble (early, mid-, or late thymocyte), or in some studies as pro-T, pre-T, cortical T or mature T [59,60]. The only distinctions

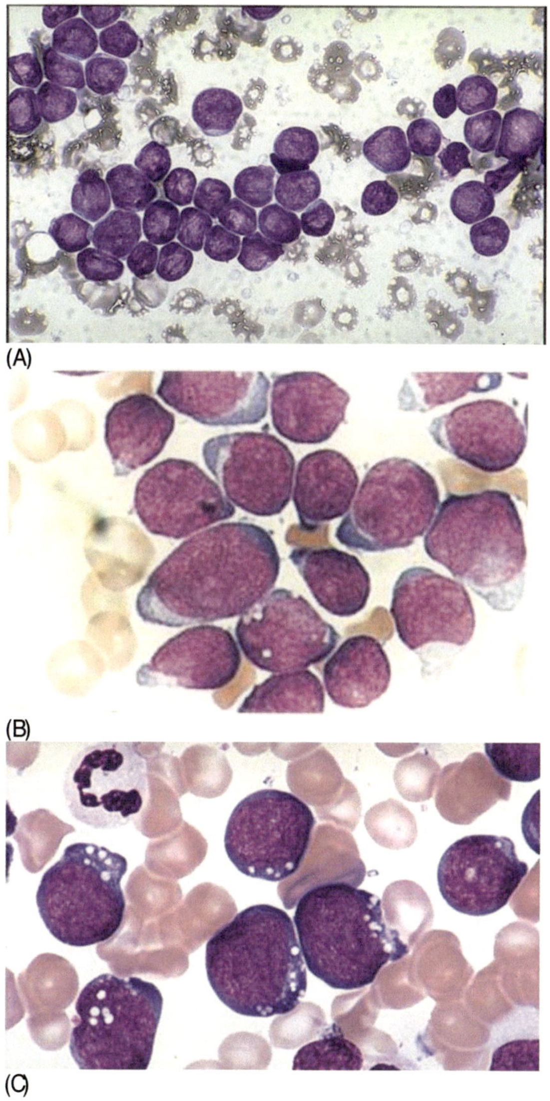

Figure 1. FAB (French American and British) morphological classification of lymphoblasts. (A) L1 lymphoblasts. (B) L2 lymphoblasts. (C) L3 lymphoblasts.

of therapeutic importance are those between T-cell, mature B, and other B-lineage (B-cell precursor) immunophenotypes [21]. The co-expression of myeloid antigens may occur on otherwise typical lymphoblasts in 5% to 30% of childhood ALL (My+ ALL). Although once thought to have an adverse prognosis, the presence of some myeloid-associated antigens in cells that predominantly mark as lymphoblasts has no prognostic significance [61,62]. By contrast, mixed-lineage leukemias represent a heterogeneous category of poorly differentiated acute leukemias that possess characteristics of both lymphoid and myeloid precursor cells. In biphenotypic leukemia a single dominant populations of blasts simultaneously coexpress both lymphoid and myeloid antigens [63]. Bilineal or biclonal leukemia is acute leukemia with two

WHO classification
Precursor B-cell ALL/LBL
Cytogenetic subgroups
t(9;22)(q34,q11),BCR/ABL
t(v;11q23);MLL rearranged
t(1;19)(q23;p13),PBX1/E2A
t(12;21)(p13;q22);TEL/AML1
Hypodiploid
Hyperdiploid, >50
Precursor T-cell ALL/LBL
Mature B-cell leukemia/lymphoma
ALL= acute lymphoblastic leukemia;
LBL= lymphoblastic lymphoma;
MLL= mixed lineage leukemia

Table 1. World Health Organization classification of acute lymphoblastic leukemia

distinct population of blasts in a single patient [64]. „Lineage switch" is the term used to describe a conversion from one phenotype at diagnosis to a different phenotype during therapy or at relapse. Mixed-lineage leukemias (biphenotypic, bilineal, and lineage switch) represent only 3% to 5% of acute leukemias occurring in patients of all ages [6,65].

4.3. Genetic classification

The role of cytogenetics in determining the biologic basis of ALL has been widely recognized. With the refinement of classic cytogenetic techniques, development of additional approaches including polymerase chain reaction (PCR) and fluorescence in situ hybridization (FISH), and merging with the molecular genetic techniques of spectral karyotyping (SKY) and comparative genomic hybridization (CGH), alterations are detected in the leukemic cells of virtually all pediatric ALL cases [66]. Cytogenetic abnormalities are important aspects of diagnosis, risk assessment, treatment and prognosis in childhood ALL. Approximately 70 percent of pediatric patients can be readily classified into therapeutically relevant subgroups based on cytogenetic and molecular genetic changes [21]. Children with hyperdiploidy (> 50 chromosomes) and the concurrent trisomies of chromosomes 4, 10, and 17 ("triple trisomies") have a favorable prognosis with a 5-year event-free survival (EFS) rate of 90% [67,68]. The presence of translocation t(12;21) is also associated with a superior EFS rate. It results in *RUNX1-ETO* fusion, formerly known as *TEL/AML1* based on the older names of the same genes fused by the breakpoint [69,70]. Hyperdiploidy accounts for one-third of newly diagnosed B-precursor ALL cases, and *TEL-AML1* for additional 25%. By contrast, hypodiploidy (< 45 chromosomes) and Philadelphia chromosome-positive (Ph+) ALL are associated with poor prognosis, with overall EFS rates generally < 50%. Hypodiploid karyotype occurs in 6% to 9% cases of pediatric ALL. The worst outcome is observed in children with near-haploid ALL (23 – 29 chromosomes), with reported EFS rates of 25% [6,21,71]. Philadelphia chromosome is a small marker chromosome present in 3% to 5% of pediatric ALL. Initially described as truncated chromosome 22, it was discovered as the result of a reciprocal translocation between c-ABL oncogene sequences on chromosome 9 and "breakpoint cluster region" (BCR) gene on chromosome 22, t(9;22)(q34;q11), resulting in the oncogenic *BCR-ABL* gene fusion [72]. Children with Ph+ ALL tend to be older, have higher initial leukocyte counts, higher frequency of central nervous system (CNS) leukemia, and respond poorly to conventional (non-tyrosine kinase inhibitor inclusive) therapy [6]. Abnormalities of the *MLL* (mixed lineage leukemia) gene at 11q23, which are seen in 5% to 10% of pediatric ALL and in up to 70% of infant leukemia, are another unfavorable cytogenetic subgroup. *MLL* rearrangements involve more than 30 different reciprocal translocations, with t(4;11)(q21;q23)(*MLL-AF4*) being the most frequent [73].

In the last decade, the application of new genome-wide screening techniques have led to the discovery of many new genetic abnormalities in childhood ALL. The exact role of these abnormalities in leukemogenesis, association with chemotherapy sensitivity or resistance and with clinical response to therapy, as well as their role as potential therapeutic targets is yet to be elucidated, but holds the promise of improving personalized therapy for every child with ALL.

5. Clinical presentation

Children with ALL often present with signs and symptoms that reflect bone marrow infiltration with leukemic blasts and the extent of extramedullary disease spread. The duration of symptoms may vary from days to months, frequently accumulating in a matter of days or weeks, and culminating in some event that brings the child to medical attention. Most of children have 3- to 4- week history of presenting symptoms. The initial presentation includes manifestations of the underlying anemia – pallor, fatigue, exercise intolerance, tachycardia, dyspnea, and sometimes congestive heart failure; thrombocytopenia – petechiae, purpura, easy bruising, bleeding from mucous membranes; neutropenia – fever whether low- or high-grade, infection, ulcerations of buccal mucosa. Anorexia is common, but significant weight loss is infrequent. Bone pain is present in one-third of patients, particularly affects long bones, and may lead to a limp or refusal to walk in young children. Bone pain reflects leukemic involvement of the periosteum, bone infarction, or expansion of marrow cavity by lymphoblasts. Joint pain and joint swelling are rarely seen [74].

Physical examination may show enlarged lymph nodes, liver and spleen. It is a common misperception that a significant lymphadenopathy and hepatosplenomegaly are hallmarks of childhood ALL. In rare cases, predominantly in patients with T-cell ALL, respiratory distress or signs of superior vena cava syndrome due to enlargement of mediastinal lymph nodes may be presenting symptoms. CNS involvement occurs in less than 5% of children with ALL at initial diagnosis. It usually presents with signs and symptoms of raised intracranial pressure (headache, vomiting, papilledema) and parenchimal involvement (seizures, cranial nerve palsies). Other rare sites of extramedullary invasion include heart, lungs, kidneys, testicles, ovaries, skin, eye or gastrointestinal tract [6,21]. Such involvement usually occurs in refractory or relapsed patients.

6. Laboratory findings

The first clue to a diagnosis of ALL is typically an abnormal result on a complete blood count. An elevated white blood cell (WBC) count (> 10.000/mm^3) occurs in approximately half of the children, with 20% showing the initial WBC greater than 50.000/mm^3. In other half of children with ALL number of WBC can be normal or low. Peripheral blood smears show blasts in most cases. In children with leukopenia, very few to none blasts are detected. Neutropenia is a common finding and is associated with an increased risk of infection. Approximately 80% of children present with anemia (hemoglobin < 10g/dL), which is usually normochromic and normocytic with low number of reticulocytes. Thrombocytopenia (platelet count < 100.000/mm^3) occurs in 75% of children at diagnosis. Spontaneous bleeding appears in patients with less than 20.000-30.000 platelets/mm^3, but severe hemorrhage is rare, provided that fever and infection are absent [6]. Rarely, transient pancytopenia may be the prodrome to childhood ALL.

To definitively establish the diagnosis of ALL, a bone marrow aspirate is generally necessary. Leukemia should be suspected in children whose marrows contain more than 5% blasts, but a minimum of 25% blast cells is required by the standard criteria before the diagnosis is confirmed [6]. More recently proposed classification systems have lowered the blast cell percentage to 20% for many leukemia types, and do not require any minimum blast cells when certain morphologic and cytogenetic features are present [53]. Usually the marrow is hyper-cellular and characterized by a homogeneous population of leukemic cells. A bone marrow aspirate may be difficult to obtain at the time of diagnosis. This is caused by the density of blasts in the marrow, but may be due to marrow fibrosis, infarction or necrosis. In such cases, bone marrow biopsy is required. Touch-preparation cytologic examination of the biopsy specimen can be helpful when aspiration is not successful [21].

A variety of other abnormal laboratory findings are frequently seen in children with ALL at diagnosis. Elevated serum uric acid levels reflect a high leukemic cells burden and the resultant increased breakdown of nucleic acids. Most patients have an elevated lactic dehydrogenase (LDH) level due to rapid cell turnover. The serum potassium level may be high in children with massive cell lysis, often together with hyperuricemia. Hypercalcemia may result from marked bone leukemic infiltration or from the production of an abnormal parathormone-like substance. Serum hypocalcemia may be secondary to hyperphosphatemia, and calcium binding phosphate released by lymphoblasts. Abnormal renal function from uric acid nephropathy and renal leukemic infiltration may be present. Liver dysfunction due to leukemic infiltration is usually mild regardless to the degree of hepatomegaly. Coagulation abnormalities may be seen but are usually not a feature of the disease, apart from a minority of patients presenting with disseminated intravascular coagulation [6].

Initial CNS involvement is found in fewer than 5% of children with ALL. CNS leukemia is most often detected in an asymptomatic child with cytologic examination of cerebrospinal fluid (CSF) after cytocentrifugation, revealing pleocytosis and the presence of blasts. Based on CSF findings, CNS involvement in ALL is defined as follows: CNS-1 status describes a patient with <5 WBC/mm^3 and without detectable blasts in the diagnostic CSF, CNS-2 status is defined as <5 WBC/mm^3 and the presence of blasts, and CNS-3 status includes patients with ≥5 WBC/

mm^3 and blasts on CSF or cranial nerve involvement or presence of cerebral mass [6,75]. Traumatic lumbar puncture (TLP) is defined as CSF with >10 red blood cells (RBC)/mm^3, with or without blasts (TLP+ or TLP-) [76]. In case of TLP+, the following formula can be helpful in defining the presence of CNS leukemia:

$$\frac{\text{CSF WBC}}{\text{CSF RBC}} > \frac{\text{Blood WBC}}{\text{Blood RBC}}$$

In symptomatic children, intracranial pressure is usually increased, and proteinorrhachia and hypoglycorrhachia are common [6,77].

7. Prognostic factors and risk classification

The identification of clinical and biologic features with prognostic value has become essential in the design of modern clinical trials. It is common practice to assign patients into different risk groups on the basis of prognostic factors, and to tailor treatment accordingly to the predicted likelihood of relapse. However, there is disagreement between large cooperative groups over the risk criteria and the terminology of defining prognostic subgroups.

Usually, childhood ALL cases are divided into standard-, intermediate- and high-risk group. Factors most often included into risk stratification are: age at diagnosis, initial WBC count, sex, race, the presence of extramedulary disease, blast immunophenotype and cytogenetics, early response to induction therapy, and minimal residual disease (MRD) [78,79].

Age at diagnosis and initial WBC count are the two features universally accepted as prognostic factors [12]. Children under 1 year and greater than 10 years of age (6 years in BFM study) have a inferior prognosis compared with children in the intermediate age group. Infants with ALL who are younger than 1 year at diagnosis have the worst prognosis [6]. There is a linear relation between initial WBC count and outcome in children with ALL; those with WBC greater than 50.000/mm^3 are recognized as having poorer prognosis [62]. Certain biologic features, e.g. T-cell ALL and infants with t(4;11), are associated with higher initial WBC counts. In most studies, girls have better prognosis than boys. This is partly due to the risk of testicular relapse, the higher incidence of T-immunophenotype and unfavourable DNA index in boys, but other genetic and endocrine effects may be present [80]. The effect of race on prognosis has been controversial, but some recent studies still report that American black children have slightly poorer outcomes when compared with white children. Asian children with ALL fare slightly better than white children [81]. The prognostic significance of cytogenetic factors and immunophenotype is discussed previously in the "Classification" section. Although early pre-B-cell ALL has better prognosis and mature T-cell ALL has a worse survival, immunophenotype is not an independent prognostic factor in the analyses of current trials [6]. Clinical features indicating the extent of extramedullary disease, i.e. the degree of hepatosplenomegaly and lymphadenopathy, presence of a mediastinal mass, and CNS disease at diagnosis, once emerged as useful prognostic indicators, disappeared as the treatment improved.

The rapidity of response to initial therapy is one of the most important prognostic indicators. BFM protocol uses the response in the peripheral blood to one week of systemic prednisone

[78,82]. Others use the response in the bone marrow after one or two weeks of induction therapy. Rapid early responders have the best EFS. Residual leukemia demonstrable in bone marrow on day 14 of induction is an independent predictor of inferior outcome. Children who do not achieve a complete remission (defined as <5% blasts in the bone marrow of normal cellularity and the absence of other evidence of leukemia) within the usual 4- to 6- week induction period have highest rate of relapse and shortened survival [6]. In recent years, measurement of MRD is incorporated in many trials. Numerous techniques have been developed to detect and quantify small amount of residual leukemic cells, with flow cytometry being the most accessible (Fluorescence activated cell sorter „FACS" analysis) [83]. The definition of remission status is also being re-examined in ongoing clinical trials. MRD levels that are undetectable or less than 10^{-4} at the end of induction therapy (or preferably earlier) are associated with the best prognosis. Conversely, day 29 induction MRD values of greater than 0.01% have a higher risk of relapse [84-86]. In the near future, gene expression profile analysis could better define distinctive genetic subclasses in childhood ALL and identify genes which may be responsible for leukemogenesis, thus leading to new targeted therapy strategies [87,88].

8. Differential diagnosis

The child with ALL typically presents with nonspecific symptoms. Thus, ALL may mimic a variety of nonmalignant and other malignant conditions. The acute onset of bleeding tendency may suggest immune thrombocytopenia. The latter disorder typically presents in an otherwise well child with a history of a preceding viral infection, and normal hemoglobin value, WBC count, and differential. Failure of other single cell lines, as seen in transient erythroblastopenia of childhood and congenital or acquired neutropenia, may lead to a suspicion of leukemia. ALL and congenital or acquired aplastic anemia may present with pancytopenia. The results of bone marrow aspiration and/or biopsy usually distinguish these two diseases. Pediatricians must also consider ALL in the differential diagnosis of patients presenting with hypereosinophilia which, in rare cases, has preceded the diagnosis of ALL or may be a presenting feature of leukemia [89]. ALL presenting with hypereosinophilia must be differentiated from eosinophilic myeloid leukemia (AML M4Eo), which is strongly associated with alterations of chromosome 16. Infectious mononucleosis and some other viral infections can be confused with ALL. Detection of atypical lymphocytes in peripheral blood smear and serologic evidence of Epstein-Barr or cytomegalovirus infection helps make a diagnosis. Children with pertussis and parapertussis may present with marked leukocytosis and lymphocytosis, but the affected cells are mature lymphocytes. Bone and joint pain in ALL may mimic juvenile rheumatoid arthritis, rheumatic fever, or osteomyelitis. These presentations also can require bone marrow aspirate if a treatment with steroids for suspected rheumatoid diseases is planned. Lastly, ALL must be distinguished from acute myelogenous leukemia and small round cell tumors that invade bone marrow including neuroblastoma, rhabdomyosarcoma, Ewing sarcoma, and retinoblastoma, but these neoplasms usually have distinct other findings [6]. By contrast, in the case of non-Hodgkin lymphoma (NHL) there may be marked overlap in clinical presentation. When staging NHL, by convention, more than 25% blast cells in the marrow establish the diagnosis of ALL, whereas a child with 5% to 25% blasts is classified as having stage IV NHL [3].

9. Treatment

Pediatric ALL is a clonal heterogeneous disease with many distinct subtypes, and a uniform approach to antileukemic treatment is no longer appropriate. Although the specific approaches to various risk groups and the terminology describing the phases of therapy may vary between clinical trials, the backbone of modern ALL treatment protocols consists of four or five main treatment elements: remission-induction phase, early intensification, consolidation/CNS preventive therapy, delayed intensification (sometimes divided into re-induction and re-consolidation phases), and maintenance or continuation therapy targeted at eliminating residual disease [21,90].

Induction Therapy. The first goal of antileukemic therapy is to induce a complete remission and restore normal hematopoiesis. Intensive induction therapy improved the remission rate to approximately 98%. Almost all protocols use glucocorticoid (prednisone/ dexamethasone), vincristine and L-asparaginase as so-called three-drug backbone plus intrathecal therapy. It is a matter of debate whether the addition of antracycline has an impact on the remission induction rate and on the duration of remission [6,91,92]. A recent meta-analysis showed that anthracyclines significantly reduced bone marrow relapse when added to standard therapy but did not increase EFS due to the concomitant increased incidence of treatment related deaths [91]. BFM protocols use prednisone as a single systemic agent in the first week of treatment and this was shown to reduce tumor load in a controlled way to avoid metabolic complications [93]. Most controversial in induction regimens is the choice of glucocorticoid, prednisone being used more frequently. It appears that the use of dexamethasone results in a lower rate of bone marrow and CNS relapse, which is probably due to higher free plasma levels and better CNS penetration of the drug [94]. There are data, however, that dexamethasone leads to more acute and long-term complications [95,96]. Three forms of L-asparaginase are available, each with different pharmacologic and pharmacokinetic profile. The specific preparation, dose, route and schedule of administration vary [97]. Pegylated form with relatively long half-life is less immunogenic and less likely to develop neutralizing antibodies, and many study groups incorporate PEG-asparaginase in current treatment protocols [98]. Failure of induction therapy occurs in about 2% of children with ALL. This may be due to early death (most often caused by infection or bleeding) or to chemoresistant leukemic cells. With institution of more intensive therapy, the overall EFS for this minor non-responsive patient population is 30% to 40% [99,100].

Early Intensification. With restoration of normal hematopoiesis, children in remission become candidates for intensification therapy. The aim of early intensification therapy, administered immediately after remission induction, is to eradicate residual leukemic cells [101,102]. There is no consensus on the best regimens and their duration. BFM protocol uses a post-induction course consisting of 6-mercaptopurine, cyclophosphamide, low-dose cytarabin plus intrathecal methotrexate. Other cooperative groups use different combinations of drugs which also lower the amount of any remaining MRD in the bone marrow [21,93].

Consolidation/ Central Nervous System Preventive Therapy. The goal of the consolidation phase is to continue to strengthen the remission in the bone marrow and to provide CNS prophylaxis. The concept of CNS prophylaxis is based on postulates that CNS is a sanctuary site for leukemic cells, which are undetected at diagnosis and are protected by the blood brain barrier from systemic chemotherapy. CNS prophylaxis can be achieved by radiation (cranial or craniospinal), intrathecal chemotherapy, high dose systemic chemotherapy, or combinations of these [103,104]. The occurrence of long-term neurologic and neuroendocrine sequelae, as well as the risk of secondary CNS neoplasms, has limited the use of cranial irradiation to a selected group of patients with an increased risk of CNS relapse [75]. Many current protocols use high-dose systemic methotrexate (four doses are given biweekly) in parallel with intrathecal chemotherapy (either intrathecal methotrexate or triple IT: methotrexate with cytarabine and hydrocortisone). The doses of intrathecally administered drugs are based on age. Effective CNS prophylactic regimens have reduced the incidence of isolated CNS relapse to less than 5% [6].

Delayed Intensification. Addition of a delayed intensification (DI) phase after standard induction/consolidation therapy has improved outcome for children with ALL [4]. The intensity of chemotherapy varies considerably depending on risk group assignment. DI mainly consists of a late repetition of the initial remission induction and early intensification phases. A 7-week DI was introduced with BFM studies in the 1980s, beginning at week 16 [105]. To minimize the development of drug resistance, cytotoxic agents were altered: prednisone was replaced with dexamethasone, doxorubicin was substituted for daunorubicin, and mercaptopurine was replaced with thioguanine [21]. Together with other drugs used in this phase, the minimal residual leukaemia cells may be further cleared up. American Children's Cancer Group included BFM backbone and also demonstrated that DI, consising of reinduction and reconsolidation, improved treatment success [106,107]. Subsequent trials have focused on augmenting DI for less favorable patient groups [108]. On most trials, children with very high-risk features, treated with multiple cycles of intensive chemotherapy during the consolidation phase, have been considered candidates for allogeneic stem cell transplantation in first remission.

Maintenance Therapy. After the completion of 6 to 12 months of more aggressive treatment, lower doses of cytotoxic drugs are used to prevent relapse. Maintenance or Continuation Therapy is unique among therapies for malignancies. The aim of the maintenance phase is to further reduce minimal residual cells that are not detectable with current techniques at this stage of treatment. Maintenance chemotherapy generally continues up to the time point of two or three years after the diagnosis or after achievement of morphological remission. On some studies, boys are treated longer than girls, while on others, there is no difference in the duration of treatment based on gender. Reduction of the duration of maintenance to less than 2 years led to an increased relapsed risk. However, patients with more aggressive leukemias who had received significantly more intensive treatment, have less benefit of maintenance therapy [21].

The usual maintenance regimen for children with ALL is a combination of mercaptopurine (6-MP) administered daily and methotrexate (MTX) administered weekly. Doses are usually adapted according to leukocyte count, using a target of 2.000 to 3.000/mm^3 [93]. There are large individual differences in the doses that are tolerated or needed to achieve the target leukocyte count. It has been shown that maintaining the highest tolerable dose of 6-MP and MTX leads to a better outcome [21]. The effect of 6-MP is better when the drug is given in the evening and without milk products [93,109]. The frequency of drug administration also may be associated with the outcome. Children who receive maintenance therapy on a continuous rather than an interrupted schedule have longer remissions. Compliance problems may diminish the efficacy of maintenance therapy. Intensification of the maintenance by the administration of vincristine/dexamethasone pulses was shown to provide no extra benefit [110].

10. Relapsed ALL

Despite current intensive front-line therapies, approximately 20% of children with ALL experience relapse, accounting for a large proportion of pediatric cancer patients [111]. Relapse is defined as the reappearance of leukemic cells at any site in the body. It may be isolated event at one site (medullary or extramedullary) or may be combined (medullary and extramedullary). Most relapsed leukemias retain their original immunophenotype and genotype, but rarely another cell lineage ("lineage switch") is observed. Molecular studies are helpful in distinguishing lineage switch from secondary leukemia, which usually occurs years later [44, 112]. In general, relapsed leukemia is less responsive and requires much more intensive treatments. Isolated extramedullary relapse is more favorable than bone marrow relapse [113]. Combined relapses have a better outcome compared to isolated medullary relapses; combined relapses in fact tend to be later and to display better response to chemotherapy [3,74].

Medullary relapse. Bone marrow remains the most common site of relapse in pediatric ALL and generally implies a poor prognosis for most patients. Later relapse is more favorable than earlier relapse [114,115]. The definition of early versus late marrow relapse varies; many groups define "early" as a marrow recurrence within 36 months from initial diagnosis, or as less than 6 months after completing the initial treatment protocol [111]. The two approaches to the treatment of medullary relapse are chemotherapy and hematopoietic stem cell transplantation (HSCT). For patients who receive only chemotherapy, a second course of CNS-directed therapy should be administered to prevent subsequent CNS relapse [21]. With aggressive multidrug reinduction therapy, second remission is achieved in 66% to 82% for early B-lineage marrow relapse, and 90% to 95% for late B-lineage marrow relapse. Second remission may be more elusive for relapsed T-cell disease. However, intensive relapse regimens generally have not resulted in improvement in salvage rates and have reached the limit of tolerability. Longer-term overall EFS rates for early relapse are 10% to 20%, compared to 40% to 50% for late marrow relapse. Outcomes for second and greater relapse are even worse. Although third remission can be achieved in approximately 40% of patients, responses are not sustained and most patients will ultimately die from their disease [74,116]. These results have given HSCT a significant role in the treatment of relapsed ALL [117]. Allogeneic HSCT is the treatment of choice in children who develop early medullary relapse [118]. Autologous transplantation offers no advantage over chemotherapy. For patients without histocompatible related donors, the options are HSCT from matched unrelated donors, umbilical cord blood transplant, and T-cell-depleted haploidentical HSCT [119,120]. In most studies, patients transplanted in earlier remissions fare significantly better than patients transplanted after multiple relapses [21].

Extramedullary relapse. Although extramedullary relapse frequently presents as an isolated finding, most occurrences are associated with MRD in the bone marrow, and it likely represents a local manifestation of systemic failure. Accordingly, these patients require intensive systemic treatment to prevent subsequent bone marrow relapse. The distinction between early and late extramedullary relapse is generally 18 months from initial diagnosis (compared with 36 months for medullary relapse) [74].

Central nervous system relapse is observed in less than 5% of children with ALL. It occurs more frequently in children with T-ALL or mature B-ALL. Intrathecal chemotherapy alone fails to cure CNS leukemia. Most regimens include intrathecal chemotherapy until CSF remission, in parallel with a systemic induction therapy, followed by consolidation chemotherapy, cranio-spinal irradiation (2.400 to 3.000 cGy cranial, and 1.200 to 1.500 cGy spinal) and maintenance intrathecal chemotherapy [6]. Factors influencing outcome include whether CNS relapse is early or late (EFS 83% and 46%, respectively), and whether the child received prior CNS irradiation [121]. For patients with earlier prophylactic irradiation, long-term secondary remission does not exceed 30%, and these patients are candidates for HSCT [6,21].

Testicular relapse occurs in less than 2% of children with ALL. Optimal therapy includes the use of systemic chemotherapy and local radiotherapy (2.400 cGy to both testes). Bilateral testicular irradiation is indicated for all patients; unilateral radiotherapy may be followed by relapse in the contralateral testis [6]. The impact of a testicular relapse on the prognosis depends whether it was early or late, and whether the recurrence is an isolated or combined event. Prolonged disease-free survival can be obtained for more than two thirds of patients with an isolated late relapse [6,122].

Leukemic relapse occasionally occurs at other extramedullary sites, including the eye, ear, ovary, uterus, kidney, bone, muscle, tonsil, mediastinum, pleura, and paranasal sinus. Optimal treatment is unclear, and may include local control measures and intensification of systemic chemotherapy.

11. Outcome

See also "Prognostic factors and risk classification"

The outcome of newly diagnosed pediatric ALL has increased significantly over the past decades. More than 95% of children achieve remission, and approximately 80% are expected to be long-term event-free survivors. The 5-year EFS varies considerably depending on risk category, from 95% (low risk) to 30% (very high risk), with infant leukemia having the worst outcomes (20% for patients younger than 90 days) [123]. An analysis of long-term survival among 21,626 people who were treated for childhood ALL in Children's Oncology Group (COG) trials from 1990-2005 found a 10-year survival of almost 84% [124].

Pediatric ALL is potentially highly curable in low-income countries, mostly due to improved supportive care with intensive chemotherapy protocols. Recent studies report overall survival rates over 60% in India [125,126], and 5-year EFS over 78% in Lebanon [127].

Similarly to frontline ALL therapy, treatment outcome for relapsed patients depends on clinical and biological characteristics of the disease. Factors indicating a poor prognosis in previously treated patients include: relapse on therapy or after a short initial remission, bone marrow involvement, T-cell immunophenotype, unfavorable cytogenetics (i.e., the presence of t(9;22) and t(4;11), and persistent levels of MRD after the first course of chemotherapy for relapse. Roughly, conventional intensive chemotherapy and radiotherapy can cure only one third of all children with relapsed ALL, with percentages ranging from 0 to 70% depending on the pattern of prognostic factors present at relapse [74,128,129].

12. Hematopoietic stem cell transplantation

HSCT has been an important treatment modality in the management of a portion of high-risk or relapsed childhood ALL. There is a need to reassess periodically the indications for HSCT, owing to the continuos improvement in chemotherapy approaches, development of novel therapeutics, precise assessment of the risk of relapse, and transplantation procedures [130].

HSCT in first remission. There is no consensus on the indications for transplantation in childhood ALL in first complete remission (CR1) among major international study groups. Historically, children with Ph+ ALL and matched sibling donor have been transplanted in CR1 [131-134]. In a recent COG study, intensive chemotherapy plus continuos imatinib exposure after remission induction therapy yielded a 3-year EFS of 80%, more than twice that of historical controls, and comparable to those of matched-related or matched-unrelated transplant [135]. Infants with *MLL*-rearranged ALL were identified early on as having a particularly poor prognosis, and universally have been considered candidates for transplantation in CR1. However, most recent COG study failed to show an advantage of HSCT over chemotherapy [136], while Interfant-99 study showed that the benefit was restricted to a very high-risk subgroup with 2 additional unfavorable prognostic features: age <6 months and either poor response to steroids or leukocyte count ≥ 300 x 10^9/L [137]. Similarly, somewhat ambiguous results have been reported from studies that attempt to compare EFS after transplant or chemotherapy for children with hypodiploid ALL [138], poor early responders [99,139], persistent MRD, and high-risk T-cell ALL [140,141]. Overall, there is no absolute indication for HSCT in children with ALL in CR1. In view of the dismal outcome of *MLL*-rearranged infant ALL, poor early responders with Ph+ ALL, and early T-cell precursor ALL, these patients are reasonable candidates for evaluation of HSCT in first remission [130].

HSCT in second or subsequent remission. The indications for relapsed or multiple relapsed ALL are less controversial among study groups. Although in the recent past HSCT would have been recommended for every child with matched-sibling donor, newer risk-based strategies suggest indications based upon the site of relapse and its timing in relation to completion of frontline therapy. Children with isolated marrow relapse on treatment or within 6 months of completion of treatment (or 36 months from diagnosis by COG definition), and those with combined marrow and extramedullary relapse within 18 months from diagnosis should be considered for HSCT [130]. The best approach for children with a late relapse is less clear-cut, as a significant proportion of them can be cured with further chemotherapy [142]. HSCT is indicated for patients with second or greater relapse, whether marrow, isolated extramedullary, or combined [130].

Donor selection and stem-cell source. Understanding how transplantation outcomes are influenced by donor source is a critical component of the therapeutic decision-making process. Matched-sibling donor is considered the gold standard for all indications [143]. Since only 20% to 25% of children with an indication for allogeneic HSCT have a MSD, for the remaining patients, a matched unrelated donor (MUD) is an alternative [130,144]. Over the past several decades, international registries have enlisted more than 18 million volunteers worldwide as potential unrelated stem cell donors. The chance of finding a suitable donor mainly depends on race/ethnicity (Caucasians being more likely to find a match), and the frequency of the HLA phenotype of the patient [145]. As a proportion of patients may not be able to rapidly identify a suitable MUD, other alternative graft sources, umbilical cord blood, haploidentical (haplo)-related donor and mismatched unrelated donor are available [146]. The outcomes of unrelated donor transplants have improved markedly in the last years, mainly due to advances in HLA typing and supportive care [147,148].

13. Novel therapies

Novel therapies in pediatric ALL are needed to improve treatment outcomes in newly-diagnosed patients with a poor prognosis and for patients with relapsed/refractory disease that have limited treatment options. New agents use a variety of approaches to selectively target leukemic cells, by altering intracellular signaling pathways, regulating gene expression, or targeting unique cell surface receptors. Use of these agents in frontline therapy provide the possibility of minimizing toxicity to normal cells [149,150].

Clofarabine is a second-generation purine nucleoside analogue approved for the treatment of pediatric patients with relapsed/refractory ALL treated with at least 2 prior regimens [151,152]. New trials are exploring the use of clofarabine in combination with cyclophosphamide and etoposide, and clofarabine in combination with cytarabine [153,154].

Imatinib mesylate (a selective inhibitor of the BCR-ABL protein kinase) has been combined with conventional chemotherapy in children with newly diagnosed and relapsed Ph+ ALL. Dramatic improvement of early EFS was achieved, with no additional toxicities [135,155]. Dasatinib, a second-generation tyrosine kinase inhibitor with potent activity against imatinib-resistant leukemic cells, is currently being tested in several phase I-III studies of pediatric Ph + ALL [156,157].

Infant ALL presents another challenge, with poor outcome particularly in children with *MLL* rearrangements. Overexpression of wild-type Fms-like tyrosine kinase (FLT3) in *MLL*-rearranged ALL is a target that is being investigated in infant ALL [158]. Lestaurtinib (CEP-701), a highly selective small molecule FLT3 tyrosine kinase inhibitor, is being combined with chemotherapy in infants with newly diagnosed ALL and *MLL* rearrangements [159].

Nelarabine (2-amino-9β-D-arabinosyl-6-methoxy-9H-guanine) is specifically cytotoxic to T-cell lineage blasts and is being studied incorporated into a frontline treatment study for children with newly diagnosed high-risk T-cell ALL [160].

Other groups of agents that have shown promising activity in the pediatric preclinical testing for ALL include a BCL-2 protein inhibitor (ABT-263), a mammalian target of rapamycin (mTOR) inhibitors (sirolimus) [161], and an aurora A kinase inhibitor (MLN8237) [162]. Monoclonal antibodies directed against a variety of specific targets such as cells expressing CD 19 (SAR3419, XMAb5574), CD 20 (rituximab) [163,164], CD22 (epratuzumab) [165], CD33 (gemtuzumab) [166] and CD52 (alemtuzumab) [167] are being developed or already in clinical trials. The major advantage of monoclonal antibody therapy is that the toxicities are limited and nonoverlapping compared with cytotoxic drugs, making them attractive candidates for combined therapy [168].

14. Late consequences

With the increasing number of children and adolescents treated of ALL, a large spectrum of adverse long-term sequelae is observed in survivors of ALL. The late effects of therapy associated with significant morbidity may include second neoplasms, neurotoxicity, cardiotoxicity, endocrine abnormalities, bone toxicity, and adverse psychosocial effects. The greatest risk for second neoplasms as well as other late consequences occurs in children who received cranial or craniospinal irradiation.

Second neoplasms. Second and subsequent neoplasms in survivors of childhood ALL are predominantly brain tumors (gliomas of varying histologic grades) and hematopoietic neoplasms (AML and myelodysplastic syndrome) [6]. The median latency period for high-grade brain tumor is 9 years but almost 20 years for low-grade tumors. Secondary AML has been linked to intensive treatment with epipodophyllotoxins and other topoisomerase II inhibitors, and has very low long-term survival rate [169]. Increasing number of solid tumors, consisting of skin, breast, bone, soft tissue, and thyroid neoplasms, have been reported. The 10-year cumulative incidence of second neoplasms is estimated at 14.6% [170,171].

Neurotoxicity. Understanding the risks of CNS toxicity is critically important in long-term follow-up of childhood ALL survivors. Although intrathecal and systemic chemotherapy or radiotherapy alone can be sufficient to induce CNS changes, the combination may be more neurotoxic. Four pathologically distinct findings of delayed CNS toxicity have been identified: cortical atrophy, necrotizing leukoencephalopathy, subacute leukoencephalopathy, and mineralizing microangiopathy [172]. Numerous studies have demonstrated abnormal CT and MRI scans in asymptomatic ALL patients who received CNS preventive therapy, as well as a significant association between these radioimaging abnormalities and neuropsychologic dysfunction [173,174]. Survivors of pediatric ALL have an increased risk for adverse psychosocial outcomes including lower cognitive functioning, executive function, depression, and decreased educational attainment [6,175].

Cardiotoxicity. Anthracyclines are the most common class of chemotherapeutic agents associated with adverse effects on the heart. Anthracycline-induced cardiomyocyte death results in hypertrophy of existing myocytes and interstitial fibrosis. The incidence of cardiomyopathy is related to the cumulative dose of anthracyclines [176]. Female and younger patients are at a higher risk. The anthracycline-induced cardiomyopathy is a progressive disorder that manifests with signs of congestive heart failure. Rapid progression of symptoms may occur with pregnancy, anesthesia, or exercise [177,178]. Dexrazoxane, a potent iron-chelating agent, provides long-term cardioprotection without compromising oncological efficacy in doxorubicin-treated children with high-risk ALL [179-181].

Endocrine abnormalities. Neuroendocrine morbidities, primarily involving the hypothalamus, have been documented in children who were treated with cranial radiotherapy. Essentially all of the hypothalamic-pituitary axes are at risk, but the principal findings are impaired growth hormone responses to provocative stimuli [6]. Growth delay is notified in some children with ALL [6,182]. Precocious puberty has been reported in some children receiving cranial irradiation, mostly in girls who receive cranial radiation in doses of 24 Gy or higher [183]. There appears to be a higher prevalence of obesity and metabolic syndrome among children who have successfully completed therapy for ALL [184,185]. Primary gonadal damage has been documented in patients of both sexes treated on cyclophosphamide-containing intensive treatment regimens. In most cases, girls with ALL retain intact reproductive function [6]. Studies of male survivors who received chemotherapy for childhood ALL showed evidence of subsequent gonadal dysfunction [186,187].

Bone toxicity. The most common chemotherapy-induced skeletal late effects are glucocorticoid-induced osteonecrosis and reduced bone mineral density. Risk factors for osteonecrosis have included adolescent age, females, white race, higher body mass index, lower albumin, and elevated cholesterol [74,188]. Limited data suggest that statins modulate cholesterol metabolism and may protect against osteonecrosis [189]. Multiple candidate gene studies have indicated several polymorphisms in genes putatively related to the development of osteonecrosis, getting conflicting results [190,191]. Reduced bone mineral density and increased fracture risk have been reported in children off chemotherapy for ALL. Routine recommendations include adequate dietary intake of calcium and vitamin D, and weight-bearing exercise. The use of bisphosphonates and other absorption-reducing agents in childhood ALL survivors remain investigational [192,193].

15. Conclusions

Pediatric ALL is a heterogeneous disease, which at present can be cured in approximately 80% of children. Improvements in long-term survival rates may have reached a plateau as further intensification of therapy may lead to a higher rate of treatment-related deaths. Therefore hope for future progress lies in the better understanding of the biology of pediatric ALL which will

http://dx.doi.org/10.5772/55655

allow for the more individualized therapy. The ultimate goals are to provide curative therapy to every child with ALL and help develop preventive measures.

Author details

Jelena Roganovic

University Children's Hospital Rijeka, Division of Hematology and Oncology, Rijeka, Croatia

References

[1] Möricke A, Zimmermann M, Reiter A, Henze G, Schrauder A, Gadner H, Ludwig WD, Ritter J, Harbott J, Mann G, Klingebiel T, Zintl F, Niemeyer C, Kremens B, Niggli F, Niethammer D, Welte K, Stanulla M, Odenwald E, Riehm H, Schrappe M. Long-term results of five consecutive trials in childhood acute lymphoblastic leukemia performed by the ALL-BFM study group from 1981 to 2000. Leukemia. 2011;24(2):265-284.

[2] Mitchell C, Richards S, Harrison CJ, Eden T. (2010) Long-term follow-up of the United Kingdom Medical Research Council protocols for childhood acute lymphoblastic leukaemia, 1980-2001. Leukemia. 2010;24(2):406-418.

[3] Conter V, Aricò M, Basso G, Biondi A, Barisone E, Messina C, Parasole R, De Rossi G, Locatelli F, Pession A, Santoro N, Micalizzi C, Citterio M, Rizzari C, Silvestri D, Rondelli R, Lo Nigro L, Ziino O, Testi AM, Masera G, Valsecchi MG; Associazione Italiana di Ematologia ed Oncologia Pediatrica. Long-term results of the Italian Association of Pediatric Hematology and Oncology (AIEOP) Studies 82, 87, 88, 91 and 95 for childhood acute lymphoblastic leukemia. Leukemia. 2010;24(2):255-264.

[4] Gaynon PS, Angiolillo AL, Carroll WL, Nachman JB, Trigg ME, Sather HN, Hunger SP, Devidas M; Children's Oncology Group.Long-term results of the children's cancer group studies for childhood acute lymphoblastic leukemia 1983-2002: a Children's Oncology Group Report. Leukemia. 2010;24(2):285-297.

[5] Tsuchida M, Ohara A, Manabe A, Kumagai M, Shimada H, Kikuchi A, Mori T, Saito M, Akiyama M, Fukushima T, Koike K, Shiobara M, Ogawa C, Kanazawa T, Noguchi Y, Oota S, Okimoto Y, Yabe H, Kajiwara M, Tomizawa D, Ko K, Sugita K, Kaneko T, Maeda M, Inukai T, Goto H, Takahashi H, Isoyama K, Hayashi Y, Hosoya R, Hanada R; Tokyo Children's Cancer Study Group. Long-term results of Tokyo Children's Cancer Study Group trials for childhood acute lymphoblastic leukemia, 1984-1999. Leukemia. 2010;24(2):383-396.

[6] Margolin JF, Rabin KR, Steuber P, Poplack DG. Acute lymphoblastic leukemia. In: Pizzo PA, Poplack DG. (eds). Principles and Practice of Pediatric Oncology, 6th ed. Philadelphia, PA: Lippincott, Williams and Wilkins 2011. p518-565.

[7] Pui CH. Recent research advances in childhood acute lymphoblastic leukemia. J Formos Med Assoc. 2010;109(11):777-787.

[8] Pui CH, Robison LL, Look AT. Acute lymphoblastic leukemia. Lancet. 2008;371(9617):1030-1043.

[9] Pui CH, Mullighan CH, Evans W, Relling MV. Pediatric acute lymphoblastic leukemia: where are we going and how do we get there? Blood. 2012;120(6):1165-1174.

[10] Scheurer ME, Bondy ML, Gourney JG. Epidemiology of childhood cancer. In: Pizzo PA, Poplack DG. (eds). Principles and Practice of Pediatric Oncology, 6th ed. Philadelphia, PA: Lippincott, Williams and Wilkins 2011. p2-16.

[11] [No authors listed]. Stat bite: Estimated new leukemia cases in 2008. J Natl Cancer Inst. 2008;100(8):531.

[12] Ribera JM, Oriol A. Acute lymphoblastic leukemia in adolescents and young adults. *Hematol Oncol Clin North Am. 2009;*23(5):1033-1042.

[13] Conter V, Rizzari C, Sala A, Chiesa R, Citterio M, Biondi A. Acute Lymphoblastic Leukemia. Orphanet Encyclopedia. 2004;1-13. http://www.orpha.net/data/patho/GB/uk-ALL.pdf (accessed 14 September 2012).

[14] Demoury C, Goujon-Bellec S, Guyot-Goubin A, Hémon D, Clavel J. Spatial variations of childhood acute leukaemia in France, 1990-2006: global spatial heterogeneity and cluster detection at 'living-zone' level. Eur J Cancer Prev. 2012;21(4):367-374.

[15] Heath CW. Community clusters of childhood leukemia and lymphoma: evidence of infection? Am J Epidemiol 2005;162(9):817-822.

[16] McNally RJ, Bithell JF, Vincent TJ, Murphy MF. Space-time clustering of childhood cancer around the residence at birth. Int J Cancer. 2009;124(2):449-455.

[17] Nyari TA, Ottóffy G, Bartyik K, Thurzó L, Solymosi N, Cserni G, Parker L, McNally RJ. Spatial clustering of childhood acute lymphoblastic leukaemia in Hungary. Pathol Oncol Res. 2012, Dec 11. [Epub ahead of print]

[18] Ross JA, Potter JD, Shu XO, Reaman GH, Lampkin B, Robison LL. Evaluating the relationships among maternal reproductive history, birth characteristics, and infant leukemia: a report from the Children's Cancer Group. Ann Epidemiol. 2007;7(3): 172-179.

[19] Caughey RW, Michels KB. Birth weight and childhood leukemia: a meta-analysis and review of the current evidence. Int J Cancer. 2009;124(11):2658-2670.

[20] Callan AC, Milne E. Involvement of the IGF system in fetal growth and childhood cancer: an overview of potential mechanisms. Cancer Causes Control. 2009;20(10): 1783-1798.

[21] Pui CH. Acute Lymphoblastic Leukemia. In: Beutler E, Lichtman MA, Coller BS, Kipps TJ, Seligsohn U: (eds.) Williams Hematology. New York: McGraw-Hill; 2001. p1141-1162. Available from: http://medtextfree.wordpress.com/2012/01/23/chapter-97-acute-lymphoblastic-leukemia/ (accessed 12 August 2012)

[22] Greaves MF, Wiemels J. Origins of chromosome translocations in childhood leukaemia. Nat Rev Cancer. 2003;3(9):639-649.

[23] Greaves M. In utero origins of childhood leukaemia. Early Hum Dev. 2005;81(1): 123-129.

[24] Wiemels J, Kang M, Greaves M. Backtracking of leukemic clones to birth. Methods Mol Biol. 2009;538:7-27.

[25] Knudson AG. Mutation and cancer: statistical study of retinoblastoma. Proc Natl Acad Sci U S A. 1971;68(4):820-823.

[26] Greaves M. Childhood leukaemia. BMJ. 2002;324(7332):283-287.

[27] Papaemmanuil E, Hosking FJ, Vijayakrishnan J, Price A, Olver B, Sheridan E, Kinsey SE, Lightfoot T, Roman E, Irving JA, Allan JM, Tomlinson IP, Taylor M, Greaves M, Houlston RS. Loci on 7p12.2, 10q21.2 and 14q11.2 are associated with risk of childhood acute lymphoblastic leukemia. Nat Genet. 2009;41(9):1006-1010.

[28] Treviño LR, Yang W, French D, Hunger SP, Carroll WL, Devidas M, Willman C, Neale G, Downing J, Raimondi SC, Pui CH, Evans WE, Relling MV. Germline genomic variants associated with childhood acute lymphoblastic leukemia. Nat Genet. 2009;41(9):1001-1005.

[29] Infante-Rivard C, Guiguet M. Family history of hematopoietic and other cancers in children with acute lymphoblastic leukemia. Cancer Detect Prev. 2004;28(2):83-87.

[30] Greaves MF, Maia AT, Wiemels JL, Ford AM. Leukemia in twins: lessons in natural history. Blood. 2003;102(7):2321-2333.

[31] Biondi A, Masera G. Molecular pathogenesis of childhood acute lymphoblastic leukemia. Haematologica. 1998;83(7):651-659.

[32] Zwaan CM, Reinhardt D, Hitzler J, Vyas P. Acute leukemias in children with Down syndrome. Hematol Oncol Clin North Am. 2010;24(1):19-34.

[33] Hasle H. Pattern of malignant disorders in individuals with Down's syndrome. Lancet Oncol. 2001;2(7):429-436.

[34] Seewald L, Taub JW, Maloney KW, McCabe ER. Acute leukemias in children with Down syndrome. Mol Genet Metab. 2012;107(1-2):25-30.

[35] Little MP. Cancer and non-cancer effects in Japanese atomic bomb survivors. J Radiol Prot. 2009;29(2A):A43-59.

[36] Wakeford R. Childhood leukaemia following medical diagnostic exposure to ionizing radiation in utero or after birth. Radiat Prot Dosimetry. 2008;132(2):166-174.

[37] Bartley K, Metayer C, Selvin S, Ducore J, Buffler P. Diagnostic X-rays and risk of childhood leukaemia. Int J Epidemiol. 2010;39(6):1628-1637.

[38] Bone CM, Hsieh GH. The risk of carcinogenesis from radiographs to pediatric orthopaedic patients. J Pediatr Orthop. 2000;20(2):251-254.

[39] Jirik V, Pekarek L, Janout V, Tomaskova H. Association between Childhood Leukaemia and Exposure to Power-frequency Magnetic Fields in Middle Europe. Biomed Environ Sci. 2012;25(5):597-601.

[40] Teepen JC, van Dijck JA. Impact of high electromagnetic field levels on childhood leukemia incidence. Int J Cancer. 2012;131(4):769-778.

[41] Laurier D, Jacob S, Bernier MO, Leuraud K, Metz C, Samson E, Laloi P. Epidemiological studies of leukaemia in children and young adults around nuclear facilities: a critical review. Radiat Prot Dosimetry. 2008;132(2):182-190.

[42] Ghirga G. Cancer in children residing near nuclear power plants: an open question. Ital J Pediatr. 2010;36:60. http://www.ncbi.nlm.nih.gov/pmc/articles/PMC2944154/pdf/1824-7288-36-60.pdf (accessed 29 November 2012)

[43] Buffler PA, Kwan ML, Reynolds P, Urayama KY. Environmental and genetic risk factors for childhood leukemia: appraising the evidence. Cancer Invest. 2005;23(1):60-75.

[44] Hijiya N, Ness KK, Ribeiro RC, Hudson MM. Acute leukemia as a secondary malignancy in children and adolescents: current findings and issues. Cancer. 2009;115(1):23-35.

[45] Alexander FE, Patheal SL, Biondi A, Brandalise S, Cabrera ME, Chan LC, Chen Z, Cimino G, Cordoba JC, Gu LJ, Hussein H, Ishii E, Kamel AM, Labra S, Magalhães IQ, Mizutani S, Petridou E, de Oliveira MP, Yuen P, Wiemels JL, Greaves MF. Transplacental chemical exposure and risk of infant leukemia with MLL gene fusion. Cancer Res. 2001;61(6):2542-2546.

[46] Infante-Rivard C, Labuda D, Krajinovic M, Sinnett D. Risk of childhood leukemia associated with exposure to pesticides and with gene polymorphisms. Epidemiology. 1999;10(5):481-487.

[47] Belson M, Kingsley B, Holmes A. Risk factors for acute leukemia in children: a review. Environ Health Perspect. 2007;115(1):138–145.

[48] Milne E, Greenop KR, Scott RJ, Bailey HD, Attia J, Dalla-Pozza L, de Klerk NH, Armstrong BK. Parental prenatal smoking and risk of childhood acute lymphoblastic leukemia. Am J Epidemiol. 2012;175(1):43-53.

[49] Smith MA, Simon R, Strickler HD, McQuillan G, Ries LA, Linet MS. Evidence that childhood acute lymphoblastic leukemia is associated with an infectious agent linked to hygiene conditions. Cancer Causes Control. 1998;9(3):285-298.

[50] Ahmed HG, Osman SI, Ashankyty IM. Incidence of Epstein-Barr virus in pediatric leukemia in the Sudan. Clin Lymphoma Myeloma Leuk. 2012;12(2):127-131.

[51] Magrath I. Epidemiology: clues to the pathogenesis of Burkitt lymphoma. Br J Haematol. 2012;156(6):744-756.

[52] Bennett JM, Catovsky D, Daniel MT, Flandrin G, Galton DA, Gralnick HR, Sultan C; French-American-British (FAB) co-operative group. Proposals for the classification of the acute leukaemias. Br J Haematol. 1976;33(4):451-458.

[53] Abdul-Hamid G. Classification of Acute Leukemia. In: Antica M. (ed.) Acute Leukemia - The Scientist's Perspective and Challenge. Rijeka: InTech;2011. p3-18. Available from: http://www.intechopen.com/books/acute-leukemia-the-scientist-s-perspective-and-challenge/classification-ofacute-leukemia

[54] Bennett JM, Catovsky D, Daniel MT, Flandrin G, Galton DA, Gralnick HR, Sultan C. The morphological classification of acute lymphoblastic leukaemia: concordance among observers and clinical correlations. Br J Haematol. 1981;47(4):553-561.

[55] Jaffe ES, Harris NL, Stein H, Vardiman JW. Pathology and Genetics of Tumours of Haematopoietic and Lymphoid Tissues. Lyon: IARC Press; 2001.

[56] Swerdlow SH, Campo E, Harris NL, Jaffe ES, Pileri SA, Stein H, Thiele J, Vardiman JW. WHO Classification of Tumours of Haematopoietic and Lymphoid Tissues. Lyon: IARC Press; 2008.

[57] Thiel E. Cell surface markers in leukemia: biological and clinical correlations. Crit Rev Oncol Hematol. 1985;2(3):209-260.

[58] Campana D, Behm FG. Immunophenotyping of leukemia. J Immunol Methods. 2000;243:59-75.

[59] Pui CH, Behm FG, Crist WM. Clinical and biologic relevance of immunologic marker studies in childhood acute lymphoblastic leukemia. Blood. 1993;82(2):343-362.

[60] Bene MC, Castoldi G, Knapp W, Ludwig WD, Matutes E, Orfao A, van't Veer MB; European Group for the Immunological Characterization of Leukemias (EGIL). Proposals for the immunological classification of acute leukemias. Leukemia. 1995, 9(10): 1783-1786.

[61] Putti MC, Rondelli R, Cocito MG, Aricó M, Sainati L, Conter V, Guglielmi C, Cantú-Rajnoldi A, Consolini R, Pession A, Zanesco L, Masera G, Biondi A, Basso G. Expression of myeloid markers lacks prognostic impact in children treated for acute lymphoblastic leukemia: Italian experience in AIEOP-ALL 88-91 studies. Blood. 1998;92(3):795-801.

[62] Pui CH, Relling MV, Downing JR. Acute lymphoblastic leukemia. N Engl J Med. 2004;350(15):1535-1548.

[63] Matutes E, Morilla R, Farahat N. Definition of acute biphenotypic leukemia. Haematologica. 1997;82(1):64–66.

[64] Weir EG, Ali Ansari-Lari M, Batista DA, Griffin CA, Fuller S, Smith BD, Borowitz MJ. Acute bilineal leukemia: a rare disease with poor outcome. Leukemia. 2007;21(11): 2264–2270.

[65] Gerr H, Zimmermann M, Schrappe M, Dworzak M, Ludwig WD, Bradtke J, Moericke A, Schabath R, Creutzig U, Reinhardt D. Acute leukaemias of ambiguous lineage in children: characterization, prognosis and therapy recommendations. Br J Haematol. 2010;149(1):84-92.

[66] Mullighan CG. The molecular genetic makeup of acute lymphoblastic leukemia. Hematology Am Soc Hematol Educ Program. 2012;2012:389-396.

[67] Trueworthy R, Shuster J, Look T, Crist W, Borowitz M, Carroll A, Frankel L, Harris M, Wagner H, Haggard M. Ploidy of lymphoblasts is the strongest predictor of treatment outcome in B-progenitor cell acute lymphoblastic leukemia of childhood: a Pediatric Oncology Group study. J Clin Oncol. 1992; 10(4):606-613.

[68] Sutcliffe MJ, Shuster JJ, Sather HN, Camitta BM, Pullen J, Schultz KR, Borowitz MJ, Gaynon PS, Carroll AJ, Heerema NA. High concordance from independent studies by the Children's Cancer Group (CCG) and Pediatric Oncology Group (POG) associating favorable prognosis with combined trisomies 4, 10, and 17 in children with NCI Standard-Risk B-precursor Acute Lymphoblastic Leukemia: a Children's Oncology Group (COG) initiative. Leukemia. 2005;19(5):734-740.

[69] Kebriaei P, Anastasi J, Larson RA. Acute lymphoblastic leukaemia: diagnosis and classification. Best Pract Res Clin Haematol. 2002;15(4):597-621.

[70] Moorman AV, Ensor HM, Richards SM, Chilton L, Schwab C, Kinsey SE, Vora A, Mitchell CD, Harrison CJ. Prognostic effect of chromosomal abnormalities in childhood B-cell precursor acute lymphoblastic leukaemia: results from the UK Medical Research Council ALL97/99 randomised trial. Lancet Oncol. 2010;11(5):429-438.

[71] Harrison CJ, Haas O, Harbott J, Biondi A, Stanulla M, Trka J, Izraeli S; Biology and Diagnosis Committee of International Berlin-Frankfürt-Münster study group. Detection of prognostically relevant genetic abnormalities in childhood B-cell precursor acute lymphoblastic leukaemia: recommendations from the Biology and Diagnosis Committee of the International Berlin-Frankfürt-Münster study group. Br J Haematol. 2010;151(2):132-142.

[72] Kurzrock R, Kantarjian HM, Druker BJ, Talpaz M. Philadelphia chromosome-positive leukemias: from basic mechanisms to molecular therapeutics. Ann Intern Med. 2003;138(10):819-830.

[73] Chowdhury T, Brady HJ. Insights from clinical studies into the role of the MLL gene in infant and childhood leukemia. Blood Cells Mol Dis. 2008;40(2):192-199.

[74] Winick NJ, Raetz EA, Ritter J, Carroll WL. Acute Lymphoblastic Leukemia. In: Caroll LW, Finlay JL (eds). Cancer in Children and Adolescents. London: Jones and Bartlett Publishers International; 2010. p161-183.

[75] Pui CH, Howard SC. Current management and challenges of malignant disease in the CNS in paediatric leukaemia. Lancet Oncol. 2008;9(3):257–268.

[76] Buerger B, Zimmermann M, Mann G, Kühl J, Löning L, Riehm H, Reiter A, Schrappe M. Diagnostic cerebrospinal fluid examination in children with acute lymphoblastic leukemia: significance of low leukocyte counts with blasts or traumatic lumbar puncture. J Clin Oncol. 2003;21(2):184–188.

[77] Lanzkowsky P. Manual of Pediatric Hematology and Oncology. London: Elsevier Inc; 2011.

[78] Möricke A, Reiter A, Zimmermann M, Gadner H, Stanulla M, Dördelmann M, Löning L, Beier R, Ludwig WD, Ratei R, Harbott J, Boos J, Mann G, Niggli F, Feldges A, Henze G, Welte K, Beck JD, Klingebiel T, Niemeyer C, Zintl F, Bode U, Urban C, Wehinger H, Niethammer D, Riehm H, Schrappe M; German-Austrian-Swiss ALL-BFM Study Group. Risk-adjusted therapy of acute lymphoblastic leukemia can decrease treatment burden and improve survival: treatment results of 2169 unselected pediatric and adolescent patients enrolled in the trial ALL-BFM 95. Blood. 2008;111(9): 4477-4489.

[79] Schultz KR, Pullen DJ, Sather HN, Shuster JJ, Devidas M, Borowitz MJ, Carroll AJ, Heerema NA, Rubnitz JE, Loh ML, Raetz EA, Winick NJ, Hunger SP, Carroll WL, Gaynon PS, Camitta BM. Risk- and response-based classification of childhood B-precursor acute lymphoblastic leukemia: a combined analysis of prognostic markers from the Pediatric Oncology Group (POG) and Children's Cancer Group (CCG). Blood. 2007;109(3):926-935.

[80] Pui CH, Boyett JM, Relling MV, Harrison PL, Rivera GK, Behm FG, Sandlund JT, Ribeiro RC, Rubnitz JE, Gajjar A, Evans WE. Sex differences in prognosis for children with acute lymphoblastic leukemia. J Clin Oncol. 1999;17(3):818-824.

[81] Kadan-Lottick NS, Ness KK, Bhatia S, Gurney JG. Survival variability by race and ethnicity in childhood acute lymphoblastic leukemia. JAMA. 2003; 290(15):2008-2014.

[82] Dordelmann M, Reiter A, Borkhardt A, Borkhardt A, Ludwig WD, Götz N, Viehmann S, Gadner H, Riehm H, Schrappe M. Prednisone response is the strongest predictor of treatment outcome in infant acute lymphoblastic leukemia. Blood. 1999;94(4):1209-1217.

[83] Campana D. Minimal residual disease monitoring in childhood acute lymphoblastic leukemia. Curr Opin Hematol. 2012;19(4):313-318.

[84] Bartram CR, Schrauder A, Köhler R, Schrappe M. Acute lymphoblastic leukemia in children: treatment planning via minimal residual disease assessment. Dtsch Arztebl Int. 2012;109(40):652-658.

[85] Borowitz MJ, MJ Devidas M, Hunger SP, Bowman WP, Carroll AJ, Carroll WL, Linda S, Martin PL, Pullen DJ, Viswanatha D, Willman CL, Winick N, Camitta BM; Children's Oncology Group. Clinical significance of minimal residual disease in childhood acute lymphoblastic leukemia and its relationship to other prognostic factors: a Children's Oncology Group study. Blood. 2008;111(12): 5477-5485.

[86] Pui CH, Campana D. New definition of remission in childhood acute lymphoblastic leukemia. Leukemia. 2000;14(5):783-785.

[87] Vrooman LM, Silverman LB. Childhood acute lymphoblastic leukemia: update on prognostic factors. Curr Opin Pediatr. 2009;21(1):1-8.

[88] Mullighan CG.Genomic profiling of B-progenitor acute lymphoblastic leukemia. Best Pract Res Clin Haematol. 2011;24(4):489-503.

[89] Sutton R, Lonergan M, Tapp H, Venn NC, Haber M, Norris MD, O'Brien TA, Alvaro F, Revesz T. Two cases of hypereosinophilia and high-risk acute lymphoblastic leukemia. Leukemia 2008; 22(7):1463-1465.

[90] Seibel NL. Treatment of acute lymphoblastic leukemia in children and adolescents: peaks and pitfalls. Hematology Am Soc Hematol Educ Program. 2008:374-380.

[91] Childhood Acute Lymphoblastic Leukaemia Collaborative Group (CALLCG). Beneficial and harmful effects of anthracyclines in the treatment of childhood acute lymphoblastic leukaemia: a systematic review and meta-analysis. Br J Haematol. 2009;145(3):376-388.

[92] van Dalen EC, Raphaël MF, Caron HN, Kremer LC. Treatment including anthracyclines versus treatment not including anthracyclines for childhood cancer. Cochrane Database Syst Rev. 2009; (1):CD006647.

[93] Schrappe M, Stanulla M. Current Treatment Approaches in Childhood Acute Lymphoblastic Leukemia. SIOP Education Book 2010; 25-38. https://www.cure4kids.org/private/courses_documents/m_382/Current-Treatment-Child-ALL.pdf (accessed 20 September 2012).

[94] Inaba H, Pui CH. Glucocorticoid use in acute lymphoblastic leukemia. Lancet Oncol. 2010;11(11):1096-1106.

[95] Hurwitz CA, Silverman LB, Schorin MA, Clavell LA, Dalton VK, Glick KM, Gelber RD, Sallan SE. Substituting dexamethasone for prednisone complicates remission induction in children with acute lymphoblastic leukemia. Cancer. 2000;88(8):1964-1969.

[96] Schrappe M, Zimmermann M, Moricke A, Mann G, Valsecchi MG, Bartram CR, Biondi A, Panzer-Grumayer R, Schrauder A, Locatelli F, Reiter A, Basso G, Niggli F, Arico M, Conter V. Dexamethasone in induction can eliminate one third of all relapses in

childhood acute lymphoblastic leukemia (ALL): results of an international randomized trial in 3655 patients (trial AIEOP-BFM ALL 2000) [abstract]. Blood (ASH Annual Meeting Abstracts) 2008;112(11):9. Abstract 7.

[97] Pieters R, Hunger SP, Boos J, Rizzari C, Silverman L, Baruchel A, Goekbuget N, Schrappe M, Pui CH. L-asparaginase treatment in acute lymphoblastic leukemia: a focus on Erwinia asparaginase. Cancer. 2011;117(2):238-249.

[98] Silverman LB, Supko JG, Stevenson KE, Woodward C, Vrooman LM, Neuberg DS, Asselin BL, Athale UH, Clavell L, Cole PD, Kelly KM, Laverdière C, Michon B, Schorin M, Schwartz CL, O'Brien JE, Cohen HJ, Sallan SE. Intravenous PEG-asparaginase during remission induction in children and adolescents with newly diagnosed acute lymphoblastic leukemia. Blood 2010;115(7):1351-1353.

[99] Oudot C, Auclerc MF, Levy V, Porcher R, Piguet C, Perel Y, Gandemer V, Debre M, Vermylen C, Pautard B, Berger C, Schmitt C, Leblanc T, Cayuela JM, Socie G, Michel G, Leverger G, Baruchel A. Prognostic factors for leukemic induction failure in children with acute lymphoblastic leukemia and outcome after salvage therapy: the FRALLE 93 study. J Clin Oncol. 2008;26(9):1496-1503.

[100] Schrappe M, Hunger SP, Pui CH, Saha V, Gaynon PS, Baruchel A, Conter V, Otten J, Ohara A, Versluys AB, Escherich G, Heyman M, Silverman LB, Horibe K, Mann G, Camitta BM, Harbott J, Riehm H, Richards S, Devidas M, Zimmermann M. Outcomes after induction failure in childhood acute lymphoblastic leukemia. N Engl J Med. 2012;366(15):1371-1381.

[101] Nachman JB, Sather HN, Sensel MG, Trigg ME, Cherlow JM, Lukens JN, Wolff L, Uckun FM, Gaynon PS. Augmented post-induction therapy for children with high-risk acute lymphoblastic leukemia and a slow response to initial therapy. N Engl J Med. 1998;338(23):1663–1671.

[102] Seibel NL, Steinherz PG, Sather HN, Nachman JB, Delaat C, Ettinger LJ, Freyer DR, Mattano LA Jr, Hastings CA, Rubin CM, Bertolone K, Franklin JL, Heerema NA, Mitchell TL, Pyesmany AF, La MK, Edens C, Gaynon PS. Early post-induction intensification therapy improves survival for children and adolescents with high-risk acute lymphoblastic leukemia and a rapid early response to induction therapy: a report from the Children's Oncology Group. Blood. 2008;111(5):2548-2555.

[103] Pui, CH. Central nervous system disease in acute lymphoblastic leukemia prophylaxis and treatment. Hematology Am Soc Hematol Educ Program. 2006:142-146.

[104] Pui CH, Thiel E. Central nervous system disease in hematologic malignancies: historical perspective and practical applications. Semin Oncol. 2009;36(4 Suppl 2):S2-S16.

[105] Henze G, Langermann HJ, Brämswig J, Breu H, Gadner H, Schellong G, Welte K, Riehm H. The BFM 76/79 acute lymphoblastic leukemia therapy study (author's transl). Klin Padiatr. 1981;193(3):145-154.

[106] Hutchinson RJ, Gaynon PS, Sather H, Bertolone SJ, Cooper HA, Tannous R, Wells LM, Heerema NA, Sailer S, Trigg ME; Children's Cancer Group/Children's Oncology Group. Intensification of therapy for children with lower-risk acute lymphoblastic leukemia: long-term follow-up of patients treated on Children's Cancer Group Trial 1881. J Clin Oncol. 2003;21(9):1790-1797.

[107] Trigg ME, Sather HN, Reaman GH, Tubergen DG, Steinherz PG, Gaynon PS, Uckun FM, Hammond GD; Children's Oncology Group. Ten-year survival of children with acute lymphoblastic leukemia: a report from the Children's Oncology Group. Leuk Lymphoma. 2008;49(6):1142-1154.

[108] Hunger SP. Development and refinement of augmented treatment regimens for pediatric high-risk acute lymphoblastic leukemia. American Society of Clinical Oncology 2012:611-615. http://www.asco.org/ASCOv2/Home/Education%20&%20Training/Educational%20Book/PDF%20Files/2012/zds00112000611.PDF (accessed 14 September 2012).

[109] Sofianou-Katsoulis A, Khakoo G, Kaczmarski R. Reduction in bioavailability of 6-mercaptopurine on simultaneous administ ration with cow's milk. Pediatr Hematol Oncol. 2006; 23(6):485-487.

[110] Conter V, Valsecchi MG, Silvestri D, Campbell M, Dibar E, Magyarosy E, Gadner H, Stary J, Benoit Y, Zimmermann M, Reiter A, Riehm H, Masera G, Schrappe M. Pulses of vincristine and dexamethasone in addition to intensive chemotherapy for children with intermediate-risk acute lymphoblastic leukaemia: a multicentre randomised trial. Lancet. 2007;369(9556):123-131.

[111] Locatelli F, Schrappe M, Bernardo ME, Rutella S. How I treat relapsed childhood acute lymphoblastic leukemia. Blood. 2012;120(14):2807-2816.

[112] Mullighan CG, Phillips LA, Su X, Ma J, Miller CB, Shurtleff SA, Downing JR. Genomic analysis of the clonal origins of relapsed acute lymphoblastic leukemia. Science. 2008;322(5906):1377-1380.

[113] Gaynon PS. Childhood acute lymphoblastic leukemia and relapse. Br J Haematol. 2005;131(5):579-585.

[114] Gaynon PS, Qu RP, Chappell RJ, Willoughby ML, Tubergen DG, Steinherz PG, Trigg ME. Survival after relapse in childhood acute lymphoblastic leukemia: impact of site and time to first relapse--the Children's Cancer Group Experience. Cancer. 1998;82(7):1387-1395.

[115] Saarinen-Pihkala UM, Heilmann C, Winiarski J, Glomstein A, Abrahamsson J, Arvidson J, Békássy AN, Forestier E, Jonmundsson G, Schroeder H, Vettenranta K, Wesenberg F, Gustafsson G. Pathways through relapses and deaths of children with acute lymphoblastic leukemia: role of allogeneic stem-cell transplantation in Nordic data. J Clin Oncol. 2006;24(36):5750-5762.

[116] Chessells JM, Veys P, Kempski H, Henley P, Leiper A, Webb D, Hann IM. Long-term follow-up of relapsed childhood acute lymphoblastic leukaemia. Br J Haematol. 2003;123(3):396-405.

[117] Martin A, Morgan E, Hijiya N. Relapsed or refractory pediatric acute lymphoblastic leukemia: Current and emerging treatments. Paediatr Drugs. 2012;14(6):377-387.

[118] van den Berg H, de Groot-Kruseman HA, Damen-Korbijn CM, de Bont ES, Schouten-van Meeteren AY, Hoogerbrugge PM. Outcome after first relapse in children with acute lymphoblastic leukemia: a report based on the Dutch Childhood Oncology Group (DCOG) relapse all 98 protocol. Pediatr Blood Cancer. 2011;57(2):210-216.

[119] Lanino E, Sacchi N, Peters C, Giardino S, Rocha V, Dini G; EBMT Paediatric, Acute Leukemia Working Parties; Eurocord. Strategies of the donor search for children with second CR ALL lacking a matched sibling donor. Bone Marrow Transplant. 2008;41 Suppl 2:S75-79.

[120] Schrauder A, von Stackelberg A, Schrappe M, Cornish J, Peters C; ALL-BFM Study Group; EBMT PD WP; I-BFM Study Group. Allogeneic hematopoietic SCT in children with ALL: current concepts of ongoing prospective SCT trials. Bone Marrow Transplant. 2008;41 Suppl 2:S71-4.

[121] Ritchey AK, Pollock BH, Lauer SJ, Andejeski Y, Barredo J, Buchanan GR. Improved survival of children with isolated CNS relapse of acute lymphoblastic leukemia: a pediatriconcology group study. *J Clin Oncol*. 1999;17(12):3745-3752.

[122] Jacobs JE, Hastings C. Isolated extramedullary relapse in childhood acute lymphocytic leukemia.Curr Hematol Malig Rep. 2010;5(4):185-91.

[123] Kanwar VS. Pediatric Acute Lymphoblastic Leukemia. Updated May 31, 2012. http://emedicine.medscape.com/article/990113-overview#aw2aab6b2b4 (accessed 3 November 2012).

[124] Hunger SP, Lu X, Devidas M, Camitta BM, Gaynon PS, Winick NJ, Reaman GH, Carroll WL. Improved survival for children and adolescents with acute lymphoblastic leukemia between 1990 and 2005: a report from the children's oncology group. J Clin Oncol. 2012;30(14):1663-1669.

[125] Bajel A, George B, Mathews V, Viswabandya A, Kavitha ML, Srivastava A, Chandy M. Treatment of children with acute lymphoblastic leukemia in India using a BFM protocol.Pediatr Blood Cancer. 2008 Nov;51(5):621-625.

[126] Arya LS, Padmanjali KS, Sazawal S, Saxena R, Bhargava M, Kulkarni KP, Adde M, Magrath I. Childhood T-lineage acute lymphoblastic leukemia: management and outcome at a tertiary care center in North India. Indian Pediatr. 2011;48(10):785-790.

[127] Muwakkit S, Al-Aridi C, Samra A, Saab R, Mahfouz RA, Farra C, Jeha S, Abboud MR. Implementation of an intensive risk-stratified treatment protocol for children

and adolescents with acute lymphoblastic leukemia in Lebanon. Am J Hematol. 2012;87(7):678-683.

[128] Einsiedel HG, von Stackelberg A, Hartmann R, Fengler R, Schrappe M, Janka-Schaub G, Mann G, Hählen K, Göbel U, Klingebiel T, Ludwig WD, Henze G. Long-term outcome in children with relapsed ALL by risk-stratified salvage therapy: results of trial acute lymphoblastic leukemia-relapse study of the Berlin-Frankfurt-Münster Group 87. J Clin Oncol. 2005;23(31):7942-7950.

[129] Nguyen K, Devidas M, Cheng SC, La M, Raetz EA, Carroll WL, Winick NJ, Hunger SP, Gaynon PS, Loh ML; Children's Oncology Group. Factors influencing survival after relapse from acute lymphoblastic leukemia: a Children's Oncology Group study. Leukemia. 2008;22(12):2142-2150.

[130] Pulsipher MA, Peters C, Pui CH. High-risk pediatric acute lymphoblastic leukemia: to transplant or not to transplant? Biol Blood Marrow Transplant. 2011;17(1 Suppl):S137-148.

[131] Aricò M, Valsecchi MG, Camitta B, Schrappe M, Chessells J, Baruchel A, Gaynon P, Silverman L, Janka-Schaub G, Kamps W, Pui CH, Masera G. Outcome of treatment in children with Philadelphia chromosome-positive acute lymphoblastic leukemia. N Engl J Med. 2000;342(14):998-1006.

[132] Balduzzi A, Valsecchi MG, Uderzo C, De Lorenzo P, Klingebiel T, Peters C, Stary J, Felice MS, Magyarosy E, Conter V, Reiter A, Messina C, Gadner H, Schrappe M. Chemotherapy versus allogeneic transplantation for very-high-risk childhood acute lymphoblastic leukaemia in first complete remission: comparison by genetic randomisation in an international prospective study. Lancet. 2005;366(9486):635-642.

[133] Sharathkumar A, Saunders EF, Dror Y, Grant R, Greenberg M, Weitzman S, Chan H, Calderwood S, Freedman MH, Doyle J. Allogeneic bone marrow transplantation vs chemotherapy for children with Philadelphia chromosome-positive acute lymphoblastic leukemia. Bone Marrow Transplant. 2004;33(1):39-45.

[134] Satwani P, Sather H, Ozkaynak F, Heerema NA, Schultz KR, Sanders J, Kersey J, Davenport V, Trigg M, Cairo MS. Allogeneic bone marrow transplantation in first remission for children with ultra-high-risk features of acute lymphoblastic leukemia: A children's oncology group study report. Biol Blood Marrow Transplant. 2007;13(2): 218-227.

[135] Schultz KR, Bowman WP, Aledo A, Slayton WB, Sather H, Devidas M, Wang C, Davies SM, Gaynon PS, Trigg M, Rutledge R, Burden L, Jorstad D, Carroll A, Heerema NA, Winick N, Borowitz MJ, Hunger SP, Carroll WL, Camitta B. Improved early event-free survival with imatinib in Philadelphia chromosome-positive acute lymphoblastic leukemia: a Children's Oncology Group Study. J Clin Oncol. 2009;27:5175–5181.

[136] Dreyer ZE, Dinndorf PA, Camitta B, Sather H, La MK, Devidas M, Hilden JM, Heerema NA, Sanders JE, McGlennen R, Willman CL, Carroll AJ, Behm F, Smith FO,

Woods WG, Godder K, Reaman GH. Analysis of the role of hematopoietic stem-cell transplantation in infants with acute lymphoblastic leukemia in first remission and MLL gene rearrangements: a report from the Children's Oncology Group. J Clin Oncol. 2011;29(2):214-222.

[137] Mann G, Attarbaschi A, Schrappe M, De Lorenzo P, Peters C, Hann I, De Rossi G, Felice M, Lausen B, Leblanc T, Szczepanski T, Ferster A, Janka-Schaub G, Rubnitz J, Silverman LB, Stary J, Campbell M, Li CK, Suppiah R, Biondi A, Vora A, Valsecchi MG, Pieters R; Interfant-99 Study Group. Improved outcome with hematopoietic stem cell transplantation in a poor prognostic subgroup of infants with mixed-lineage-leukemia (MLL)-rearranged acute lymphoblastic leukemia: results from the Interfant-99 Study. Blood. 2010;116(15):2644-2650.

[138] Nachman JB, Heerema NA, Sather H, Camitta B, Forestier E, Harrison CJ, Dastugue N, Schrappe M, Pui CH, Basso G, Silverman LB, Janka-Schaub GE. Outcome of treatment in children with hypodiploid acute lymphoblastic leukemia. Blood. 2007;110(4): 1112-1115.

[139] Balduzzi A, Valsecchi MG, Uderzo C, De Lorenzo P, Klingebiel T, Peters C, Stary J, Felice MS, Magyarosy E, Conter V, Reiter A, Messina C, Gadner H, Schrappe M. Chemotherapy versus allogeneic transplantation for very-high-risk childhood acute lymphoblastic leukaemia in first complete remission: comparison by genetic randomisation in an international prospective study. Lancet. 2005;366(9486):635-642.

[140] Krance R. Transplantation for children with acute lymphoblastic leukemia. Bone Marrow Transplant. 2008;42 Suppl 1:S25-S27.

[141] Inukai T, Kiyokawa N, Campana D, Coustan-Smith E, Kikuchi A, Kobayashi M, Takahashi H, Koh K, Manabe A, Kumagai M, Ikuta K, Hayashi Y, Tsuchida M, Sugita K, Ohara A. Clinical significance of early T-cell precursor acute lymphoblastic leukaemia: results of the Tokyo Children's Cancer Study Group Study L99-15. Br J Haematol. 2012;156(3):358-365.

[142] Davies SM, Mehta PA. Pediatric acute lymphoblastic leukemia: is there still a role for transplant? Hematology Am Soc Hematol Educ Program. 2010;2010:363-367.

[143] Miano M, Labopin M, Hartmann O, Angelucci E, Cornish J, Gluckman E, Locatelli F, Fischer A, Egeler RM, Or R, Peters C, Ortega J, Veys P, Bordigoni P, Iori AP, Niethammer D, Rocha V, Dini G; Paediatric Diseases Working Party of the European Group for Blood and Marrow Transplantation. Haematopoietic stem cell transplantation trends in children over the last three decades: a survey by the paediatric diseases working party of the European Group for Blood and Marrow Transplantation. Bone Marrow Transplant. 2007;39(2):89-99.

[144] Spellman SR, Eapen M, Logan BR, Mueller C, Rubinstein P, Setterholm MI, Woolfrey AE, Horowitz MM, Confer DL, Hurley CK; National Marrow Donor Program; Center for International Blood and Marrow Transplant Research. A perspective on the selec-

tion of unrelated donors and cord blood units for transplantation. Blood. 2012;120(2): 259-265.

[145] Pidala J, Kim J, Schell M, Lee SJ, Hillgruber R, Nye V, Ayala E, Alsina M, Betts B, Bookout R, Fernandez HF, Field T, Locke FL, Nishihori T, Ochoa JL, Perez L, Perkins J, Shapiro J, Tate C, Tomblyn M, Anasetti C. Race/ethnicity affects the probability of finding an HLA-A, -B, -C and -DRB1 allele-matched unrelated donor and likelihood of subsequent transplant utilization. Bone Marrow Transplant. 2012 Aug 6. doi: 10.1038/bmt.2012.150. [Epub ahead of print]

[146] Ballen KK, Koreth J, Chen YB, Dey BR, Spitzer TR. Selection of optimal alternative graft source: mismatched unrelated donor, umbilical cord blood, or haploidentical transplant. Blood. 2012;119(9):1972-1980.

[147] Perez LE. Outcomes from unrelated donor hematopoietic stem cell transplantation. Cancer Control. 2011;18(4):216-221.

[148] González-Vicent M, Molina B, Andión M, Sevilla J, Ramirez M, Pérez A, Díaz MA. Allogeneic hematopoietic transplantation using haploidentical donor vs. unrelated cord blood donor in pediatric patients: a single-center retrospective study. Eur J Haematol. 2011;87(1):46-53.

[149] Lech-Maranda E, Mlynarski W. Novel and emerging drugs for acute lymphoblastic leukemia. Curr Cancer Drug Targets. 2012;12(5):505-521.

[150] Lee-Sherick AB, Linger RM, Gore L, Keating AK, Graham DK. Targeting paediatric acute lymphoblastic leukaemia: novel therapies currently in development. Br J Haematol. 2010;151(4):295-311.

[151] Harned TM, Gaynon PS. Treating refractory leukemias in childhood, role of clofarabine. Ther Clin Risk Manag. 2008; 4(2): 327–336.

[152] Hijiya N, Barry E, Arceci RJ. Clofarabine in pediatric acute leukemia: current findings and issues. Pediatr Blood Cancer. 2012;59(3):417-22.

[153] Hijiya N, Thomson B, Isakoff MS, Silverman LB, Steinherz PG, Borowitz MJ, Kadota R, Cooper T, Shen V, Dahl G, Thottassery JV, Jeha S, Maloney K, Paul JA, Barry E, Carroll WL, Gaynon PS. Phase 2 trial of clofarabine in combination with etoposide and cyclophosphamide in pediatric patients with refractory or relapsed acute lymphoblastic leukemia. Blood. 2011;118(23):6043-9.

[154] Advani AS, Gundacker HM, Sala-Torra O, Radich JP, Lai R, Slovak ML, Lancet JE, Coutre SE, Stuart RK, Mims MP, Stiff PJ, Appelbaum FR. Southwest Oncology Group Study S0530: a phase 2 trial of clofarabine and cytarabine for relapsed or refractory acute lymphocytic leukaemia. Br J Haematol. 2010;151(5):430-4.

[155] Biondi A, Schrappe M, De Lorenzo P, Castor A, Lucchini G, Gandemer V, Pieters R, Stary J, Escherich G, Campbell M, Li CK, Vora A, Aricò M, Röttgers S, Saha V, Valsecchi MG. Imatinib after induction for treatment of children and adolescents with

Philadelphia-chromosome-positive acute lymphoblastic leukaemia (EsPhALL): a randomised, open-label, intergroup study. Lancet Oncol. 2012;13(9):936-945.

[156] Aplenc R, Blaney SM, Strauss LC, Balis FM, Shusterman S, Ingle AM, Agrawal S, Sun J, Wright JJ, Adamson PC. Pediatric phase I trial and pharmacokinetic study of dasatinib: a report from the children's oncology group phase I consortium. J Clin Oncol. 2011;29(7):839-844.

[157] Koo HH. Philadelphia chromosome-positive acute lymphoblastic leukemia in childhood. Korean J Pediatr. 2011; 54(3):106-110.

[158] Brown P, Small D. FLT3 inhibitors: a paradigm for the development of targeted therapeutics for paediatric cancer. Eur J Cancer. 2004;40(5):707-721.

[159] Brown P, Levis M, McIntyre E, Griesemer M, Small D. Combinations of the FLT3 inhibitor CEP-701 and chemotherapy synergistically kill infant and childhood MLL-rearranged ALL cells in a sequence-dependent manner. Leukemia. 2006;20(8): 1368-1376.

[160] Dunsmore KP, Devidas M, Linda SB, Borowitz MJ, Winick N, Hunger SP, Carroll WL, Camitta BM. Pilot study of nelarabine in combination with intensive chemotherapy in high-risk T-cell acute lymphoblastic leukemia: a report from the Children's Oncology Group. J Clin Oncol. 2012;30(22):2753-2759.

[161] Houghton PJ, Morton CL, Gorlick R, Lock RB, Carol H, Reynolds CP, Kang MH, Maris JM, Keir ST, Kolb EA, Wu J, Wozniak AW, Billups CA, Rubinstein L, Smith MA. Stage 2 combination testing of rapamycin with cytotoxic agents by the Pediatric Preclinical Testing Program. Mol Cancer Ther. 2010;9(1):101-112.

[162] Carol H, Boehm I, Reynolds CP, Kang MH, Maris JM, Morton CL, Gorlick R, Kolb EA, Keir ST, Wu J, Wozniak AE, Yang Y, Manfredi M, Ecsedy J, Wang J, Neale G, Houghton PJ, Smith MA, Lock RB. Efficacy and pharmacokinetic/pharmacodynamic evaluation of the Aurora kinase A inhibitor MLN8237 against preclinical models of pediatric cancer. Cancer Chemother Pharmacol. 2011;68(5):1291-1304.

[163] Griffin TC, Weitzman S, Weinstein H, Chang M, Cairo M, Hutchison R, Shiramizu B, Wiley J, Woods D, Barnich M, Gross TG; Children's Oncology Group. A study of rituximab and ifosfamide, carboplatin, and etoposide chemotherapy in children with recurrent/refractory B-cell (CD20+) non-Hodgkin lymphoma and mature B-cell acute lymphoblastic leukemia: a report from the Children's Oncology Group. Pediatr Blood Cancer. 2009;52(2):177-181.

[164] Meinhardt A, Burkhardt B, Zimmermann M, Borkhardt A, Kontny U, Klingebiel T, Berthold F, Janka-Schaub G, Klein C, Kabickova E, Klapper W, Attarbaschi A, Schrappe M, Reiter A; Berlin-Frankfurt-Münster group. Phase II window study on rituximab in newly diagnosed pediatric mature B-cell non-Hodgkin's lymphoma and Burkitt leukemia. J Clin Oncol. 2010;28(19):3115-3121.

[165] Raetz EA, Cairo MS, Borowitz MJ, Blaney SM, Krailo MD, Leil TA, Reid JM, Goldenberg DM, Wegener WA, Carroll WL, Adamson PC; Children's Oncology Group Pilot Study. Chemoimmunotherapy reinduction with epratuzumab in children with acute lymphoblastic leukemia in marrow relapse: a Children's Oncology Group Pilot Study. J Clin Oncol. 2008;26(22):3756-3762.

[166] Cooper TM, Franklin J, Gerbing RB, Alonzo TA, Hurwitz C, Raimondi SC, Hirsch B, Smith FO, Mathew P, Arceci RJ, Feusner J, Iannone R, Lavey RS, Meshinchi S, Gamis A. AAML03P1, a pilot study of the safety of gemtuzumab ozogamicin in combination with chemotherapy for newly diagnosed childhood acute myeloid leukemia: a report from the Children's Oncology Group. Cancer. 2012;118(3):761-769.

[167] Angiolillo AL, Yu AL, Reaman G, Ingle AM, Secola R, Adamson PC. A phase II study of Campath-1H in children with relapsed or refractory acute lymphoblastic leukemia: a Children's Oncology Group report. Pediatr Blood Cancer. 2009;53(6): 978-983.

[168] Barth M, Raetz E, Cairo MS. The future role of monoclonal antibody therapy in childhood acute leukaemias. Br J Haematol. 2012;159(1):3-17.

[169] Rihani R, Bazzeh F, Faqih N, Sultan I. Secondary hematopoietic malignancies in survivors of childhood cancer: an analysis of 111 cases from the Surveillance, Epidemiology, and End Result-9 registry. Cancer. 2010;116(18):4385-4394.

[170] Meadows AT, Friedman DL, Neglia JP, Mertens AC, Donaldson SS, Stovall M, Hammond S, Yasui Y, Inskip PD. Second neoplasms in survivors of childhood cancer: Findings from the Childhood Cancer Survivor Study cohort. J Clin Oncol. 2009;27(14):2356–2362.

[171] Friedman DL, Whitton J, Leisenring W, Mertens AC, Hammond S, Stovall M, Donaldson SS, Meadows AT, Robison LL, Neglia JP. Subsequent neoplasms in 5-year survivors of childhood cancer: The Childhood Cancer Survivor Study. J Natl Cancer Inst. 2010;102(14):1083-1095.

[172] Ochs J, Mulhern R, Fairclough D, Parvey L, Whitaker J, Ch'ien L, Mauer A, Simone J. Comparison of neuropsychologic functioning and clinical indicators of neurotoxicity in long-term survivors of childhood leukemia given cranial radiation or parenteral methotrexate: a prospective study. J Clin Oncol. 1991;9(1):145-151.

[173] Cole PD, Kamen BA. Delayed neurotoxicity associated with therapy for children with acute lymphoblastic leukemia. Ment Retard Dev Disabil Res Rev. 2006;12(3): 174-83.

[174] Daams M, Schuitema I, van Dijk BW, van Dulmen-den Broeder E, Veerman AJ, van den Bos C, de Sonneville LM. Long-term effects of cranial irradiation and intrathecal chemotherapy in treatment of childhood leukemia: a MEG study of power spectrum and correlated cognitive dysfunction. BMC Neurol. 2012;12(1):84. Published online 2012 August 28. doi: 10.1186/1471-2377-12-84 (accessed 3 November 2012).

[175] Edelstein K, D'agostino N, Bernstein LJ, Nathan PC, Greenberg ML, Hodgson DC, Millar BA, Laperriere N, Spiegler BJ. Long-term neurocognitive outcomes in young adult survivors of childhood acute lymphoblastic leukemia. J Pediatr Hematol Oncol. 2011;33(6):450-458.

[176] Sorensen K, Levitt GA, Bull C, Dorup I, Sullivan ID. Late anthracycline cardiotoxicity after childhood cancer: a prospective longitudinal study. *Cancer. 2003;*97(8): 1991-1998.

[177] Lipshultz SE. Exposure to anthracyclines during childhood causes cardiac injury. Semin Oncol. 2006;33(3 Suppl 8):S8-14.

[178] Iarussi D, Indolfi P, Galderisi M, Bossone E. Cardiac toxicity after anthracycline chemotherapy in childhood. Herz. 2000;25(7):676-88.

[179] Elbl L, Hrstkova H, Tomaskova I, Blazek B, Michalek J. Long-term serial echocardiographic examination of late anthracycline cardiotoxicity and its prevention by dexrazoxane in paediatric patients. Eur J Pediatr. 2005;164(11):678-684.

[180] Harake D, Franco VI, Henkel JM, Miller TL, Lipshultz SE. Cardiotoxicity in childhood cancer survivors: strategies for prevention and management. Future Cardiol. 2012;8(4):647-670.

[181] Trachtenberg BH, Landy DC, Franco VI, Henkel JM, Pearson EJ, Miller TL, Lipshultz SE. Anthracycline-associated cardiotoxicity in survivors of childhood cancer. Pediatr Cardiol. 2011;32(3):342-353.

[182] Chow EJ, Friedman DL, Yasui Y, Whitton JA, Stovall M, Robison LL, Sklar CA. Decreased adult height in survivors of childhood acute lymphoblastic leukemia: a report from the Childhood Cancer Survivor Study. J Pediatr. 2007;150(4):370-375.

[183] Duffner PK. Long-term effects of radiation therapy on cognitive and endocrine function in children with leukemia and brain tumors. Neurologist. 2004;10(6):293-310.

[184] Skoczen S, Surmiak M, Strojny W. Survivors of acute lymphoblastic leukemia and body mass changes. Expert Opin Drug Saf. 2010;9(1):65-77.

[185] Oudin C, Simeoni MC, Sirvent N, Contet A, Begu-Le Coroller A, Bordigoni P, Curtillet C, Poirée M, Thuret I, Play B, Massot MC, Chastagner P, Chambost H, Auquier P, Michel G. Prevalence and risk factors of the metabolic syndrome in adult survivors of childhood leukemia. Blood. 2011;117(17):4442-4448.

[186] Krawczuk-Rybak M, Solarz E, Wysocka J, Matysiak M, Gadomski A, Kazanowska B, Sega-Pondel D. Testicular function after treatment for acute lymphoblastic leukemia (all) in prepubertal and pubertal boys. Pediatr Hematol Oncol. 2009;26(7):504-514.

[187] Romerius P, Ståhl O, Moëll C, Relander T, Cavallin-Ståhl E, Wiebe T, Giwercman YL, Giwercman A. High risk of azoospermia in men treated for childhood cancer. Int J Androl. 2011;34(1):69-76.

[188] Kadan-Lottick NS, Dinu I, Wasilewski-Masker K, Kaste S, Meacham LR, Mahajan A, Stovall M, Yasui Y, Robison LL, Sklar CA. Osteonecrosis in adult survivors of childhood cancer: a report from the childhood cancer survivor study. J Clin Oncol. 2008;26(18):3038-45.

[189] Sheen C, Vincent T, Barrett D, Horwitz EM, Hulitt J, Strong E, Grupp SA, Teachey DT. Statins are active in acute lymphoblastic leukaemia (ALL): a therapy that may treat ALL and prevent avascular necrosis. Br J Haematol. 2011;155(3):403-407.

[190] French D, Hamilton LH, Mattano LA Jr, Sather HN, Devidas M, Nachman JB, Relling MV; Children's Oncology Group. A PAI-1 (SERPINE1) polymorphism predicts osteonecrosis in children with acute lymphoblastic leukemia: a report from the Children's Oncology Group. Blood. 2008;111(9):4496-4499.

[191] Relling MV, Yang W, Das S, Cook EH, Rosner GL, Neel M, Howard S, Ribeiro R, Sandlund JT, Pui CH, Kaste SC. Pharmacogenetic risk factors for osteonecrosis of the hip among children with leukemia. J Clin Oncol. 2004;22(19):3930-3936.

[192] Lethaby C, Wiernikowski J, Sala A, Naronha M, Webber C, Barr RD. Bisphosphonate therapy for reduced bone mineral density during treatment of acute lymphoblastic leukemia in childhood and adolescence: a report of preliminary experience. J Pediatr Hematol Oncol. 2007;29(9):613-616.

[193] Leblicq C, Laverdière C, Décarie JC, Delisle JF, Isler MH, Moghrabi A, Chabot G, Alos N. Effectiveness of pamidronate as treatment of symptomatic osteonecrosis occurring in children treated for acute lymphoblastic leukemia. Pediatr Blood Cancer. 2012 Sep 21. doi: 10.1002/pbc.24313. [Epub ahead of print] (accessed 20 October 2012).

Chapter 3

Acute Leukemia Clinical Presentation

Gamal Abdul Hamid

Additional information is available at the end of the chapter

http://dx.doi.org/10.5772/53531

1. Introduction

Acute leukemias are highly malignant neoplasms and are responsible for a large number of haematopoietic cancer-related deaths (Jemal et al 2006). Although the survival rates have improved remarkably in the younger age group, the prognosis in older patients is still poor (Redaelli et al 2003).

The clinical presentation of acute leukemia results from infiltration of bone marrow or extramedullary sites by blasts. As a result, initial symptoms may be due to the presence of anemia, neutropenia, or thrombocytopenia. Patients generally present with nonspecific complaints including weakness, lethargy, fatigue, dyspnea, fever, weight loss, or bleeding. Blasts may also infiltrate organs or lymph nodes, resulting in hepatosplenomegaly or adenopathy. Bone marrow infiltration with blasts can result in bone pain. Mucosal bleeding, petechiae, ecchymosis, and fundal hemorrhages may occur as a result of thrombocytopenia.

Patients with acute promyelocytic leukemia (APL) characteristically present with coagulopathy and signs of disseminated intravascular coagulation (DIC). It should be noted, however, that rapid cell turnover can result in DIC in any form of acute leukemia.

In acute monocytic leukemia the common findings are weakness, bleeding and a diffuse erythematous skin rash. There is a high frequency of extramedulary infiltration of the lungs, colon, meninges, lymphnodes, bladder and larynx and gingival hyperplasia.

The clinical onset of acute lymphoblastic leukemia (ALL) is most often acute, although a small percentage of cases may evolve insidiously over several months (Pui 2006). The presenting symptoms and signs correlate with the leukemic cell burden and the degree of bone marrow replacement, leading to cytopenias.

1. Marrow failure due to infiltration	
– Fatigue, pallor,	– Anemia
– spontaneous bruising	– Thrombocytopenia
– Infections, sepsis	– Neutropenia
2.*Infiltration of other organs*	
– liver, spleen, lymph nodes (particularly in ALL)	
– Lymphadenopathy	
– Hepatosplenomegaly	
– Mediastinal masses (T-ALL)	
– Gums	
– Gum hypertrophy (monocytic subtype of acute myeloblastic leukemia)	
– Bone pain, especially in children with ALL	
– Skin -Leukemia cutis	
– Soft tissue -Chloromas	
– Testis	
– Central nervous system (CNS)	
– Solid organs	
3. *Leukostasis*(only seen with WBC > 50 x 10^9/L)	
– CNS -Strokes	
– Lungs -Pulmonary infiltrates, hypoxemia	
4. *Constitutional symptoms*	
– Fevers, sweats are common	
– Weight loss uncommon	
5. *Other*	
– Exposure of substances that can initiate coagulation can cause DIC	

Table 1. Pathophysiology of the clinical manifestations of acute leukemias

2. Signs, symptoms and laboratory features of Acute Myeloblastic Leukemia (AML)

Clinical manifestations of AML result either from the proliferation of leukaemic cells or from bone marrow failure that leads to decrease in normal cells. Leukaemic cells can infiltrate tissues, leading to hepatomegaly, splenomegaly, skin infiltrates and swollen gums. As an indirect effect of the leukaemic proliferation leading to high cell destruction, hyperuricaemia and occasionally renal failure may occur. The haematopoiesis suppression leads to clinical features of anaemia, neutropenia and thrombocytopenia. Signs and symptoms that signal the onset of AML include pallor, fatigue, weakness, palpitations, and dyspnea on exertion. They reflect the development of anemia; however, weakness, loss of sense of wellbeing, and fatigue on exertion may be disproportionate to the severity of anemia. (Gur et al 1999). Easy bruising, petechiae, epistaxis, gingival bleeding, conjunctival hemorrhages, and prolonged bleeding from skin injuries reflect thrombocytopenia and are frequent early manifestations of the disease. Very

http://dx.doi.org/10.5772/53531

infrequently gastrointestinal, genitourinary, bronchopulmonary, or central nervous system bleeding can occur at the onset of the disease. Neutropenia translates into infectious manifestations. Pustules or other minor pyogenic infections of the skin and of minor cuts or wounds are most common. Major infections such as pneumonia, pyelonephritis, and meningitis are uncommon as presenting features of the disease, in part because absolute neutrophil counts under 500/μl (0.5×10^9/L) are uncommon until chemotherapy is begun. Anorexia and weight loss are frequent findings. Fever is present in many patients at the time of diagnosis. Myeloid (granulocyte) sarcoma (MS) is an extramedullary tumor that occurs in 2 to 14% of cases of AML (John et al 2004); and is composed of immature and mature granulocytes or monocytes (Brunning et al 2001). These neoplasms are known by a variety of names in the literature, including granulocytic sarcoma, monocytic sarcoma, extramedullary myeloid cell tumor, myelosarcoma, myeloblastoma, and chloroma (Carneiro et al. 1984, Valbuena et al 2005). Virtually any extramedullary site can be involved by MS. Most patients with MS have a history of a myeloid neoplasm, most often AML and less often a myelodysplastic or myeloproliferative disease (Brunning et al 2001). Alternatively, MS can be the initial manifestation of AML that subsequently involves blood and bone marrow (Schmitt-Graff et al 2002). Very rarely, MS can be the only site of disease. MS is relatively more common in patients who have leukemias with prominent monocytic differentiation, such as acute myelomonocytic or monocytic leukemia and chronic myelomonocytic leukemia (Menasce et al 1999, Elenitoba et al 1996). MS manifesting as a testicular mass is uncommon and only rarely has occurred as an isolated mass. The tumors are usually localized ; they often involve bone, periostium, soft tissues, lymph nodes, or skin. Common sites of myeloid sarcoma are orbit and paranasal sinuses. However, it should be noted that according to the WHO classification the infiltrates of any site of the body by myeloid blasts in AML patients are not classified as myeloid sarcoma unless they present with tumor masses in which the tissue architecture is effaced (Pileri et al 2008).

Blasts may infiltrate organs or lymph nodes, resulting in adenopathy or hepatosplenomegaly. Palpable splenomegaly and hepatomegaly occur in about one third of patients. Testicular infiltration is less common in AML than ALL, with an incidence of 1 to 8 % (Wiernik et al 2001). Meningeal involvement has been reported in 5 to 20% of children and up to 16% of adults with AML (John et al 2004). Leukemic blast cells circulate and enter most tissues in small numbers. Occasionally biopsy or autopsy will uncover marked aggregates or infiltrates of leukemic cells, and less frequently collections of such cells may cause functional disturbances.

3. Signs, symptoms and laboratory features of Acute Promyelocytic Leukemia (APL)

Acute promyelocytic leukaemia (APL) is a distinctive sub-type of acute myeloid leukaemia that has distinct biologic and clinical features.

According to the older French-American-British (FAB) classification of AML, based solely on morphology as determined by the degree of differentiation along different cell lines and the extent of cell maturation (Cheson et al 1990), APL is sub-typed as AML-M3. The new World

Health Organization (WHO) classification of AML incorporates and interrelates morphology, cytogenetics, molecular genetics, and immunologic markers and is more universally applicable and prognostically valid (Brunning et al 2001). APL exists as 2 types, hypergranular or typical APL and microgranular (hypogranular) APL. APL comprises 5% to 8% of cases of AML and occurs predominately in adults in midlife (Büchner et al. 1999). Both typical and microgranular APL are commonly associated with DIC (Karp et al. 1987, Gollard et al 1996, Davey et al 1986, Tobelem et al 1980). The severe bleeding diathesis associated with APL has a specific sensitivity to treatment with all-trans retinoic acid (ATRA), which acts as a differentiating agent (Licht et al 1995). High complete remission rates in APL may be obtained by combining ATRA treatment with chemotherapy (Brunning et al 2001).

4. Signs, symptoms and laboratory features of Acute Myelomonocytic (AML-M4) and Acute Monoblastic/Monocytic Leukemia (AML-M5)

Acute myelomonocytic (M4) and monoblastic/monocytic leukemia (M5), are the morphologic subtype of acute myelogenous leukemia that are most commonly characterized by weakness, bleeding and a diffuse erythematous skin rash and frequently presents with extramedullary involvement, including liver, spleen, lymph nodes, gingiva, skin, eyes, larynx, lung, bladder, meninges and the central nervous system. Involvement of the gastrointestinal tract is rare, the mouth, rectum and anal canal being the most affected sites (Lichtman et al 1995). By contrast, leukemic infiltration of the stomach has been very rarely described, and when it has, it has been mainly in children (Kasantikul et al 1989 ; Kontny et al. 1995; Domingo-Domenech et al 2000). Serum and urinary muramidase levels are often extremely high.

Neurological symptoms may occur such as, headache, nausea, vomiting, photophobia, cranial nerve palsies, pupil edema and/ or nuchal rigidity. These symptoms may result from leuko-stasis, but may also reveal meningeal invasion by myeloblasts or be the presenting symptoms of a "chloroma". These chloromas often have an orbital or periorbital localization, or may arise around the spinal cords causing paraparesis or " Cauda equine" syndrome. CNS leukemic infiltration occurs in 6-16% of AML (Abbott et al 2003), especially in AML-M4.

Renal insufficiency occurs seldom. It is caused by hyperuriccuria and / or hyperphosphaturia, leading to obstructing tubular deposits and oliguria/ anuria.

5. Signs, symptoms and laboratory features of Acute Lymphoblastic Leukemia (ALL)

The clinical presentation of ALL may range from insidious nonspecific symptoms to severe acute life-threatening manifestations, reflecting the extent of bone marrow involvement and degree of extramedullary spread (Pui et al 2006) (Table 2). The symptoms at onset are primarily produced by the detrimental effects of the expanding cell population on bone marrow, and secondarily by the infiltration of other organs and by metabolic disturbances (Henderson et al 1990, Gur et al. 1999). In younger patients the anemia-induced fatigue may be the only presenting feature. Dyspnea, angina, dizziness, and lethargy may reflect the degree of anemia in older patients presenting with ALL. Approximately half of all patients may present with fever attributable to the pyrogenic cytokines, such as IL-1, IL-6, TNF, released from the leukemic cells, infections, or both. Arthralgia and bone pain due to bone marrow expansion by the leukemic cells and occasionally necrosis can be observed, although less commonly in adults compared to children. Pallor, petechiae, and ecchymosis in the skin and mucous membranes due to thrombocytopenia, DIC, or a combination of the above may be observed. ALL may present with either leukopenia (~20%) or moderate (50%–5–25 × 10^9/L) and severe leukocytosis (10%–>100 ×10^9/L) with hyperleukocytosis (>100 x 10^9 /L) present in approximately 15% of the pediatric patients (Pui et al 2006). Neutropenia (less than 500 granulocytes per mm^3) is a common phenomenon and is associated with an increased risk of serious infection. Hypereosinophilia, generally reactive, may be present at diagnosis. The majority of patients present with platelet counts less than 100 × 10^9/L (75%), while 15% have platelet counts of less than 10 × 10^9/L. Decreased platelet counts (median, 50x10^9/L) are usually present at diagnosis and can be readily distinguished from immune thrombocytopenia, as isolated thrombocytopenia is rare in leukemia. Severe hemorrhage is uncommon, even when platelet counts are as low as 20x10^9/L, and infection and fever are absent. Coagulopathy, usually mild, can occur in T-cell ALL and is only rarely associated with severe bleeding. More than 75% of the patients presents with anemia, which is usually normochromic and normocytic and associated with a normal to low reticulocyte count. Anemia or thrombocytopenia is often mild (or even absent) in patients with T-cell ALL. Pancytopenia followed by a period of spontaneous hematopoietic recovery may precede the diagnosis of ALL in rare cases and must be differentiated from aplastic anemia.

Bone marrow is usually infiltrated with >90% blast cells. Infiltration with less than 50% blasts represents only 4% of cases. Though the distinction between lymphoblastic leukaemia and lymphoma is still arbitrary, for many treatment protocols 25% bone marrow blasts is used as threshold for defining leukaemia (Borowitz & Chan 2008). Normal trilineage haematopoiesis is consequently decreased. The classical triad of symptoms related to bone marrow failure are the following: (1) fatigue and increasing intolerance to physical exercise (caused by anaemia), (2) easy bruising and bleeding from mucosal surfaces and skin (caused by thrombocytopenia especially when platelets are <20 × 10^9 /L), and (3) fever with infections (40% of all cases, caused by absolute granulocytopenia). Hyperleukocytic leukaemias with >100 x 10^9 /L blast cells rarely lead to the leukostasis syndrome and catastrophic early bleeding (Porcu et al 2000). Also malaise, lethargy, weight loss, fevers, and night sweats are often present but typically are not severe. Compared to AML, patients with ALL experience more bone and joint pain. Rarely, they may present with asymmetric arthritis, low back pain, diffuse osteopenia, or lytic bone lesions [Gur et al 1999]. Children experience these symptoms more frequently than adults. Young children may have difficulties in walking due to bone pain [Farhi et al 2000]. Lymphadenopathy, splenomegaly, and hepatomegaly are more common than in AML and affect half of the adults with ALL. CNS involvement is also more common in ALL compared to AML.

Signs and symptoms	Clinical and laboratory findings
Pallor, fatigue, exertional dyspnea, CHF	Anemia
Fever (~50%), infection (<30%	Neutropenia
Petechiae, ecchymosis, retinal hemorrhages	Thrombocytopenia
Hepatomegaly, splenomegaly (~50%), lymphadenopathy	Leukocytosis (10% of patients with WBC > 100,000)
Bone pain and joint pain (5–20%)	
Leukemia cutis	Leukostasis
Dyspnea, hypoxia, mental status changes, Cough, dyspnea, chest pain	Mediastinal Mass (80% of patients with T-cell ALL)
Headache, diplopia, cranial neuropathies, Particularly cranial nerves VI, VIII, papilledema, nausea, vomiting	CNS involvement (<10%)
Painless testicular/scrotal enlargement	Testicular involvement (<1%)
Intracranial bleeding, DIC	Elevated prothrombin time (PT), partial thromboplastin time (PTT), low fibrinogen
Tumor lysis syndrome	Acute renal failure (uncommon), acidosis, hypekalemia, hyperphosphatemia, hypocalcemia, elevated serum LDH and, uric acid level

Table 2. Clinical features of adult acute lymphocytic leukemias

Patients may present with cranial neuropathies (most often involving the 6th and 7th cranial nerves). Nausea, vomiting, headache, or papilledema may result from meningeal infiltration and obstruction of the outflow of cerebrospinal fluid (CSF) leading to a raised intracranial pressure. Testicular involvement, presenting as a painless, unilateral mass, is noted at diagnosis in approximately 2% of boys. It is associated with infant or adolescent age, hyperleukocytosis, splenomegaly, and mediastinal mass [Farhi et al 2000]. The diagnosis of testicular involvement is made by wedge biopsies. Bilateral biopsies are necessary due to the high incidence of contralateral testicular disease [Amendola et al 1985.[

6. Central nervous system involvement

The incidence of CNS involvement in patients with AML is considerably less common than CNS involvement in both adults and children with ALL (Charles et al 2012). Early CNS leukemia occurs in 8% of patients at the time of the first diagnosis while the percentage of relapsing CNS leukemia is 10%. (Hardiono et al 2001).

Patients with CNS involvement may be asymptomatic or may have symptoms related to increased intracranial pressure (headache, nausea, vomiting, irritability). All patients newly diagnosed with ALL should have a lumbar puncture for cytologic analysis of the cerebrospinal fluid; for AML, however, this is performed only in patients with symptoms indicative of CNS involvement (Pavlovsky et al 1973). There is an association of central nervous system involvement and diabetes insipidus in AML with monosomy 7, abnormalities of chromosome 3 and inversion of chromosome 16. (Glass et al 1987; Lavabre-Bertrand et al. 2001; Harb et al 2009).

Central nervous system hemorrhage and infection are reported to cause 80% (Lazarus et al 2006) of all deaths in patients with leukemia. The intracerebral hemorrhages that are often related to intravascular leukostases and leukemic nodules, and associated with leukocyte counts more than $100x10^9/L$ in peripheral blood (Phair et al 1964).

6.1. Leukemic parenchymal tumor

CNS may be affected as a solid tumors consisting of myeloid leukemic blasts called granulocytic sarcomas or chloromas (Recht et al 2003, Teshima et al 1990). The term chloroma results from the greenish color of these tumors caused by the presence of myeloperoxidase. Chloromas usually have a dural attachment although parenchymal tumors have rarely been reported. These tumors are hypercellular and avidly enhance with either cranial magnetic resonance imaging (MRI) or cranial computed tomography (CT). Neurologic findings are dependent upon location. Chloromas most often occur in bone that may result in epidural spinal cord compression, the orbit that may result in proptosis and a restrictive ophthalmopathy, or dura, which may simulate a meningioma.

6.2. Intracranial hemorrhage

Hemorrhagic complications are common in patients with acute leukemia (approximately 20%) and constitute the second most common cause of death in such patients (20% of all leukemic deaths result from intracranial hemorrhage) (Kim et al 2004, Kawanami et al 2002). Intracranial hemorrhage (ICH) is the most common hemorrhagic complication in acute promyelocytic leukemia and is not infrequent in AML and ALL (ranging in occurrence from 2-18% of all patients with acute leukemia). ICH may occur at the time of diagnosis (early hemorrhage) or subsequent to diagnosis and following initial treatment (late hemorrhage) (Cortes et al 2001). DIC, disseminated aspergillosis or mucormycosis, leukemic cell infiltration, thrombocytopenia or L-asparaginase chemotherapy-related consequences, are the most common etiologies for ICH. Both DIC (especially common in the M3 subtype of AML) and thrombocytopenia typically result in a solitary often-massive ICH whereas disseminated fungal infection and ICH occurring during neutropenia and is a result of hemorrhagic infarction. Leukemic cell infiltration occurs with extreme leukocytosis (defined as $>300x10^9$ leukemic cells/L and increase the risk of multiple intracranial hemorrhages in acute leukaemia(Bunin et al 1985). L-asparaginase may induce hyperfibrinogenemia and result in cortical vein or sinus thrombosis complicated with venous infarction. Fungal-related mycotic aneurysms may also lead to ICH and would be a consideration in a patient with blood culture positive for fungus. Topographically the majority of ICH is intraparenchymal with cerebral hemorrhage more common than cerebellar. (Wolk et al 1974).

Subarachnoid hemorrhage occurs in the context of ICH, either in isolation or more frequently as more diffuse hemorrhage secondary to DIC. Spinal subarachnoid hemorrhage may occur in the context of DIC and acute promyelocytic leukemia and present primarily with back pain that migrates rostrocaudally.

Risk - factor analysis revealed that female gender, APL, leukocytosis, thrombocytopenia and prolonged PT were the risk factors for fatal intracranial hemorrhages, while other reports have suggested the significance of serum fibrinogen (Wide et al 1990).

6.3. Leukemic meningitis

Meningeal leukemia appears more often in patients with ALL than in those with AML (Lazarus et al 2006). The manner in which leukemia cells enter the CNS is a subject of controversy, but the likely source include hematogenous spread or direct spread from adjacent infiltrated bone marrow.

Meningitis in leukemia may result from leptomeningeal infiltration of tumor (LM), subarachnoid hemorrhage, chemical (treatment-related following intra-CSF instillation of chemotherapy) or infection (bacterial or fungal) (Cash et al 1987, Dekker et al 1985). The presence or absence of LM always needs to be ascertained as if diagnosed, prognosis is profoundly affected. Chemical meningitis (typically due to intra-CSF cytarabine or methotrexate and most often given intraventricularly) is temporally related to intra-CSF chemotherapy. Chemical meningitis begins one to two days after intra-CSF chemotherapy administration, It is transient typically lasting less than five days and demonstrates no evidence of infection by CSF culture. Like other meningitis syndromes, patients complain of headache, fever, nausea, vomiting, photophobia and meningismus. Notwithstanding an inflammatory CSF, chemical meningitis rapidly abates and is mitigated by oral steroids. Infectious meningitis occurs in leukemia due to immunosuppression both as a result of the underlying disease and its treatment. *Listeria, Candida* and *Aspergillus* are common infectious etiologies however clinical presentation differs. *Listeria* presents as a meningitise syndrome whereas *Candida* presents with a diffuse encephalopathy and multiple small brain abscesses and *Aspergillus* presents with progressive hemorrhagic stroke confined to a single vascular territory (Gerson et al 1985, Winston et al 1993).

6.4. Cerebrospinal fluid in leukemic patients

The cerebrospinal fluid findings in leukemic patients must be carefully evaluated since bacterial meningitis, abscess formation or fungal disease occur with increased frequency. Cerebrospinal fluid pleocytosis, chemical abnormalities (elevated protein and low sugar) and elevated pressure may be present in these potential complications of the disease or its therapy. Appropriate cultures and stains, are often helpful in diagnosis. Abscesses can often be detected by brain scans, electroencephalograms and arteriography.

6.4.1. Categories of CNS status at diagnosis of acute leukemia

Patients who have nontraumatic diagnostic lumbar punctures at diagnosis may be placed into 3 categories according to white blood cells (WBCs) per microliter and the presence or absence of blasts on the cytospin: central nervous system 1 (CNS1) refers to CSF with <5 WBCs per microliter with cytospin negative for blasts; Cxlink refers to CSF with <5 WBCs per microliter with cytospin positive for blasts; CNS3 refers to CSF with >5 WBCs per microliter with cytospin

http://dx.doi.org/10.5772/53531

positive for blasts. Children with ALL who presents with CNS disease at diagnosis (CNS3) are at high risk for treatment failure compared with patients not meeting the criteria of the CNS disease at diagnosis. Patients with Cxlink may be at an increased risk of CNS relapse, although this may not apply to all treatment regimens and can be overcome by more intensive intrathecal treatment (Burger et al 2003).

7. Testicular involvement

Involvement of the testis - one of the most common sites of relapse in acute lymphoblastic leukemia usually presents with painless enlargement of one or both testis. Testicular involvement occurs in 10% to 23% of boys during the course of the disease at a median time of 13 months from diagnosis. Occult testicular involvement is recognized in 10% to 33% of boys undergoing bilateral wedge biopsies performed during the first 3 years of treatment or at any time after cessation of the therapy (Lanzkowsky et al. 1985). In a study in which biopsies were done in boys with newly diagnosed ALL, microscopic testicular involvement was reported to be 21% (Neimeyer et al 1993). Testicular involvement of the endothelial side of the interstitium of one or both testis, leads to increased testicular size and firmness [Kay et al 1983]. Hydrocele resulting from lymphatic obstruction may also present with painless scrotal enlargement and is readily identified by ultrasonography. Overt testicular involvement may occur in any form of acute lymphoblastic leukemia, most commonly in common C-ALL, but also in T-ALL and B-ALL. Rarely it is present when ALL is first diagnosed, but most often it is a late complication and, as with meningeal leukemia, the higher the initial blood blast count is, the earlier the discovery of testicular disease is likely (Nesbit et al 1980).

8. Superior vena cava syndrome

Superior vena cava syndrome comprises the signs and symptoms associated with compression or obstruction to the superior vena cava. Patients with ALL (particularly T-ALL), may present with symptoms of cough, dyspnea, stridor, or dysphagia from tracheal and esophageal compression by a mediastinal mass (15% of patients). Compression of the great vessels by a bulky mediastinal mass also may lead to the life threatening superior vena cava syndrome (Marwaha et al 2011). A child with leukemia may experience anxiety, confusion, drowsiness and sometimes unconsciousness (Salsali et al 1969). There is facial edema, plethora, cyanotic faces. Venous engorgement of neck, chest and arm with collateral vessel and some sign of pleural effusion and pericardial effusion may be present (Rice et al 2006).

9. Skin involvement

Various cutaneous lesions can be observed in patients with acute leukemias. These include specific cutaneous lesions resulting from infiltration of the skin by the leukemic cells, characteristic diseases such as pyoderma gangrenosum and Sweet syndrome, cutaneous signs of infection or hemorrhage resulting from the bone marrow dysfunction induced by the malignant process or chemotherapy.

Skin involvement may be of three types: nonspecific lesions, leukemia cutis, or granulocytic sarcoma of skin and subcutis. Nonspecific lesions include macules, papules, vesicles, pyoderma gangrenosum, or vasculitis (Bourantas et al. 1994, Nambiar Veettil et al 2009), neutrophilic dermatitis (Sweet's syndrome) (Cho K-H et al 1997, Philip R Cohen 2007), cutis vertices gyrata, or erythema multiforme or nodosum (Byrd et al 1995). Leukemia cutis lesions usually appear at the time of diagnosis of systemic disease or thereafter, but occasionally can occur before peripheral blood or bone marrow involvement (aleukemic leukemia cutis). (Christos Tziotzios et al 2011, Márcia Ferreira et al 2006). T-cell ALL may show epidermotropism and monocytic leukemia often involves the entire dermis and the superficial panniculus (Yalcin et al 2004).

10. The gastrointestinal tract

Gastrointestinal (GI) manifestations of leukemia occur in up to 25% of patients at autopsy, generally during relapse. Its presence varies with the type of leukemia and has been decreasing over time due to improved chemotherapy. Gross leukemic lesions are most common in the stomach, ileum, and proximal colon. Leukemia in the esophagus and stomach includes hemorrhagic lesions from petechiae to ulcers, leukemic infiltrates, pseudomembranous esophagitis, and fungal esophagitis. (Dewar et al. 1981) The mouth, colon, and anal canal are sites of involvement that most commonly lead to symptoms. Oral manifestations may bring the patient to the dentist; gingival or periodontal infiltration and dental abscesses may lead to an extraction followed by prolonged bleeding or an infected tooth socket. (Dean et al. 2003). The gingival hyperplasia is most commonly seen with the AML subtypes acute monocytic leukemia M5 (67%), acute myelomonocytic leukemia M4 (18.5%) and acute myelocytic leukemia M1-M2 (3.7%) (Cooper et al 2000). Enterocolitis, a necrotizing inflammatory lesion involving the terminal ileum, cecum, and ascending colon, can be a presenting syndrome or can occur during treatment. Fever, abdominal pain, bloody diarrhea, or ileus may be present and occasionally mimic appendicitis. Intestinal perforation, an inflammatory mass, and associated infection with enteric gram-negative bacilli or clostridial species are often associated with a fatal outcome. Isolated involvement of the gastrointestinal tract is rare.(Tim et al 1984).. Neutropenic enterocolitis (NE), which is a fulminant necrotizing process is a well-recognized complication of neutropenia in patients dying from hematologic malignancies especially acute leukemia as indicated by various autopsy series (Steinberg et al 1973). Proctitis, especially common in the monocytic variant of AML, can be a presenting sign or a vexing problem during periods of severe granulocytopenia and diarrhea.(Christos Tziotzios et al. 2011)

11. Respiratory tract involvement

Infectious and noninfectious pulmonary complications represent a critical problem for patients with leukemia, which itself can be the direct cause of pulmonary leukostasis, pulmonary leukemic infiltration (PLI), and leukemic cell lysis pneumopathy. These disorders are usually more frequent in patients with hyperleukocytic leukemia. Pulmonary leukostasis is characterized by occlusion of the pulmonary capillaries and arterioles by leukemic cells. Leukemic infiltration may lead to laryngeal obstruction, parenchymal infiltrates, alveolar septal infiltration, or pleural seeding. Each of these events can result in severe symptoms and radiologic findings (Potenza et al 2003, Wu et al 2008).

Pulmonary disease in leukaemia is frequent and often lethal. Lung involvement in leukaemia is primarily due to (a) leukostasis of vessels and (b) true leukaemic infiltration of interstitium and alveoli. (Majhail et al 2004, Porcu et al 2000) Clinically, leukostasis in leukaemia should be suspected in patients with unexplained fever and cardiopulmonary or cerebral dysfunction. Pulmonary leukostasis was found in about40% of autopsy series. (Mark et al 1987). Maile *et al* 1983 noted parenchymal opacities on 90% of chest radiographs obtained shortly before death in adult patients with leukaemia. These radiologic opacities on autopsy were attributed to infections, haemorrhages, leukaemic infiltrations and edema. In addition, drug induced pulmonary infiltrates and leukoagglutinin transfusion reactions were also reported (Mark et al 1987). In spite of the above data, pulmonary leukostasis in leukaemia has been mentioned only incidentally as a cause of abnormalities on chest radiography.

12. Cardiac complications

Cardiac complications of the patients with acute leukemia are common. Most of the cardiac complications may be due to chemotherapeutics such as antracyclins, besides anemia, infections, or direct leukemic infiltrations of the heart. Symptomatic pericardial infiltrates, transmural ventricular infiltrates with hemorrhage, and endocardial foci with associated intracavitary thrombi can, on occasion, cause heart failure, arrhythmia, and death. Infiltration of the conducting system or valve leaflets or myocardial infarction may occur. (Ashutosh et al 2002, Fernando et al 2004). Cardiac and other tissue damage as a consequence of release of eosinophil granule contents can occur in patients with leukemia, associated with eosinophilia (Kocharian et al 2006). Cardiac damage is a major determinant of the overall prognosis.

13. Urogenital involvement

The urogenital organs can also be affected. The kidneys are infiltrated with leukemic cells in a high proportion of cases, but functional abnormalities are rare. Hemorrhages in the pelvis or the collecting system are frequent, however, cases of vulvar, bladder neck, prostatic, or testicular involvement have been described.. (Quien et al 1996).

14. Musculoskeletal system

Musculoskeletal manifestations are the presenting complaint in up to 20% of patients with pediatric leukemia,(Andreas et al 2007). The main clinical osteoarticular manifestations in early leukemia include limb pain, nighttime pain, arthralgia, and arthritis. Skeletal manifestations of acute leukaemia (bone or back pain, arthritis or radiographical abnormalities of skeleton) are well described in children (Barbosa et al 2002). Arthritis can occur at any time during the course of acute leukaemia. It may lead to delay in diagnosis and therapy and any delay in therapy is associated with poor prognosis (Sandeep et al 2006). The most common clinical presentation of leukaemic arthritis is additive or migratory asymmetrical oligoarticular large joint arthritis and in some cases juvenile idiopathic arthritis. (Evans et al. 1994, Mirian et al. 2011). The joints most commonly involved are the knee, followed by the ankle, wrist, elbow, shoulder and hip. Onset of arthritis may be sudden or insidious, and parallel the course of acute leukaemia (Sandeep et al. 2006).

Arthritis as the first manifestation of acute leukaemia is however extremely uncommon in adults.

15. Hyperleukocytosis and leukostasis

Leukostasis is a syndrome, caused by clumping of leukocytes in the vasculature of the lungs and brain, often resulting in hypoxia, dyspnea, confusion, and coma, and may be fatal.

Leukapheresis is indicated in the initial management of leukostasis in patients with hyperleukocytosis in acute leukemias, particularly myeloid leukemias, or in patients who are at high risk of developing such a complication.

Adult T-cell leukemia/lymphoma is a distinct form of ALL that presents with progressive lymphadenopathy, hepatosplenomegaly, and hypercalcemia. It involves the skin, lungs, bone marrow, intestinal tract, and CNS. This disease is associated with HTLV-1 and is endemic in the Caribbean, southeastern United States, Africa, and Japan. Circulating tumor cells have a characteristic "cloverleaf"-shaped nucleus.

The risk factors for leukostasis are acute the leukaemia itself, younger age (most common in infants), certain types of leukaemia like acute promyelocytic (microgranular variants), acute myelomonocytic, acute monocytic leukaemia and T cell type of ALL. Cytogenetic abnormalities – 11q23 translocations and presence of Philadelphia chromosome are also associated with leukostasis (Porcu et al 2000). The pathogenesis of leukostasis is determined by: - 1) sluggish flow with stasis, 2) aggregation of leukaemic cells, 3) formation of microthrombi, 4) release of toxic granules, 5) endothelial damage, 6) oxygen consumption by leukocytes, 7) tissue invasion (Litchman et al 1987). Leukostasis is usually associated with counts of >100 x 10^9 but acute monocytic leukaemia may present with leukostasis with counts of 50 x 10^9/L. 5-13% of patients of AML and 10-30% of patients of ALL will manifest with hyperleukocytosis. Earlier leukostasis was thought to be due to the presence of critical leukocrit (fractional leukocyte volume) and increased viscosity. Although hyperleukocytosis is also common presenting feature in patients with ALL, particularly with T-cell phenotype, 11q23, and t(9;22) chromosomal rearrangements, symptomatic leukostasis is exceedingly rare [Porcu et al 2000]. While WBC count is a major factor contributing to microvessel occlusion seen with leukostasis, other features, such as activation of adhesion cell surface markers and mechanical properties of the leukemic blasts, are likely to be important. For example, the stiffness of myeloid blasts, as measured by atomic force microscopy, is 18 times that of lymphoid blasts [Rosenbluth et al 2006]. This difference in deformability of the cells may at least partially explain the increased frequency of leukostasis in AML compared to than in ALL. Presence of symptoms suggestive of leukostasis, such as headache, blurred vision, dyspnea, hypoxia, constitute a medical emergency and efforts should be made to lower the WBC rapidly. However, the role of leukapheresis to reduce tumor burden in patients with ALL and leukocytosis remains controversial.

16. Metabolic complications

Hyperuricemia and hyperphosphatemia with secondary hypocalcemia are frequently encountered at diagnosis, even before chemotherapy is initiated, especially in patients with B-cell or T-cell ALL with high leukemic cell burden. Severe metabolic abnormalities may accompany the initial diagnosis of ALL and AML (Haralampos et al 1999). Patients with high leukemic burden are at risk of developing acute tumor lysis syndrome (ATLS). Such metabolic changes may lead to the development of oliguric renal failure due to the tubular precipitation of urate and calcium phosphate crystals, fatal cardiac arrhythmias, hypocalcemic tetany, and seizures (Jeha 2001).

17. Lactic acidosis

Lactic acidosis (LA), as the presenting manifestation of acute leukemia, is rare, but potentially fatal complication of acute leukemia (Grossman et al 1983), characterized by low arterial pH due to the accumulation of blood lactate. It has been suggested that LA occurring in the setting of hematological malignancy is associated with an extremely poor prognosis [Sillos et al 2001]. Lactate, the end product of anaerobic glycolysis, is metabolized to glucose by the liver and kidneys. Because leukemic cells have a high rate of glycolysis even in the presence of oxygen and produce a large quantity of lactate, LA may result from an imbalance between lactate production and hepatic lactate utilization [Sillos et al 2001]. Several factors may contribute to the high rate of glycolysis. Overexpression or aberrant expression of glycolytic enzymes, such as hexokinase, the first rate-limiting enzyme in the glycolytic pathway [Mazurek et al 1997] allows leukemic blasts to proliferate rapidly and survive for prolonged periods [Mathupala et al 1997]. Although insulin normally regulates the expression of this enzyme, insulin-like growth factors (IGFs) that are overexpressed by malignant leukemic cells, can mimic insulin activity [Werner 1996,]. LA is frequently associated with acute tumor lysis syndrome (ATLS) and its extent is correlated with the severity of ATLS.

Typically, the patient with lactic acidosis presents with weakness, tachycardia, nausea, mental status changes, hyperventilation, and hypotension, which may progress to frank shock as acidosis worsens. Laboratory studies show a decreased blood pH (<7.37), a widened anion gap (>18), and a low serum bicarbonates.

HCT-CI weighted scores	Definitions of comorbidities included in the new HCT-CI	Comorbidity
1	Atrial fibrillation or flutter, sick sinus syndrome, or ventricular arrhythmias	Arrhythmia
1	Coronary artery disease - one or more vessel-coronary artery stenosis requiring medical treatment, stent, or bypass graft, congestive heart failure, myocardial infarction, or EF ≤ 50%	Cardiac
1	Crohn disease or ulcerative colitis	Inflammatory bowel disease
1	Requiring treatment with insulin or oral hypoglycemics but not diet alone	Diabetes
1	Transient ischemic attack or cerebrovascular accident	Cerebrovascular disease
1	Depression or anxiety requiring psychiatric consult or treatment	Psychiatric disturbance
1	Chronic hepatitis, bilirubin > ULN to 1.5 × ULN, or AST/ALT > ULN to 2.5 × ULN	Hepatic, mild
1	Patients with a body mass index > 35 kg/m2	Obesity
1	Requiring continuation of antimicrobial treatment after day 0	Infection
2	SLE, RA, polymyositis, mixed CTD, or polymyalgia rheumatica	Rheumatologic
2	Requiring treatment	Peptic ulcer
2	Serum creatinine > 2 mg/dL, on dialysis, or prior renal transplantation	Moderate/severe rena
2	DLco and/or FEV1 66%-80% or dyspnea on slight activity	Moderate pulmonary
3	Treated at any time point in the patient's past history, excluding nonmelanoma skin cancer	Prior solid tumo
3	Except mitral valve prolapse	Heart valve disease
3	DLco and/or FEV1 ≤ 65% or dyspnea at rest or requiring oxygen	Severe pulmonary
3	Liver cirrhosis, bilirubin > 1.5 × ULN, or AST/ALT > 2.5 × ULN	Moderate/severe hepatic

Table 3. Definitions of comorbidities and HCT-CI scores included in the HCT-CI

18. Comorbidity

Many factors have been studied to predict outcome and allocate treatment in acute leukemia. The best established prognostic factors are karyotype and age. However, comorbidity may play an important role in the outcome.

A comprehensive assessment including performance status, evaluation of comorbidities and abilities to perform activities of daily living, geriatric depression scale in elderly patients has been proven to be useful in detecting treatment-related changes in older cancer patients and has been recommended to be incorporated into clinical outcome analysis. An index developed specifically for patients with hematologic malignancies has been developed: the Hematopoietic Cell Transplantation-Specific Comorbidity Index (HCT-CI) presented in Table 3 (Sorror ML et al 2005). This index captures comorbidities that predict non-relapse mortality in patients considered for allogeneic transplant and also proved to be a helpful tool for defining comorbid conditions in elderly untreated AML patients. (Novotny J et al 2009; Sorror ML et al 2007). Modifications such as modified EBMT risk score have been developed and evaluated for ALL patients (Terwey T et al, 2010).

Comorbidity scoring is currently still under the investigation in many cooperative groups. It is important to bear in mind that when translating the results from clinical trials into treatment decision-making for the individual patient, many patients with e.g. „unacceptable" renal, cardial or hepatic abnormalities are generally not included into clinical trials. By such approach at least 20-30% of younger patients and more than 50% of elderly patients with AML are excluded and have not been reported in any results. Because of that it would be important to propose comorbidity score for all leukemia patients and to evaluate how many of the patients are able to receive standard therapy and stem cell transplantation, how many of them are candidate for low-intensity treatment and supportive care.

While acute leukemia patients depend on the expert recommendations from their physicians, knowledge of clinical presentation and patient's related prognostic factors can help to improve treatment decision and to identify patients who would benefit most from either intensive or low-intensive treatment or even best supportive care alone.

Author details

Gamal Abdul Hamid

Faculty of Medicine, University of Aden, Yemen

References

[1] Abbott, B. L, Rubnitz, J. E, Tong, X, Srivastava, D. K, Pui, C. H, et al. Clinical significance of central nervous system involvement at diagnosis of pediatric acute myeloid leukemia; Leukemia (2003). , 17, 2090-96.

[2] Amendola, B, Hutchinson, R, Crossmann, H. B, & Amendola, M. A. Isolated testicular leukemic relapse; Urology (1987). i Volume XXX, , 3(3), 240-243.

[3] Andreas, H. Gomoll, Childhood Leukemia Presenting as Sternal Osteomyelitis, The American Journal of Orthopedics, Am J Orthop. (2007). EE150., 148.

[4] Ashutosh HardikarPrem Shekar. Cardiac Involvement in a Case of Acute Lymphoblastic Leukemia, Ann Thorac Surg (2002). , 73, 1310-2.

[5] Barbosa, C. M, Nakamura, C, Terreri, M. T, et al. Musculoskeletal manifestation as the onset of acute leukemias in childhood]. Pediatr (Rio J) (2002). Portuguese., 78, 481-4.

[6] Borowitz, M. J. Chan JKC. B lymphoblastic leukemia/lymphoma, not otherwise specified. In: WHO Classification of Tumours of Haematopoietic and Lymphoid Tissues (eds S.H. Swerdlow, E. Campo, N.L. Harris, E.S. Jaffe, S.a. Pileri, H. Stein, J. thiele & J.W. Vardiman), IARC, Lyon, (2008). , 127-129.

[7] Bourantas, K, Malamou-mitsi, V, Christou, L, et al. Cutaneous vasculitis as the initial manifestation in acute myelomonocytic leukemia. Ann Intern Med (1994).

[8] Brunning, R. D, Matutes, E, Flandrin, G, et al. Acute myeloid leukemia not otherwise categorized: myeloid sarcoma. In: Jaffe ES, Harris NL, Stein H, et al, eds. World Health Organization Classification of Tumours: Pathology and Genetics of Tumours of Haematopoietic and Lymphoid Tissues. Lyon, France: IARC Press; (2001). , 2001, 104-105.

[9] Brunning, R. D, Matutes, E, Harris, N. L, et al. Acute myeloid leukaemia: introduction. In: Jaffe ES, Harris NL, Stein H, et al., eds.: Pathology and Genetics of Tumours of Haematopoietic and Lymphoid Tissues. Lyon, France: IARC Press, (2001). World Health Organization Classification of Tumours, 3., , 77-80.

[10] Büchner, T, Hiddemann, W, Wörmann, B, et al. Double induction strategy for acute myeloid leukemia: the effect of high-dose cytarabine with mitoxantrone instead of standard-dose cytarabine with daunorubicin and thioguanine: a randomized trial by the German AML Cooperative Group. Blood (1999). , 6.

[11] Bunin, N. J, & Pui, C. H. Differing complications of hyperleukocytosis in children with acute lymphoblastic and nonlymphoblastic leukemia. J clin Oncol (1985). , 3, 1590-1595.

[12] Burger, B, Zimmermann, M, Mann, G, et al. Diagnostic cerebrospinal fluid examination in children with acute lymphoblastic lymphoma: significance of low leukocyte counts with blast or traumatic lumpar puncture. J Clinoncol. (2003). , 21, 184-8.

[13] Byrd, J. C, Edenfield, W. J, & Shields, D. J. and Dawson NA; Extramedullary myeloid cell tumors in acute nonlymphocytic leukemia: a clinical review. *JCO* Jul 1, (1995).

[14] Carneiro, P. C, Amico, D, & Naves, E. JB, et al. Granulocytic sarcoma (chloroma): spinal cord compression and testicular involvement. Rev Hosp Clin Fac Med Sao Paulo. (1984)., 39, 248-250.

[15] Cash, J, Fehir, K. M, & Pollack, M. S. Meningeal Involvement in Early Stage Chronic Lymphocytic Leukemia. Cancer (1987)., 59, 798-800.

[16] Charles A SchifferRichard A Larson et al, Involvement of the central nervous system with acute myeloid leukemia, Up-to-date Jan 25, (2012).

[17] Cheson, B. D, Cassileth, P. A, Head, D. R, et al. Report of the National Cancer Institute-sponsored workshop on definitions of diagnosis and response in acute myeloid leukemia. J Clin Oncol (1990)., 8(5), 813-9.

[18] Cho, K-H, Han, K-H, Sim, S-W, et al. Neutophilic dermatoses associated with myeloid malignancy. Clin Exp Dermatol (1997).

[19] Christos TziotziosAreti Makrygeorgou, The Clinical Picture Leukemia cutis, Cleveland clinic journal of medicine (2011). (4)

[20] Cooper, C. L, Loewen, R, & Shore, T. Gingival hyperplasia complicating acute myelomonocytic leukemia. J. Can. Dent. Assoc (2000)., 66, 78-79.

[21] Cortes, J. Central nervous system involvement in adult acute lymphocytic leukemia. HematolOncolClin North Am. (2001)., 15, 145-162.

[22] Davey, D. D, Fourcar, K, & Burns, C. P. Goekin JA: Acute myelocytic leukemia manifested by prominent generalized lymphadenopathy. Am J Hematol (1986).

[23] Dean, ., Acute leukaemia presenting as oral ulceration to a dental emergency service. Australian Dental Journal 2003;48:3..

[24] Dekker, A. W, Elderson, A, Punt, K, & Sixma, J. J. Meningeal Involvement in Patients With Acute Nonlymphocytic Leukemia. Cancer (1985)., 56, 2078-2082.

[25] Dewar, G. J, Lim, C-N. H, & Michalyshyn, B. Akabutu J: Gastrointestinal complications in patients with acute and chronic leukemia. Can J Surg (1981).

[26] Djunic, I, Virijevic, M, Novkovic, A, Djurasinovic, V, Colovic, N, Vidovic, A, Suvajdzic-vukovic, N, & Tomin, D. Pretreatment risk factors and importance of comorbidity for overall survival, complete remission, and early death in patients with acute myeloid leukemia. Hematology. (2012). Mar;, 17(2), 53-8.

[27] Domingo-domènech, E, Boqué, C, Narváez, J. A, Romagosa, V, Domingo-clarós, A, & Grañena, A. Acute monocytic leukemia in the adult presenting with associated extramedullary gastric infiltration and ascites. Haematologica (2000)., 85(8), 875-7.

[28] Elenitoba-johnson, K, Hodges, G. F, King, T. C, et al. Extramedullary myeloid cell tumors arising in the setting of chronic myelomonocytic leukemia: a report of two cases. Arch Pathol Lab Med. (1996)., 120, 62-67.

[29] Evans, T. I, Nercessian, B. M, & Sanders, K. M. Leukemic arthritis. Semin Arthritis Rheum. (1994). Aug;, 24(1), 48-56.

[30] Farhi, D. C, & Rosenthal, N. S. Acute lymphoblastic leukemia. Clin Lab Med (2000). vii, 20(1), 17-28.

[31] Fernando, P. Chaves,* Karen Quillen, Pericardial Effusion: A Rare Presentation of Adult T-Cell Leukemia/Lymphoma, American Journal of Hematology (2004). , 77, 381-383.

[32] Gerson, S. L, et al. Invasive pulmonary aspergillosis in adult acute leukemia: clinical clues to its diagnosis. J Clin Oncol, (1985). , 1109-1116.

[33] Glass, J. P, Vantassel, P, Keating, M. J, et al. Central nervous system complications of a newly recognized subtype of leukemia: AMML with a pencentric inversion of chromosome 16. Neurology (1987).

[34] Gollard, R. P, Robbins, B. A, & Piro, L. Saven A: Acute myelogenous leukemia presenting with bulky lymphadenopathy. Acta Haematol (1996).

[35] Grossman, L, Holloway, R, Costa, D, Roncari, M, Lazarovits, D, & Baker, A. M, et al. Lactic acidosis in a patient with acute leukemia. Clin Invest Med (1983). , 6, 85-8.

[36] Gur, H, Koren, V, Ehrenfeld, M, Ben-bassat, I, & Sidi, Y. Rheumatic manifestations preceding adult acute leukemia: Characteristics and implication in course and prognosis. Acta Haematol (1999). , 101(1), 1-6.

[37] Harb, A, Tan, W, Wilding, G. E, Battiwalla, M, Sait, S. N, Wang, E. S, & Wetzler, M. Acute myeloid leukemia and diabetes insipidus with monosomy 7. Cancer Genet Cytogenet (2009). , 190(2), 97-100.

[38] Haralampos, J. Milionis, Constantinos L. Bourantas, Kostas C. Siamopoulos, Moses S. Elisaf. Acid-Base and Electrolyte Abnormalities in Patients With Acute Leukemia; American Journal of Hematology, (1999). , 62, 201-207.

[39] Hardiono, D, et al. Clinical features and survival pattern of central nervous system leukemia in children with acute lymphoblastic leukemia, PaediatrIndones (2001). , 41, 247-252.

[40] Henderson, E. S, & Afshani, E. Clinical manifestation and diagnosis. In: Henderson ES, Lister TA, editors. Leukemia. 5th ed. Philadelphia: WB Saunders. (1990). , 291-359.

[41] Jeha, S. Tumor lysis syndrome. Seminars in Hematology (2001). Suppl 10), 4-8.

[42] Jemal, A, Siegel, R, & Ward, E. Cancer statistics, (2006). CA Cancer J Clin. 2006; , 56, 106-130.

[43] John, P, Greer, M, Maria, R, & Marsha, C. Acute Myeloid Leukemia in Adults. In: Wintrobe's Clinical Hematology. Lippincott Williams & Wilkins, A wolters Kluwer Company Philadelphia 11th edition (2004). , 2097-2142.

[44] Karp, J. E, Merz, W. G, Hendricksen, C, et al. Oral norfloxacin for prevention of gram-negative bacterial infections in patients with acute leukemia and granulocytopenia. A randomized, double-blind, placebo controlled trial. Ann Intern Med (1987). , 106(1), 1-7.

[45] Kasantikul, V, Shuangshoti, S, & Phanthumchinda, K. Subacute combined degeneration of the spinal cord in acute monoblastic leukemia. J Med Assoc Thai (1989). , 72, 474-7.

[46] Kawanami, T, Kurita, K, Yamakawa, M, Omoto, E, & Kato, T. Cerebrovascular disease in acute leukemia: a clinicopathological study of 14 patients. Intern Med. (2002). , 41(12), 1130-4.

[47] Kay, H. E. Testicular infiltration in acute lymphoblastic leukaemia. British Journal Haematology (1983).

[48] Kim, H, Lee, J-H, Choi, S-J, et al. Analysis of fatal intracranial hemorrhage in 792 acute leukemia patients. Haematologica (2004). , 89, 622-624.

[49] Kocharian, A, & Izadyar, M. Cardiac Involvement in a Patient with Eosinophilia and Inversion of Chromosome 16(A Case of Chronic Eosinophilic Leukemia or AML-M4EO?, Archive of SID (2006). , 13q22.

[50] Kontny, U, Gutjahr, P, & Schumacher, R. Unusual pattern of gastric and hepatic infiltration in an infant with acute monocytic leukemia. Pediatr Radiol (1995). , 25(1), 19-20.

[51] Lanzkowsky PhilipLeukemias. In Manual of Pediatric Hematology and Oncology. Churchill Livingstone, New York, Edinburgh, London, Madrid, Melbourne, Milan, Tokyo. (1985). , 295.

[52] Lavabre-bertrand, T, Bourquard, P, Chiesa, J, Berthéas, M. F, Lefort, G, Taïb, J, Lavabre-bertrand, C, Navarro, M, & Bureau, J. P. Diabetes insipidus revealing acute myelogenous leukaemia with a high platelet count, monosomy 7 and abnormalities of chromosome 3: a new entity? Eur J Haematol (2001). , 66(1), 66-9.

[53] Lazarus, H. M, Richards, S. M, Chopra, R, et al. Central nervous system involvement in adult acute lymphoblastic leukemia at diagnosis: results from the international ALL trial MRC UKALL-XII/ECOG E2993. Blood. (2006). , 108, 465-472.

[54] Licht, J. D, Chomienne, C, Goy, A, et al. Clinical and molecular characterization of a rare syndrome of acute promyelocytic leukemia associated with translocation (11;17). Blood (1995).

[55] Lichtman, M. A. Acute myelogenous leukemia. In: Beutler E, Lichtman MA, Coller BS, Kipps TJ, eds. Williams Hematology. New York: McGraw-Hill;(1995)., 272-298.

[56] Litchman, M. A, Heal, J, & Rowe, J. M. Hyperleukocytic leukaemia. Rheological and clinical features and management. Ballier's Clinical Haematology (1987)., 1, 725-46.

[57] Maile, C. W, Moore, A. V, Ulreich, S, & Putman, C. E. Chest radiographic pathologic correlation in adult leukemia patients. Invest Radiol (1983)., 18, 495-9.

[58] Majhail, N. S, & Lichtin, A. E. Acute leukemia with a very high leukocyte count: confronting a medical emergency. Cleveland Clin J Med (2004)., 71, 633-7.

[59] Márcia FerreiraMónica Caetano et al, Leukemia cutis resembling a flare-up of psoriasis, Dermatology Online Journal (2006)., 12(3)

[60] Mark, A. Van Buchem, Wondergem JH, Schultze LJ, teVelde J, Kluin PM, Bode PJ, et al. Pulmonary leukostasis: Radiologic- Pathologic study. Radiology (1987). , 165, 739-41.

[61] Marwaha, R. K, & Kulkami, K. P. Superior vena cava obstruction in childhood acute lymphoblastic leukemia; Indian Ped J. (2011). Jan (48)(1) 78-9

[62] Mathupala, S. P, Rempel, A, & Pedersen, P. L. Aberrant glycolytic metabolism of cancer cells: Aremarkable coordination of genetic, transcriptional, post-translational, and mutational events that lead to a critical for type II hexokinase. J Bioenerg Biomembr. (1997). Aug;, 29(4), 339-43.

[63] Mazurek, S, Boschek, C. B, & Eigenbrodt, E. The role of phosphometabolites in cell proliferation, energy metabolism, and tumor therapy. Journal of Bioenergetics and Biomembranes.(1997).

[64] Menasce, L. P, Banerjee, S. S, Beckett, E, et al. Extra-medullary myeloid tumor (granulocytic sarcoma) is often misdiagnosed: a study of 26 cases. Histopathology. (1999)., 34, 391-398.

[65] Mirian, S. Tamashiro,INa′dia Emi Aikawa et al Discrimination of acute lymphoblastic leukemia from systemic-onset juvenile idiopathic arthritis at disease onset, CLINICS (2011)., 66(10), 1665-1669.

[66] Nambiar VeettilJoe THOMAS et al, Cutaneous vasculitis as a presenting manifestation of acute myeloid leukemia, International Journal of Rheumatic Diseases (2009)., 12, 70-73.

[67] Neimeyer, C. M, & Sallah, S. E. Acute Lympholastic Leukemia. Hematology of infancy and childhood. (Ed. D. Nathan and Oski) Sounders comp. Philadelphia, London, Toronto, Montreal, Sydney, Tokyo. (1993)., 1258-1259.

[68] Nesbit, M. E. Jr, Robison LL, Ortega JA, Sather HN, Donaldson M, Hammond D. Testicular relapse in childhood acute lymphoblastic leukemia: association with pretreat-

ment patient characteristics and treatment. A report for Childrens Cancer Study Group. Cancer. (1980). Apr 15;, 45(8), 2009-2016.

[69] Novotny, J, Aisenbrey, A, Nückel, H, & Dührsen, U. Comorbidity Is An Independent Prognostic Factor in AML: Comparison of Two Comorbidity Scores.; Blood (ASH Annual Meeting Abstracts), Nov (2009).

[70] Pavlovsky, S, & Eppinger-helft, M. Murill FS: Factors that influence the appearance of central nervous system leukemia. Blood (1973).

[71] Phair, J. P, & Anderson, R. E. Namiki H: The central nervous system in leukemia. Ann Int Med (1964).

[72] Philip R CohenSweet's syndrome- a comprehensive review of an acute febrile neutrophilic dermatosis, Orphanet Journal of Rare Diseases (2007).

[73] Pileri, S. A, Orazi, A, & Falini, B. Myeloid sarcoma. In: WHO Classification of Tumours of Haematopoietic and Lymphoid Tissues (eds S.H. Swerdlow, E. Campo, N.L. Harris, E.S. Jaffe, S.a. Pileri, H. Stein, J. thiele & J.W. Vardiman), (2008). IARC, Lyon.Porcu P, Cripe LD, Ng EW,, 127-129.

[74] Porcu, P, Cripe, L. D, Ng, E. W, Bhatia, S, Danielson, C. M, Orazi, A, et al. Hyperleukocytic leukemias and leukostasis: a review of pathophysiology, clinical presentation and management. Leuk Lymphoma (2000). , 1-18.

[75] Potenza, L, Luppi, M, Morselli, M, et al. Leukaemic pulmonary infiltrates inadult acute myeloid leukaemia: a high-resolution computerized tomography study. Br J Haematol. (2003).

[76] Pui, C. H. Acute lymphoblastic leukemia. In: Pui CH, editor. Childhood leukemias. New York: Camridge University Press; (2006). , 439-472.

[77] Quien, E. T, Wallach, B, Sandhaus, L, et al. Primary extramedullary leukemia of the prostate. Am J Hematol, (1996).

[78] Recht, L, & Mrugala, M. Neurologic complications of hematologic neoplasms. Neurol Clin N Am. (2003). , 2003(21), 87-105.

[79] Redaelli, A, Lee, J. M, Stephens, J. M, & Pashos, C. L. Epidemiology and clinical burden of acute myeloid leukemia, Expert Rev. Anticancer Ther. (2003). , 3, 695-710.

[80] Rice, T. W, Rodriguez, R. M, & Light, R. W. The superior vena cava syndrome: clinical characteristics and evolving etiology. *Medicine (Baltimore).* Jan (2006). , 85(1), 37-42.

[81] Rosenbluth, M. J, Lam, W. A, & Fletcher, D. A. Force microscopy of nonadherent cells: a comparison of leukemia cell deformability. Biophys J (2006). , 90, 2994-3003.

[82] Salsali, M, & Cliffton, E. E. Superior vena cava obstruction in carcinoma of lung. *N Y State J Med.* Nov 15 (1969). , 69(22), 2875-80.

[83] Sandeep, C, Telhan, A, et al. Acute differentiated leukemia in an adult presenting as arthritis, Singapore Med J (2006).

[84] Schmitt-graff, A, Wickenhauser, C, Kvasnicka, H. M, et al. Extramedullary initial manifestations of acute myeloid leukemia (AML) [in German]. Pathologe. (2002). , 23, 397-404.

[85] Sillos, E. M, et al. Lactic acidosis: A metabolic complication of hematologic malignancies: Case report and review of the literature. Cancer (2001).

[86] Sorror, M. L, Maris, M. B, Storb, R, Baron, F, Sandmaier, B. M, Maloney, D. G, & Storer, B. Hematopoietic cell transplantation (HCT)-specific comorbidity index: a new tool for risk assessment before allogeneic HCT. Blood. (2005). Oct 15;, 106(8), 2912-9.

[87] Sorror, M. L, Sandmaier, B. M, Storer, B. E, Maris, M. B, Baron, F, Maloney, D. G, Scott, B. L, Deeg, H. J, Appelbaum, F. R, & Storb, R. Comorbidity and disease status based risk stratification of outcomes among patients with acute myeloid leukemia or myelodysplasia receiving allogeneic hematopoietic cell transplantation. J Clin Oncol. (2007). Sep 20;, 25(27), 4246-54.

[88] Steinberg, D, Gold, J, & Brodin, A. Necrotizing enterocolitis in leukemia. Arch Int Med (1973).

[89] Tan, A. W, et al. Extensive calcinosis cutis in relapsed acute lymphoblastic leukaemia. Annals of the Academy of Medicine, Singapore (2004).

[90] Terwey, T. H, Hemmati, P. G, Martus, P, Dietz, E, Vuong, L. G, Massenkeil, G, Dörken, B, & Arnold, R. A modified EBMT risk score and the hematopoietic cell transplantation-specific comorbidity index for pre-transplant risk assessment in adult acute lymphoblastic leukemia. Haematologica. (2010). May;, 95(5), 810-8.

[91] Teshima, T, Akashi, K, Shibuka, T, et al. Central Nervous System Involvement in Adult T-Cell Leukemia/Lymphoma. Cancer (1990). , 65, 327-332.

[92] Thiede, C, Koch, S, Creutzig, E, et al. Prevalence and prognostic impact of NPM1 mutations in 1485 adult patients with acute myeloid leukemia (AML). Blood. (2006). , 107, 4011-4020.

[93] Tim, B. Hunter, John C. Bjelland, Gastrointestinal Complications of Leukemia and Its Treatment, rican Roentgen Ray Society,AJR (1984).

[94] Tobelem, G, Jacquillat, C, Chastang, C, et al. Acute monoblastic leukemia: a clinical and biologic study of 74 cases. Blood (1980).

[95] Valbuena, J. R, Admirand, J. H, Gualco, G, et al. Myeloid sarcoma involving the breast. Arch Pathol Lab Med. (2005). , 129, 32-38.

[96] Virappane, P, Gale, R, Hills, R, et al. Mutation of the Wilm's Tumor 1 gene is a poor prognostic factor associated with chemo-resistance in normal karyotype acute myeloid leukemia. J Clin Oncol. (2008). Jul 7.

[97] Weirnik, P. H. Extramedullary manifestations of adult leukemia. In: American cancer society atlas of clinical oncology adult leukemias. London : BC Decker Inc, (2001). , 2001, 275-292.

[98] Werner, H. LeRoith, D. The role of the insulin-like growth factor system in human cancer. Advances in Cancer Research (1996). , 1996(68), 183-223.

[99] Wide, J. T, & Davies, J. M. Hemostasis problems in acute leukemia. Blood Rev (1990). , 4, 245-251.

[100] Winston, D. J, Chandrasekar, P. H, Lazarus, H. M, Goodman, J. L, Silber, J. L, Horowitz, H, Shadduck, R. K, Rosenfeld, C. S, Ho, W. G, Islam, M. Z, & Buell, D. N. Fluconazole prophylaxis of fungal infections in patients with acute leukemia. Results of a randomized placebo-controlled, double-blind, multicenter trial. Ann Intern Med, (1993). , 495-503.

[101] Wolk, R. W, Masse, S. R, Conklin, R, & Freireich, E. J. The incidence of central nervous system leukemia in adults with acute leukemia. Cancer (1974). , 33, 863-71.

[102] Wu, Y. K, Huang, Y. C, Huang, S. F, et al. Acute respiratory distress syndrome caused by leukemic infiltration of the lung. J Formos Med Assoc. (2008).

[103] Yalcin, A. D, Keskin, A, & Calli, N. Monocytic Acute Non-Lymphocytic Leukemia Presenting As A Malign-Appearing Cutaneous Eruption. Internet J of Dermatol (2004).

Chapter 4

Therapy-Related Acute Myeloid Leukemias

Margarita Guenova, Gueorgui Balatzenko and
Georgi Mihaylov

Additional information is available at the end of the chapter

http://dx.doi.org/10.5772/52459

1. Introduction

Therapy-related acute myeloid leukemia (t-AML) is a heterogeneous group of myeloid neoplasms occurring as an overwhelming complication in patients receiving previous cytotoxic chemotherapy and/or radiation therapy used to treat haematopoietic or solid malignancies or associated with immunosuppressive treatment for non-neoplastic rheumatologic/autoimmune diseases or solid organ transplantation (Offman et al., 2004; Kwong, 2010). T-AML is an increasingly recognized condition included in the category of therapy-related myeloid neoplasms in the revised WHO classification of tumours of haematopoietic and lymphoid tissues, together with therapy-related myelodysplastic syndrome (t-MDS) and myelodysplastic/myeloproliferative neoplasm, that constitute a unique clinical syndrome (Vardiman et al., 2009).

The average age of the population in the developed countries is increasing, and cancer incidence increases with age. Both improved early detection of first malignancies and primary oncologic therapy have led to enhanced survival rates, and the risk of t-AML has consequently risen over the last few decades (Travis, 2006; Ries et al., 2008). Thus patients are, in a sense, the fortunate victims of our own success. Secondary leukemias challenge both the understanding of leukemogenesis and the clinical management of these conditions. The disease offers a unique opportunity to study leukaemic transformation by relating specific genetic and molecular abnormalities to the biologic effects of particular agents. The detailed insights into pathogenetic mechanisms will eventually help to establish a more differentiated clinical approach to successfully treat, but hopefully also prevent, these often fatal consequences of cytotoxic therapies. Despite that t-AMLs share common phenotypic features with de novo AML, the prognosis is generally unfavorable.

In general, t-AML are of particular importance to study for several reasons: (i) they represent the most serious long-term complications to current cancer therapy and the understanding would help to identify patients at risk in order to tailor therapy; (ii) they can be directly induced by chemically well-defined agents or irradiation with well-known cellular effects; (iii) they present the same chromosome aberrations and gene mutations as de novo AML, allowing for extrapolation of results from one to the other type of disease thus clarifying the biological processes leading to leukemogenesis; (iv) an early stage of MDS with refractory cytopenia is often diagnosed in therapy-related diseases, because most patients are followed thoroughly after intensive chemotherapy or irradiation, while in *de novo* AML, such information is often lacking; (v) there is still no consensus on the therapeutic management.

2. Epidemiology

The proportion of therapy-related AMLs varies from 5% to higher than 10% out of all cases of AMLs depending on the primary disease and the applied treatment in regard to chemical structure and dose of the used compounds, as well as to the type and intensity of used physical agent (Schneider et al., 1999). The GIMEMA registry reports an incidence of 5% of AML occurring as a second malignancy in Italy, however this registry includes only patients in whom treatment is feasible. Similarly, t-AML account for about 6% of all new AML cases in the UK, thus corresponding to an incidence rate at around 0.2/100 000/year (reviewed in Seedhouse & Russell, 2007). For a 12-years period, the review of our own data also showed that in 26 out of 407 consecutive cases of adult AML diagnosed and treated in our institution had a history for a previous malignancy treated with chemotherapy and/or radiotherapy which accounts for 6,1% (Balatzenko & Guenova, 2012). Higher values were reported by others as the pooled analysis of a consecutive series of 372 Swedish adult AML cases compared to 4230 unselected cases reported in the literature 1974 – 2001 revealed an incidence of 13% and 14%, respectively (Mauritzson et al.,2002).

2.1. Age

All age groups are affected - both children and adults develop AML following treatment with antineoplastic agents. However, children deserve particular consideration, taking into account the long life-expectancy of oncological patients cured by chemo and radiotherapy (Le Deley et al., 2003). As demonstrated in the published literature, the risk of developing AML following chemotherapy is not reliably correlated with the age of the pediatric patient. There is no consistent evidence that indicates that younger children will be at increased risk; in fact, some studies suggest that younger children might actually display a decreased susceptibility. Unlike secondary solid tumors such as breast, central nervous system, bone, and thyroid cancer which are highly dependent on the age of the patient at time of diagnosis and treatment; an age dependency for t-AML risk was not observed in the same pediatric patient populations (reviewed in Pyatt et al., 2007). In addition, though in the Guidelines for Carcinogen Risk Assessment (2005), presented at the Risk Assessment Forum U.S. Environmental

Protection Agency a 10-fold higher risk attributable to early-life carcinogenic exposure was assumed, leading to a reasonable expectation that children can be more susceptible to many carcinogenic agents, the available scientific and medical literature does not support the hypothesis that children necessarily possess an increased risk of developing AML following leukemogenic chemical exposure (Pyatt et al., 2007, Barnard et al, 2005).

In adult patients there is a higher risk and shorter latency period for the development of t-AML (Dann et al., 2001). In general, there is no convincing evidence for gender predisposition (Pagano et al., 2001; Smith et al. 2003).

2.2. Primary malignancies

Due to decreasing overall death rates in cancer there is an increasing number of cured patients at risk of developing t-AML. The review of reports on long follow-up of high numbers of patients treated with relatively uniform protocols comprising cytotoxic drugs, growth factors and radiation therapy individually or in combination highlights the major trends, with the greatest likelihood of developing therapy-related myeloid neoplasms following treatment of hematopoietic malignancies and breast cancer in adults, ALL and central nervous system tumors in children, germ cell tumours, lung cancer, etc. A significant proportion of t-AMLs nowadays involve patients treated for non-neoplastic disorders, and those treated with high-dose chemotherapy followed by autologous stem cell transplantation (Mauritzson et al., 2002; Suvajdžić et al. 2012; Ramadan et al., 2012). Representative studies are summarised in Table 1 demonstaring the incidence of t-AML in different primary diseases.

2.2.1. Hematologic malignancies

Up to 10% of patients with a preceeding lymphoid neoplasm treated with conventional chemotherapy and especially high-dose therapy and autologous stem cell transplantation may develop a t-AML within 10 years following primary therapy (Table 1). In patients with Hodgkin lymphoma (HL), the risk of t-AML has been reported to range between 1% and 10%, depending on the type of therapy administered, the study population size, and the follow-up duration. In patients with non-Hodgkin's lymphoma (NHL), an increased risk of secondary malignancies including therapy-related myeloid neoplasms has been reported, in particular when fludarabine-containing regimens or SCT are used. Significant risk factors were older age at the time of diagnosis, male sex, and fludarabine- or nucleoside analogs-containing therapy or SCT.Interestingly, leukemia cases are rarely or never seen in patients treated with radiotherapy alone (Mudie et al. 2006). Secondary carcinogenesis remains a major late complication in patients with acute lymphoblastic leukemia, particularly in children. A retrospective study of the cumulative incidence of secondary neoplasms after childhood ALL over 30 years showed that the risk of t-AML is higher in ALL children who receive a high cumulative dose and prolonged epipodophyllotoxin therapy in weekly or bi-weekly schedules, with short-term use of G-CSF and central nervous system irradiation as additive risk factors (Hijiya et al.,2007).

Primary Disease	Number of patients in the study	Number of patients with t-AML	Therapy	Median Latency	References
Hematological Malignancies					
Acute lymphoblastic leukemia (adults)	641	6 (0.9%)	CT	32 months	Verma et al.,2009
Acute lymphoblastic leukemia (children)	733	13 (1.8%)	CT	3 years	Pui et al.,1989
Acute lymphoblastic leukemia (children)	1290	37 (2,9%)	CT	3.8 years	Hijiya et al., 2007
Acute lymphoblastic leukemia	1494	6 (0.4%)	CT	1.3 years	Tavernier et al.,2007
CLL	521	3 (0.6%)	CT	34 months	Morrison et al.,2002
B-NHL; T-NHL; Hodgkin's lymphoma	1347	11 (0.8%)	HDCT± MoAbs		Tarella et al.,2011
NHL	230	11 (4.8%)	HD CT + RT	4.4 years	Micallef et al.,2000
NHL	29153	29 (0.1%)	RT ± CT; other	61 months	Travis et al.,1991
Hodgkin's lymphoma	5411	36 (0.7%)	RT ± CT	5 years	Josting et al.,2003
Hodgkin's lymphoma	2676	17 (0.6%)	RT; CT; RT +CT	79.9 months	Devereux et al.,1990
Hodgkin's lymphoma	29552	143 (0.5%)	RT; CT; RT +CT	ND	Kaldor et al.,1990
Hodgkin's lymphoma	947	23 (2.4%)	RT; CT; RT +CT	58 months	Cimino et al. ,1991
Hodgkin's lymphoma	32591	169 (0.5%)	RT; CT; RT +CT	ND	Dores et al.,2002
Hodgkin's lymphoma (children)	1380	24 (1.7%)	RT; CT; RT +CT	ND	Bhatia et al.,1996
Hodgkin's lymphoma	794	8 (1.0%)	RT; RT+CT	5 years	Mauch et al., 1996
Multiple Myeloma	8740	39* (0.4%)	CH, HDM-ASCT, IMiDs	45.3 months	Mailankody et al.,2011
Multiple Myeloma	2418	5 (0.2%)	CH, HDM-ASCT, IMiDs	ND	Barlogie et al.,2008
APL	77	3 (3.9%)	CT ± ATRA		Latagliata et al.,2002
Solid Tumors					
Small cell lung carcinoma	158	3 (1.9%)		2.7 years	Chak et al.,1984
Germ-cell tumours	212	4 (1.9%)	CT	ND	Pedersen-Bjergaard et al.,1991

http://dx.doi.org/10.5772/52459

Primary Disease	Number of patients in the study	Number of patients with t-AML	Therapy	Median Latency	References
Germ-cell tumours	442 174 124	3 (0.7%) 3 (1.7%) 0	CT RT+CT RT	ND	Schneider et al.,1991
Germ-cell tumors (children)	716 416	6 (0.84%) 0	CT+RT RT or S	101 weeks	Schneider et al.,1999
Ovarian Cancer	63359	109 (0.2%)	CT	4 years	Vay et al.,2011
Ovarian Cancer	99113	95 (0.1%)	RT; CT; RT +CT	4-5 years	Kaldor et al.,1990
Ovarian Cancer	28971	1 (0.003%) 65 (0.2%) 25 (0.09%)	RT CT RT+CT	3.3 years	Travis et al.,1999
Breast Cancer	5299 646	27 (0.5%) 5 (0.8%)	CT RT	ND	Fisher et al.,1985
Breast Cancer	82700	74 (0.09%)	CT; RT; CT +RT	5 years	Curtis et al.,1992
Breast Cancer	1474	14 (0.9%)	CH ± RT	66 months	Diamandidou et al., 1996
Testicular Cancer	1909	3 1 2	CT RT RT+CT	7.7 years	van Leeuwen et al., 1993
Testicular Cancer	28843	27 (0.09%)	CH; RT	ND	Travis et al.,1997
Prostate Cancer	487	3 (0.6%)	CH	48 months	Flaig et al.,2008
Prostate Cancer	168612	184 (0.1%)	RT		Ojha et al., 2010
Auto-immune diseases					
Reumatoid arthritis	53067	68 (SIR=2,4)		ND	Askling et al. 2005
Reumatoid arthritis	4160	0 (SIR=0)	TNF antagonist	NA	Askling et al. 2005
Multiple sclerosis	2854	21(SIR=1,84)		NA	Martinelli et al. 2009
Systemic lupus erythematodis	5715	8(OR=1,2)		ND	Loststrone et al. 2009
Wegener's granulomatosis	293	(SIR=19,6)		6,8-18,5 yrs	Faaurschou et al. 2008
Ulcerative colitis	2012	(OR=3,8)		ND	Johnson et al. 2012

Legend: * including terapy-related MDS; ND – no data; CT – chemotherapy; RT – radio therapy; IMiDs – Immunomodulatory drugs; MoAbs – monoclonal antibodies; HD – high dose; ASCT - autologous stem cell transplantation; ND – no data; S – surgery; ATRA - all-trans retinoic acid; NHL – non-Hodgkin's lymphoma; APL – acute promyelocytic leukaemia; OR – odds ratio; SIR – standardized incidence ratio.

Table 1. Representative studies of the incidence of t-AML in different primary diagnoses.

2.2.2. *Solid tumours*

In most studies, an increased risk of t-AML was reported in breast cancer patients treated with chemoradiotherapy ± radiotherapy. Besides, an increased incidence of t-MDS/AML in patients treated with surgery alone and in patients with a family history of breast cancer suggests a possible association between the two diseases.

When looking at solid tumors, an increased risk of t-AML has been reported in breast cancer patients treated with chemoradiotherapy ± radiotherapy (Table 1). Praga et al. analyzed 9796 breast cancer patients treated in 19 randomized trials (Praga et al., 2005). The cumulative 8-year risk of t-AML showed wide variability between patients treated with standard or high cumulative doses of epirubicin (0.37% vs 4.97%, respectively). In almost 400,000 breast cancer patients, significant risk factors were also younger age at the time of breast cancer diagnosis, advanced stage disease with distal involvement and treatment using radiotherapy (Martin et al., 2009).A large proportion of patients with testicular cancer can be cured by radiochemotherapy, including topoisomerase II inhibitors and cisplatin, but t-MDS/AML represents a major problem with a mean cumulative risk of 1.3 to 4.7% at 5 years (Travis et al., 2000). An increased incidence of AML was found in children with non-testicular germ cell tumors after chemoradiotherapy, with a cumulative incidence in patients treated with combined chemotherapy and radiotherapy. No cases of leukemia were found in patients treated with radiotherapy or surgery only (Schneider et al.,1999).

2.2.3. *Hematopoietic stem cell trasplantation*

An increased risk of therapy-related myelodysplastic syndrome and t-AML after high-dose therapy and autologous stem-cell transplantation (ASCT) for malignant lymphoma has been described by several studies, reporting a highly variable incidence ranging from 1-3% (Lenz et al., 2004; Howe et al., 2003) to 12% (Micallef et al., 2000). The incidence of therapy-related myeloid neoplasms after SCT is related to the type of conditioning regimens, as patients receiving the combination of TBI and alkylating agents seem to have an especially increased risk, but also to the type of previous chemotherapy, its effects on harvested hematopoietic stem cells and the use of growth factors. The development of t-MN after SCT has been shown to be associated with and preceded by markedly altered telomere dynamics in hematopoietic cells, which may reflect increased clonal proliferation and/or altered telomere regulation in premalignant cells (Chakraborty et al., 2009). In the allogeneic bone marrow or hematopoietic stem cell transplantation setting, donor cell–derived leukemias (DCL) and myelodysplastic neoplasms represent a rare but intriguing form of leukemogenesis. DCL represents a unique form of leukemogenesis in which normal donor cells become transformed into an aggressive leukemia or MDS following engraftment in a foreign host environment (Wang et al., 2011; Sala-Torra et al., 2006).

2.2.4. *Auto-immune diseases*

The risk of developing therapy-related AML also applies to patients with non-malignant conditions, such as autoimmune diseases treated with cytotoxic and/or immunosuppressive agents. There is considerable evidence to suggest an increased occurrence of hematologic malignancies in patients with autoimmune diseases compared to the general population, with a further increase in risk after exposure to cytotoxic therapies. Unfortunately, studies have failed to reveal a clear correlation between leukemia development and exposure to individual agents used for the treatment of autoimmune diseases. The association of t-AML and autoimmune diseases was clearly demonstrated in a recent study reporting for an odds ratio of AML OR=1,29 (95% CI, 1.2–1.39) by comparing 13,486 patients aged over 67 years with myeloid malignancies to 160,086 population-based matched controls using the SEER-Medicare database of Hematopoietic Malignancy Risk Traits (SMAHRT). Specifically, AML was associated with rheumatoid arthritis (OR 1.28), systemic lupus erythematosus (OR 1.92), polymyalgia rheumatica (OR 1.73), autoimmune haemolytic anaemia (OR 3.74), systemic vasculitis (OR 6.23), ulcerative colitis (OR 1.72) and pernicious anaemia (OR 1.57) (Anderson et al., 2009). This was confirmed in a recent study by Kristinsson et al. that included 9,219 patients with AML and 42,878 matched controls from population-based central registries in Sweden and reported for a 1.7-fold (95% CI, 1.5–1.9) increased risk of AML (Kristinsson et al., 2011).

In summary, certain inflammatory medical conditions and a personal history of cancer, independent from therapy, are associated with an increased risk of myeloid leukemia. According to the WHO classification, the distinction of t-AMLs from de novo leukemias is solely based on the patient's history but not on the specific biomarkers. Interestingly, it has been observed that 20–30% of acute leukemias, occurring as second malignancy, developed in the absence of previous chemo and/or radiotherapy exposure suggesting that besides the proven leukemogenic mechanisms of chemo and immunosuppressive therapy and ionizing radiations, other factors such as genetics, chronic immune stimulation and environment could favour the onset of multiple neoplastic diseases (Pagano et al., 2001; Johnson et al., 2012). We have to admit that there is insufficient evidence to label leukemias that develop in patients who are exposed to cytotoxic agents as 'therapy-related leukemias'. Further investigation of the underlying mechanisms and defects, including defects in immunity, DNA repair, and apoptosis in these patients are warranted rather than studying only drug mechanisms that lead to leukemogenesis .

3. Risk factors for the development of t-AML

Despite that it has been suggested that chemotherapy (CT) and radiotherapy (RT) are associated with a considerable increase in the risk for the development of t-AML compared to the general population, it still only occurs in a relatively small number of patients. The actuarial risk varies from study to study, but an increase in the risk of AML of 0.25 to 1 % per year has been generally observed. The risk is dose dependent and increases exponentially with age after the age of 40 years, paralleling the risk of primary AML in the general population (Pedersen-Bjergaard J., 2005).

It is important to identify risk factors that may confer susceptibility to the development of the condition, including life style, environmental and occupational, as well as host factors, such as differences in drug catabolism, membrane transport or inefficient DNA repair that could explain the predisposition to leukemia. In general chemotherapy confers a greater risk while involved field radiation is associated with very little or no increased risk of leukemia. Characteristic features often relate to the type of previous therapy; alkylating agents or RT; drugs binding to the enzyme DNA-topoisomerase, or antimetabolites.

3.1. Host factors

Lichtman (2007) after a review of 463 618 cases of cancer patients treated with chemotherapy and radiotherapy, reported 741 cases of AML/MDS, or less than 1%. These data clearly demonstrate, that after exposure to chemotherapy and/or radiotherapy only a small proportion of patients develop t-AMLs, which supports the idea, that a host predisposition to the leukemogenic potential of chemotherapy and radiotherapy probably exits (Czader & Orazi, 2009). Understanding individual susceptibility factors is important not only to identify patients at risk in order to tailor therapy, but also to clarify the biological processes leading to leukemogenesis (Leone et al.,2007).

3.1.1. Cancer susceptibility conditions

During the last years, a number of factors were identified, that might cause a predisposition to both de novo and t-AML, including several cancer susceptibility syndromes (Knoche et al., 2006). **Neurofibromatosis type 1 (NF1)** results from a mutation in or deletion of the *NF1* gene. The gene product neurofibromin serves as a tumor suppressor; and the decreased production of this protein results in the myriad of clinical features. Children with *NF1* are at increased risk of developing benign and malignant solid tumors as well as hematologic malignancies, including acute myelogenous leukemia. The normal *NF1* allele is frequently deleted in the bone marrow cells from NF1 patients with hematologic malignancies, suggesting a pathogenic role in primary leukemogenesis. The idea that NF1 is essential to regulate the growth of myeloid cells and functions as a tumor suppressor gene raises the possibility that children with NF1 might be susceptible to the development of secondary leukemias. (Maris et al.,1997)

Similarly, **germline p53 mutations** may predispose some children to therapy-related leukemia and myelodysplasia. Several reports described the occurrence of t-AML in single cases but no consistent association has been reported to date (Felix et al., 1996; Talwalkar et al., 2010; reviewed in Sill et al., 2011).

Some observation also suggest that individuals with constitutional genetic variation in the p53 pathway such as certain allelic variants within the *MDM2* and *TP53* genes – both involved in the *TP53* DNA damage response pathway – wereat significantly increased risk for chemotherapy-related AML. Analysis of associations between patients with t-AML and 2 common functional p53-pathway variants, the *MDM2* SNP309 and the *TP53* codon 72 polymorphism revealed that, an interactive effect was detected such that *MDM2* TT *TP53* Arg/Arg double homozygotes, and individuals carrying both a *MDM2* G allele and a *TP53* Pro allele, were at increased risk of t-AML. This interactive effect was observed in patients previously treated with chemotherapy but not in patients treated with radiotherapy, and in patients with loss of chromosomes 5 and/or 7. In addition, there was a trend toward shorter latency to t-AML in *MDM2* GG versus TT homozygotes in females but not in males, and in younger but not older patients.These data indicate that the *MDM2* and *TP53* variants interact to modulate responses to genotoxic therapy and are determinants of risk for t-AML (Ellis et al., 2008).

The ***RUNX1/AML1* gene** is the most frequent target for chromosomal translocation in leukemia. Besides, point mutations in the *RUNX1* gene are another mode of genetic alteration in development of leukemia. Monoallelic germline mutations in *RUNX1* result in familial platelet disorder predisposed to acute myelogenous leukemia (Osato M., 2004). Among therapy-related myeloid neoplasms after successful treatment for acute promyelocytic leukemia, leukaemia transformation of myeloproliferative neoplasms has been reported to have a strong association with *RUNX1* mutations. The mutations occur in a normal, a receptive, or a disease-committed hematopoietic stem cell (Harada & Harada, 2011).

Recently, an oncogenic germline ***C-RAF*** mutations were described in patients with t-AML. Besides, analysis of blast cells from patients with *C-RAF* germline mutations revealed loss of the tumor and metastasis suppressor *RAF kinase inhibitor protein* (RKIP) as a functional somatic event in carriers of C-RAF germline mutations, which contributes to the development of t-AML (Zebisch et al., 2009).

Over the last years, **genome-wide association studies** were also conducted in the attempt to increase the knowledge of susceptibility factors for t-AML. A recent study of Knight et al., 2009, represents an important step toward the translational goal of identifying persons at risk for t-AML at the time of their original cancer diagnosis so that their initial cancer therapy can be modified to minimize this risk. The major findings were that the effect of genetic factors contributing to cancer risk are potentiated and more readily discernable in t-AML compared with sporadic cancer. Even in a small sample set, this enrichment allowed for the identification and replication of likely t-AML–predisposing genetic variants, each of which may contribute significantly to overall risk. Distinct subsets of patients with t-AML may have distinct inherited susceptibilities toward t-AML (Knight et al., 2009).

A novel concept addresses **epigenetic modifications** as an important factor in conferring disease susceptibility, including global hypomethylation resulting in chromosomal instability and loss of genetic integrity, and promoter specific DNA hypermethylation which leads to silencing of tumor suppressor genes. Recent studies by Voso et al., 2010 demonstared that gene promoter methylation is a common finding in t-MDS/AML and has been associated to a shorter latency period from the treatment of the primary tumor. Among the studied genes, p15 methylation correlated to monosomy/deletion of chromosome 7q, suggesting that it could be a relevant event in alkylating agent-induced leukemogenesis.

DAPK1 was more frequently methylated in t-MDS/AML when compared to de novo MDS and AML (39% vs 15.3% and 24.4%, p=0.0001). Besides, the methylation pattern appeared to be related to the primary tumor, with DAPK1 more frequently methylated in patients with a previous lymphoproliferative disease (75% vs 32%, p=0.006). In patients studied for concurrent methylation of several promoters, t-MDS/AML were significantly more frequently hypermethylated in 2 or more promoter regions than de novo MDS or AML suggesting that promoter hypermethylation of genes involved in cell cycle control, apoptosis and DNA repair pathways is a frequent finding in t-MDS/AML and may contribute to secondary leukemogenesis. These studies support the hypothesis that chemotherapy and individual genetic predisposition have a role in t-MDS/AML development, and the identification of specific epigenetic modifications may explain complexity and genomic instability of these diseases and give the basis for targeted-therapy. The significant association with previous malignancy subtypes may underlie a likely susceptibility to methylation of specific targets and a role for constitutional epimutations as predisposing factors for the development of therapy-related myeloid neoplasm. However, how the epigenetic machinery is disrupted after chemo/radiotherapy and during secondary carcinogenesis is still unknown, warranting further studies (Voso et al., 2010; Greco et al., 2010).

3.1.2. Detoxification pathways

Another probable mechanisms that predispose to t-AML could be related to accumulation of reactive species that escape detoxification mechanisms or are produced in excess due to drug metabolizing enzymes polymorphisms, or due to DNA damage which is inefficiently repaired because of defective DNA-repair (Seedhouse et al., 2004).

Drug or xenobiotic metabolizing enzymes play key roles in the detoxification of xenobiotics, as well as of a number of commonly used chemotherapeutics. Besides, drug metabolizing enzymes display a high degree of polymorphism in the general population. The potential role of the polymorphisms of most of these genes in the etiology of primary or t-AML has been suggested (Perentesis, 2001).

One of the most important compounds of CYP system is a *CYP3A* that takes part in the metabolism of various chemotherapeutics, such as epipodophyllotoxins, etoposide and teniposide, as well as cyclophosphamide, ifosphamide, vinblastine, and vindesine. It has been reported that a polymorphism in the 5' promoter region of the *CYP3A4* gene (*CYP3A4*-V) may decrease production of a precursor of the potentially DNA-damaging quinone (Felix et al., 1998), therefore the variant gene showed a protective effect against the development of t-AML (Rund et al., 2005). In contrast, individuals with the *CYP3A4*-wild type genotype are at increased risk for t-AML. Often, polymorphic variants in detoxification enzymes may cooperate in modulating the individual's risk of AML. The absence of polymorphism variants *CYP1A1*2A*, del{GSTT1} and *NQO1*2* is associated with a 18-fold lower risk of t-AML, whereas the presence of only *NQO1*2* or all three polymorphisms enhances the risk of t-AML (Bolufer et al., 2007).

Glutathione S-transferases (GSTs) detoxify potentially mutagenic and DNA-toxic metabolites of several chemotherapeutic agents, such as adriamycin, BCNU, bleomycin, chlorambucil, cisplatin, etoposide, melphalan, mitomycin C, mitoxantrone, vincristine, cyclophosphamide, etc. The variant allele of *GSTP1* gene, with a substitution of isoleucine to valine at amino acid codon 105, is associated with a decreased activity of the enzyme and is over-represented in t-AML cases compared with de novo AML, particularly among those with prior exposure to known *GSTP1* substrates, but not among patients exposed to radiotherapy alone (Allan et al., 2001).

An increased risk of developing t-AML has been observed in breast cancer patients with a 677T/1298A haplotype in *MTHFR*, the gene encoding methylene tetrahydrofolate reductase involved in methotrexate metabolism, as well as in patients with 677C/1298C haplotype treated for a primary hematopoietic malignancy with a cyclophosphamide-including regimes (Guillem et al., 2007).

3.1.3. DNA repair

Another mechanism implicated into the t-AML development includes defects of the individual DNA-repair machinery which is genetically determined and is believed to be the result of combinations of multiple genes, each of which may display subtle differences in their activities. Double-strand breaks in DNA lead either to cell death or loss of genetic material resulting in chromosomal aberrations. Insufficient repair results in acquisition and persistence of mutations, whereas elevated levels of repair can inhibit the apoptotic pathway and enable a cell with damaged DNA, attempting repair, to misrepair and survive (Leone et al., 2007).

There is accumulating evidence suggesting a role for **mismatch repair (MMR)** in susceptibility to t-AML. MMR is functionally reflected as microsatellite instability which has been reported in a significant number of t-AML patient presentation samples (reviewed in Seedhouse et al, 2007). However, **double strand breaks (DSBs)** in DNA are arguably the most important class of DNA damage because they may lead to either cell death or loss of genetic material, resulting in chromosome aberrations. High levels of DSBs arise following ionising irradiation and chemotherapy drug exposure. Therefore, DSB repair seems to be critical for t-AML susceptibility. The *RAD51* gene plays a key role in DNA-repair process and its variant *RAD51*-G135C is associated with a 2.66-fold increased risk of t-AML compared to a control group (Jawad et al., 2006). If variants of more than one DNA-repair genes are present, for example RAD51-135C and XRCC3-241Met, the risk of t-AML development is even higher (OR 8.11), presumably because of the large genotoxic insult these patients receive after their exposure to radiotherapy or chemotherapy (Seedhouse et al., 2004). Interestingly, it seems that polymorphic variants in DNA-repair and detoxification enzymes may co-operate, thus having a synergistic effect that leads to modulation of the individual's risk of AML.The risk of development of AML is further increased (OR 15.26) in patients in which the burden of DNA damage is increased when a deletion of the GSTM1 gene is present (Seedhouse et al., 2004). Similarly, carriers of both the RAD51-G135C and CYP3A4-A-290G variants are at highest AML risk (Voso et al., 2007). Besides, the genetic interaction between an increased DNA repair capacity in patients with *RAD51*-G135C, associated with suppressed apoptosis, and affected stem cell numbers due to a *HLX1*-homeobox gene polymorphism, may increase the number of genomes at risk during cancer therapy and results in an increased risk of t-AML up to 9.5-fold (Jawad et al., 2006).

Another possible mechanisms might involve the **base excision repair (BER) pathway, which** corrects individually damaged bases, occuring as the result of endogenous processes, ionising irradiation and exogenous xenobiotic exposure; and the **nucleotide excision repair (NER)** that removes structurally unrelated bulky damage induced by ultra violet radiation, environmental factors and endogenous processes and repairs a significant amount of DNA damage caused by chemotherapeutic agents. A few studies addressed the possible role of polymorphisms of DNA repair genes encoding the X-ray cross-complementing group 1 (XRCC1) protein which plays an important role in excision and ligation of oxidized DNA bases and strand breaks, in cooperation with other enzymes in the base excision repair (BER) pathway, as well as NER polymorphisms, particularly *ERCC2* (XPD) Lys751Gln SNP. Polymorphisms of these genes are associated with decreased DNA repair rates and increased genotoxic damage, measured by single-strand breaks and chromosomal aberrations. It might be speculated that compromised repair activity may lead to accumulation of DNA damage and predispose to secondary cancers and increased treatment-related toxicity to normal tissues. There is a large set of data implying the functional importance of the *XRCC1*-399 polymorphism with the variant Gln allele being associated with a decreased capacity to repair DNA damage and a consequent increased level of DNA damage (reviewed in Seedhouse & Russel, 2007). Evidence has been provided that the variant glutamine allele of XPD Lys751Gln SNP has been associated with an increased risk of t-AML (Kuptsova-Clarkson et al., 2010). Interestingly, Seedhouse et al., 2002 demonstrated that the presence of variant *XRCC1*-399Gln was protective for t-AML hypothesising that when haematopoietic progenitor cells in the bone marrow are damaged by therapy, cells with the *XRCC1*-399Gln allele (reduced BER capacity) are likely to be driven towards apoptosis, whilst those wild type cells are more likely to attempt repair, harbour mutations and initiate clonal disease resulting in t-AML (Seedhouse et al., 2002).

3.2. Previous therapy

By definition t-AMLs occur as late complications of cytotoxic chemotherapy and/or radiation therapy administered for a prior neoplastic or non-neoplastic disorder (Vardiman et al., 2008). Chemotherapy and ionizing radiation cause extensive DNA damage and affect unfortunately not only neoplastic but also normal cells. Presumably if genes controlling growth and differentiation of haematopoietic stem cells are affected, a neoplastic myeloid clone may arise. Further, repeated therapies may facilitate the selection of such a clone due to the inevitable immunosupression.

Mechanism of action	Agent	References
Alkylating agents	Busulfan	Dastugue et al., 1990
	Carboplatin	Miyata et al., 1996
	Carmustine	Perry et al., 1998

http://dx.doi.org/10.5772/52459

Mechanism of action	Agent	References
	Chlorambucil	Rosenthal et al., 1996
	Cisplatin	Samanta et al., 2009
	Cyclophosphamide	Au et al., 2003
	Dacarbazine	Collins et al., 2009
	Dihydroxybusulfan	Pedersen-Bjergaard et al.,1980
	Lomustine	Perry et al., 1998
	Mechlorethamine	Metayer et al., 2003
	Melphalan	Kyle et al., 1070; Yang et al., 2012
	Mitolactol	Bennett et al., 1994
	Mitomycin C	Nakamori et al., 2003
	Procarbazine	Travis et al., 1994
	Semustine	Boice et al., 1983
	Temozolomide	Noronha et al., 2006
Topoisomerase II inhibitors	4-Epidoxorubicin	Riggi et al., 1993
	Bimolane	Xue et al., 1997
	Dactinomycin	Scaradavou et al., 1995
	Daunorubicin	Blanco et al., 2001
	Doxorubicin	Yonal et al., 2012
	Etoposide	Haupt et al., 1994
	Mitoxantrone	Colovic et al., 2012
	Razoxane	Bhavnani et al., 1994
	Teniposide	Ezoe et al. 2012
Antimetabolites	5-fluorouracil	Turker et al., 1999
	Fludarabine	Smith et al., 2011
	6-Mercaptopurine	Bo et al., 1999
	Methotrexate	Kolte et al., 2001
Antimicrotubule agents	Docetaxel	Griesinger et al., 2004
	Paclitaxel	See et al., 2006
	Vinblastine - leukemogenic effects were not confirmed	Carli et al., 2000
	Vincristine - leukemogenic effects were not confirmed	Carli et al. 2000
Growth factors	Granulocyte colony-stimulating factor	Relling et al., 2003
	Granulocyte-macrophage colony-stimulating factor	Hershman et al., 2007
Immunomodulators	Azathioprine	Kwong et al.,2010

Table 2. Cytotoxic agents implicated in t-AML.

Although increased risk of t-AML has been observed after chemotherapy or radiotherapy alone or in combination, chemotherapy generally confers greater risk. Radiation alone is rarely associated with increased risk of t-AML. However, cytotoxic drugs are often given in complex schedules and sometimes in combination with radiotherapy, making it difficult to assess the tumorigenic role of each drug. The most common cytotoxic drugs commonly implicated are listed in the Table 2.

3.2.1. Alkylating agents

Alkylaing agents were the first chemotherapeutics to be associated with secondary leukaemia development after successful treatment of other solid or haematopoietic neoplasms (Kyle et al., 1970; Smit & Meyler, 1970). The mechanisms of DNA damage include either methylation or DNA inter-stand crosslinking formation. Monofunctional alkylating agents (incl. dacarbasine, procarbasine, temozolomide) have one reactive moiety and generally induce base lesions by transferring alkyl groups (-CH_3 or CH_2-CH_3) to oxygen or nitrogen atoms of DNA bases, resulting in highly mutagenic DNA base lesions (reviewed in Drablos et al., 2004). In contrast, bifunctional alkylating agents (incl. melphalan, cylophosphamide, chlorambucil) have two reactive sites and in addition to DNA base lesions, intra- and inter-strand crosslinks can be formed by attacking two bases within the same or on opposing DNA strands which furtheron could result in translocations, inversions, insertions and loss of heterozygosity (reviewed in Helleday et al., 2008).

The latency between treatment and t-MN is generally long, between 5 and 7 years, and overt leukemia is frequently preceeded by a dysplastic phase. These cases are generally characterized by loss or deletion of chromosome 5 and/or 7 [-5/del(5q), -7/del(7q)]. In the University of Chicago's series of 386 patients with t-MDS/t-AML, 79 patients (20%) had abnormalities of chromosome 5, 95 patients (25%) had abnormalities of chromosome 7, and 85 patients (22%) had abnormalities of both chromosomes 5 and 7. t-MDS/t-AML with a -5/del(5q) is associated with a complex karyotype, characterized by trisomy 8, as well as loss of 12p, 13q, 16q22, 17p (*TP53* locus), chromosome 18, and 20q. In addition, this subtype of t-AML is characterized by a unique expression profile (higher expression of genes) involved in cell cycle control (*CCNA2, CCNE2, CDC2*), checkpoints (*BUB1*), or growth (*MYC*), loss of expression of *IRF8*, and overexpression of *FHL2*. Haploinsufficiency of the *RPS14, EGR1, APC, NPM1*, and *CTNNA1* genes on 5q has been implicated in the pathogenesis of MDS/AML (Qian et al., 2010). Cases with−7/7q−, but normal chromosome 5 often have methylation of the *CDKN4B* gene promoter and somatic mutations of the *RUNX1* gene (Christiansen et al., 2004). Thus, two major patterns of t-AML after alkylating agents have been identified (Pedersen-Bjergaard et al., 2006).

3.2.2. Topoisomerase II inhibitors

Commonly used topoisomerase inhibitors bind to the enzyme/DNA complex at the strand cleavage stage of the topoisomerase reaction, interacting with topoisomerase I (topotecan) or II(doxorubicin, epipodophyllotoxin, e.g. etoposide and teniposide). Topoisomerase II inhibitors block the enzymatic reaction through religation and enzyme release, leaving the DNA with a permanent strand break. Chromosomal breakpoints have been found to be preferential sites of topoisomerase II cleavage, which are believed to be repaired by the nonhomologous end-joining DNA repair pathway to generate chimaeric oncoproteins that underlie the resultant leukaemias (reviewed in Joannides & Grimwade, 2010).

T-AMLs occur after a shorter latency time, ranging between 1 and 3 years from the primary treatment, usually arising without a previous dysplastic phase. Several factors, such as the schedule and the concurrent use of asparaginase, dexrazoxane or G-CSF, are considered very important in determining the relative risk. Exposure to topoisomerase II inhibitors is predominantly associated with t-AML characterized by reciprocal translocations with as many as 40 different partner genes, such as t(9;11), t(19;11) or t(4;11) in 80% of the cases, as well as with internal duplications, deletions, and inversions translocations of the *MLL* gene on chromosome band 11q23 Other less frequent genetic alterations are t(8;21), t(3;21), t(16;21), t(17;21), inv(16), t(8;16), t(9;22), t(15;17) (Cowell et al., 2012; Salas et al., 2011, Yin et al., 2005; Felix, 1998).

3.2.3. *Antimetabolites*

Antimetabolites (e.g. azathioprine, 6-thioguanine, fludarabine) share structural similarities with nucleotides, and can be incorporated into DNA or RNA, thereby interfering with replication and causing inhibition of cell proliferation. Once placed in the newly synthesized DNA strand, metabolites are prone to methylation and formation of the highly mutagenic base lesions that closely resemble the induced by alkylating agents. Cell cycle arrest and cell death after treatment are triggered by the DNA MMR machinery. However, MMR-deficient cells can tolerate methylated lesions, potentially forming a leukaemic clone (Offman et al., 2004). In line with the cytogenetic aberrations found with alkylating agents, patients with t-AML after antimetabolites treatment frequently harbour partial or complete loss of chromosomes 5 and 7 (Morrison et al., 2002; Smith et al., 2011).

3.2.4. *Granulocyte-colony stimulating factor (G-CSF)*

Since some of G-CSF effects include stimulation of the proliferation of granulocytic progenitors and premature release of neutrophils from the bone marrow enhancing their capacity for phagocytosis, ROS (reactive oxygen species) generation and bacterial cell killing, two mechanisms have been implicated in the G-CSF-mediated promotion of therapy-related myeloid neoplasms (Beekman & Touw, 2010). First, G-CSF-induced production and release of ROS by bone marrow neutrophils may result in increased DNA damage and mutation rates in Human hematopoietic stem and progenitor cells (Touw & Bontenbal, 2007). Second, repeated application of G-CSF results in a continuous leaving of these cells from their protective bone marrow niche, which may render them more susceptible to genotoxic stress (Trumpp et al., 2010). In an attempt to evaluate the risk of acute myeloid leukemia or myelodysplastic syndrome in patients receiving chemotherapy with or without G-CSF, Lyman et al., 2010 systematically reviewed 25 randomized controlled trials and identified 6058 and 6746 patients were randomly assigned to receive chemotherapy with and without initial G-CSF support, respectively. An absolute risk of 0.43% was determined, however, the administration of G-CSF showed benefits for a substantial proportion of patients and outweighs the increased risk of secondary leukemias.

3.2.5. Ionizing radiation

The risk of leukemia following radiation is considerably smaller than after chemotherapy, with a relative peak at the 5th to 9th year after radiotherapy exposure showing a slow decline afterwards. The underlying mechanisms refer to the formation of reactive oxygen species through radiolysis of water molecules resulting from the exposure of cells to ionizing radiation, which are highly reactive and capable of oxidizing or deaminating DNA bases and increasing the frequency of DNA double strand breaks (Rassool et al., 2007), on one hand, or can also directly induce strand breaks by disruption of the sugar phosphate backbone of DNA, potentially leading to the formation of large scale chromosomal rearrangements (Klymenko et al., 2005). The radiation-related leukemia risk depends on the dose given to the active bone marrow, the dose rate, and the extent of exposed marrow (Travis L., 2006). Due to cell killing at higher doses the risk of t-AML is considerably larger at low doses: patients in whom high radiation doses to limited fields have been given are associated with little or no increased risk of leukemia (UNSCEAR 2000 Report), while exposure of extended fields of radiotherapy as well as low-dose total body irradiation may result in considerably higher risks (Travis et al., 1996; Travis et al., 2000) of leukemia.

4. Molecular pathogenesis

It has been suggested, that t-AML are a direct consequence of mutational events induced by chemotherapy, radiation therapy, immunosuppressive therapy, or a combination of these modalities (Godley & Larson, 2008). Similarly to de novo AML, t-AMLs are complex genetic diseases, requiring cooperating mutations in interacting pathways for disease initiation and progression. Establishing a leukaemic phenotype requires acquisition of crucial genetic aberrations, such as point mutations, fusion genes formation or gene rearrangements, deletion or inactivation of tumor-suppressor genes, or changes in the expression of critical oncogenes or growth factor receptor genes (Larson, 2004). Most probably, multiple events are involved in which DNA damage from exposure to genotoxic stress leads to the secondary abnormalities that cause t-AML (Pedersen-Bjergaard, 2001). A major difference between t-AML and de novo AML is that high doses of mutagenic chemo-/radiotherapy impact on the DNA of haematopoietic stem and precursor cells in the socondary myeloid neoplasms. In contrast, chronic exposure to low doses of occupational/environmental agents over extended periods of time may be operational in the development of high-risk de novo MDS/AML (Sill et al., 2011).

However, these differences are not apparent in all cases and there is a clinical and biological overlap between t-AML and high-risk de novo myelodysplastic syndromes and acute myeloid leukaemia suggesting similar mechanisms of leukaemogenesis. Recently, similarities in therapy-related and elderly acute myeloid leukemia were found in terms of the similar clinical and molecular aspects and unfavorable prognosis. In older individuals prolonged exposure to environmental carcinogens may be the basis for these similarities (D'Alò et al., 2011). On the other hand, a recently published study reported that AML diagnosed in the past decade in patients after receiving radiotherapy alone differ from therapy-related myeloid neoplasms occurring after cytotoxic chemotherapy/combined-modality therapy and share genetic features and clinical behavior with de novo AML/MDS, suggesting that post-radiotherapy MDS/AML may not represent a direct consequence of radiation toxicity (Nardi et al., 2012). Therefore, other factors might be involved such as genetic variants conferring predisposition to the primary malignacy that may also be of relevance for therapy-related leukaemogenesis and account for subtle biologic differences between t-MNs and high-risk de novo MDS/AML (Sill et al., 2011). Besides, the nature of the causative agent has an important bearing upon the characteristics, biology, time to onset and prognosis of the resultant leukaemia (Joannides & Grimwade, 2010).

Various pathogenetic mechanisms have been elucidated so far and different genetic pathways for the multistep development of t-MDS/t-AML have been proposed, in which particular mechanisms of DNA damage that lead either to chromosomal deletions, balanced translocations or induction of defective DNA-mismatch repair could promote survival of misrepaired cells giving rise to the leukemic clone (Leone at al., 2007). Multiple tumor suppressor genes or oncogenes may need to be mutated to ultimately transform a cell resulting in impaired differentiation of hematopoietic cells and/or in proliferative and survival advantage. Different molecular pathways may cooperate in the genesis of leukemia and at least 8 alternative genetic pathways have been defined based on characteristic recurrent chromosome abnormalities(Pedersen-Bjergaard et al., 2007).

Interestingly, analysis of gene expression in CD34+ cells from patients who developed t-MDS/AML after autologous hematopoietic cell transplantation revealed altered gene expression related to mitochondrial function, metabolism, and hematopoietic regulation and the genetic programs associated with t-MDS/AML are perturbed long before disease onset (Li et al., 2011). Similarly, the gene expression profiles in diagnostic acute lymphoblastic leukemic cells from children treated on protocols that included leukemogenic agents, revealed a signature of 68 probes, corresponding to 63 genes, that was significantly related to risk of t-AML. The distinguishing genes included transcription-related oncogenes (*v-Myb*, *Pax-5*), cyclins (*CCNG1*, *CCNG2* and *CCND1*) and histone *HIST1H4C*. Common transcription factor recognition elements among similarly up- or downregulated genes included several involved in hematopoietic differentiation or leukemogenesis (*MAZ*, *PU.1*, *ARNT*). This approach has identified several genes whose expression distinguishes patients at risk of t-AML, and suggests targets for assessing germline predisposition to leukemogenesis (Bogni et al., 2006).

The comparison of samples from t-AML and de novo AML patients using high resolution array CGH revealed more copy number abnormalities (CNA) in t-AML than in de novo AML cases: 104 CNAs with 63 losses and 41 gains (mean number 3.46 per case) in t-AML, while in de novo-AML, 69 CNAs with 32 losses and 37 gains (mean number of 1.9 per case). The authors suggested that CNA can be classified into several categories: abnormalities common to all AML; those more frequently found in t-AML and those specifically found in de novo AML (Itzhar et al., 2011).

Recently, a growing amount of data suggests that DNA methylation abnormalities may contribute to a multistep secondary leukemogenesis. Two distinct alterations of normal DNA methylation patterns may occur in cancer: (i) a global hypomethylation resulting in chromosomal instability and loss of genetic integrity, and (ii) promoter specific DNA hypermethylation which leads to silencing of tumor suppressor genes. Cytotoxic drugs and radiation have been shown to affect tissue DNA methylation profile. Radiation is able to induce a stable DNA hypomethylation in both target and bystander tissues. Gene promoter methylation is a common finding in t-MDS/AML and has been associated to a shorter latency period from the treatment of the primary tumor. Among the studied genes, *p15* methylation correlated to monosomy/deletion of chromosome 7q, suggesting that it could be a relevant event in alkylating agent-induced leukemogenesis. Besides, a frequent methylation of *DAPK* in the t-MDS/AML group was observed, especially in patients with a previous lymphoproliferative disease. In patients studied for concurrent methylation of several promoters, t-MDS/AML were significantly more frequently hypermethylated in 2 or more promoter regions than de novo MDS or AML suggesting that promoter hypermethylation of genes involved in cell cycle control, apoptosis and DNA repair pathways is a frequent finding in t-MDS/AML and may contribute to secondary leukemogenesis. However, how the epigenetic machinery is disrupted after chemo/radiotherapy and during secondary carcinogenesis is still unknown (Voso et al., 2010).

5. Clinical features

Similarly to de novo AML, therapy-related AMLs comprise an extremely heterogeneous group of biologically different hematologic malignancies and their clinical presentation varies in a significant degree from cases to case, depending on applied chemo- and or radiotherapy for the primary disorder as well as on other factors.

As expected, the most frequent complaints at the presentation of patients with t-AMLs include: fatigue, weakness, and occasionally fever, bleeding complications caused by thrombocytopenia, anemia, and leukopenia. Features that are fairly common in de novo acute leukemia, such as hepatomegaly, splenomegaly, lymphadenopathy, gingival hyperplasia, skin rash, or neurological complications, are notably absent from the presentations of patients with t-MDS/t-AML. Bone marrow biopsies typically reveal hypercellularity with some degree of marrow fibrosis, although hypocellular and even aplastic marrows can be seen (Godley & Le Beau, 2007).

Morphologically, t-AML can present in the broad spectrum of myeloid leukemias. Mostly in patients after previous therapy with alkylating agents multilineage dysplasia can be observed. However, dysplasia can be seen in some patients with balanced translocations as well. Dysgranulopoiesis includes hypogranular neutrophils, with hypo- or hyperlobulated nuclei, nuclear excrescences, and pseudo-Pelger-Huet nuclei. Red cell morphology in most

http://dx.doi.org/10.5772/52459

cases is characterised by macrocytosis and poikilocytosis, periodic acid-Schiff-positive normoblasts, dyserythropoiesis with megaloblastoid changes, erythroid hyperplasia, ringed sideroblasts, nuclear budding, karyorrhexis, binuclearity, and nuclear bridging. Megakaryocyte dysplasia within the bone marrow includes micromegakaryocytes, abnormal nuclear spacings, mononuclear forms, giant compound granules, and hypogranular cytoplasm. Cases of therapy-related myeloid neoplasms related to treatment with topoisomerase II inhibitors typically present as overt acute myeloid leukemia without a myelodysplastic prephase. Morphologic features are not unique in therapy-related cases. Although monocytic and monoblastic differentiation is often present, the appearance may be that of de novo cases, including those with recurrent cytogenetic abnormalities (Godley & Le Beau, 2007; Vardiman et al., 2008).

Immunophenotypic studies are not used to distinguish t-AML from de novo cases but rather to clarify abnormal populations, reflecting the heterogeinety of the underlying morphology. The phenotype findings are similar to their de novo counterparts. The myeloblasts are characteristically CD34-positive and express pan-myeloid markers (CD13, CD33) and flow cytometry may be helpful in assessing the proportion of myeloid blasts, as well as aberrant antigenic expression, such as CD7, CD56, CD19, etc. Immunophenotypic maturation patterns of the myeloid and erythroid lineages may also be evaluated. The maturing myeloid cells may show abnormal patterns of antigen expression and/or light scatter properties. However, the relevance of such findings is similar to that in de novo cases (Wood B., 2007; Vardiman et al., 2008).

Clinical and laboratory features of patients with t-AML with recurrent genetic abnormalities have been of particular interest. In some studies, hematologic characteristics of patients with t-AML with t(8;21) and inv(16), are identical to those of de novo AML with the same karyotypes (Quesnel et al., 1993). Simmilarly, according to Duffield et al., 2012, t-APL and de novo APL had abnormal promyelocytes with similar morphologic and immunophenotypic features, comparable cytogenetic findings, and comparable rates of FMS-like tyrosine kinase mutations (Duffield et al., 2012). Interestingly, compared with patients with t-APL, those with de novo APL had a greater median body mass index-BMI (31.33 vs. 28.48), incidence of obesity (60.4% vs. 27.3%), and history of hyperlipidemia (45.3% vs. 18.2%), suggesting that abnormalities in lipid homeostasis may in some way be of pathogenic importance in de novo APL (Elliott et al., 2012). t-AML-t(8;21) shares many features with de novo AML-t(8;21)(q22;q22), however patients with t-AML-t(8;21) are older and had a lower WBC count, substantial morphologic dysplasia, Auer rods are detected only certain patients, an increase in eosinophils is uncommon (Gustafson et al., 2009). The detection of morphologic features characteristic of t(8;21) with associated multilineage dysplasia is fairly unique to t(8;21) t-AML/MDS (Arber et al., 2002). Despite that, some studies reported that t-AML/MDS with t(8;21) may have a high frequency of expression of CD19 and CD34 (Arber et al., 2002), this was not confirmed by others (Gustafson et al., 2009).

Rearrangements involving the *MLL* gene on chromosome band 11q23 are a hallmark of therapy-related acute myeloid leukemias following treatment with topoisomerase II poisons (Libura et al., 2005). French-American-British (FAB) subtype distribution of cases with

11q23/*MLL* rearrangement does not differ between de novo AML and t-AML (Schoch et al., 2003). In adults, patients with t-AML and t(9;11)(p21-22;q23) are more likely to be women and older, without other statistically significant differences with regard to clinical features; immunophenotype; morphologic, cytogenetic, and molecular genetic features; or miRNA expression, compared to de novo AML cases (Chandra et al., 2010). Pediatric patients with t(9;11) positive secondary AML are older at diagnosis, have higher hemoglobin levels, and central nervous system leukemia or hepatosplenomegaly is less frequent. Whereas the t(9;11)(p21;q23) occurred exclusively in the FAB M5 subtype in de novo AML, the FAB M0 and M4 subtypes were also represented in secondary cases (Sandoval et al., 1992).

Chromosome/ Molecular Aabnormality	GIMEMA 2001 n=127	**G-A AML SG 2011 n=200**	Serbia 2012 n=42	Our data 2012 n=26	De novo AML, 2011 n= 2653
Age – mean (range) years	58 (21-87)	57.8 (18.6-79.4)	56.07 (23-84)	53.5 (22-83)	53.2 (16.2-85)
Male %/female %	44/56	32/68	29/71	46/54	53/47
Latency median (range) months	52 (2-379)	48.5 (4-530)	54.62 (6-243)	48 (3-216)	NA
WBC – mean x10^9/L	6.7	7.4	27.2	24.4	12.5
CR rate %	55	63	23.8	42	67
Median OS months	7	12	5.94	6	20
Reference	Pagano et al, 2001	Kayser et al, 2011	Suvajdžić et al, 2012	Balatzenko et al., 2012	Kayser et al, 2011

Table 3. Major clinical data in t-AML patients' cohorts.

The analysis of 179 t-AML patients from the GIMEMA Archive of Adult Acute Leukaemia, including 41 treated with surgery only, allowed for the distinction of some differences compared to de novo AML cases. The median age of t-AML was significantly higher than that of other AML (63 years vs. 57 years), the number of men was significantly lower than the number of women [4.8% vs. 7.4%) most probably due to the high incidence in breast cancer patients; as was the number of patients aged <65 years [5.3% vs. 7.5%]. Interestingly, an increased incidence of cancer was observed among first-degree relatives of patients with AML occurring after a primary malignancy [36.9% vs. 27.2% in de novo AML]. Prevalent types of primary malignancies were breast cancer, lymphoma and Hodgkin's disease (Pagano et al., 2001). Higher WBC count and females predominance in t-AML had also been observed by others (Schoch et al., 2004).

http://dx.doi.org/10.5772/52459

6. Genetic and molecular features

It is widely accepted, that the spectrum of chromosome aberrations is comparable in t-AML and de novo AML, however the frequencies of distinct cytogenetic categories is different depending on the characteristics of the analyzed patient cohort (reviewed in Schoch et al., 2004). Two are the most striking features of t-AML: the extremely high frequency of abnormal clonal karyotype up to 75%-96% compared to 50%-59% in de novo AML (Schoch et al., 2004; Godley & Larson, 2008; Grimwade et al., 2010; Mauritzson et al., 2002); and a clear predominance of unfavorable cytogenetics, such as deletion or loss of chromosomes 5 and/or 7 or a complex karyotype (Godley & Larson, 2008). However, the frequency and the spectrum of abnormal karyotypes varies depending on the nature of the applied antecedent anti-neoplastic therapy (Rund et al., 2004).

Unbalanced chromosome aberrations such as abnormalities of chromosomes 5 and/or 7 account for 76% of the cases with an abnormal karyotype.Complex karyotypes are seen in 26.9% of t-AML as compared to 11.30% of de novo AML (Schoch et al., 2004). Recurring balanced rearrangements account for 11% of cases (Larson & Le Beau, 2005), with a specific over-presentation of 11q23 abnormalities – 12.9% vs. 3.7% in de novo AML (Schoch et al., 2004). Comparative data on chromosome/molecular aberrations in t-AML and de novo AML are presented in Table 4.

6.1. Unbalanced chromosome aberrations

Generally, t-AMLs with unbalanced chromosome abnormalities are developed after exposure to alkylating agents and/or ionizing radiation. This group is considered as a biologically distinct form and the most frequent type of t-AML accounting for approximately 75% of cases. The disease usually follows a long period of latency generally occuring 5–10 years after the drug exposure and is characterized frequently by a preleukemic phase and tri-lineage dysplasia. Typical cytogenetical aberrations comprise loss or deletion of chromosome 5 and/or 7 [-5/del(5q), -7/del(7q)]. Frequently, abnormalities of chromosome 5 are part of a complex karyotype, that additionally includes trisomy 8, as well as loss of 12p, 13q, 16q22, 17p (*TP53* locus), chromosome 18, and 20q (Qian et al., 2010).

The complex and hypodiploid karyotypes with unbalanced chromosome changes results in multiple severe molecular abnormalities with a gene-dosage effect for some of the genes that depend on the nature of the primary chromosome aberration. The loss of the coding regions for tumor suppressor genes from hematopoietic progenitor cells is a particularly unfavorable event, since the remaining allele becomes susceptible to inactivating mutations leading to the leukemic transformation (Leone et al., 2001; Joannides & Grimwade, 2011).

Interestingly, significant proportion of older patients are diagnosed with leukaemia with no antecedent history of exposure, and some of these cases show a remarkably similar phenotype to classic therapy-related leukaemia (D'Alò et al., 2011). The specific cytogenetic abnormalities common to MDS, alkylating-agent-related AML and poor-prognosis AML [3q-, -5/5q-, -7/7q-, +8, +9, 11q-, 12p-, -18, -19, 20q-, +21, t(1;7), t(2;11)], probably reflect a common pathogenesis distinct from that of other de novo AMLs. Possibly, tumour suppressor genes are implicated and genomic instability may be a cause of multiple unbalanced chromosomal translocations or deletions. Typically, these patients are either elderly or have a history of exposure to alkylating agents or environmental exposure 5-7 years prior to diagnosis (Dann & Rowe, 2001).

Chromosome/Molecular Aabnormality	De novo AML	Therapy-related AML
BRAF	1.5%	6%
CEBPA mutations	7% - 15%	0 – 6%
c-KIT mutations	2% - 5%	1% - 4%
DNMT3A mutations	18% - 22%	16%
*FLT3*internal tandem duplications	22% - 35%	7% - 12%
FLT3 – tyrosine kinase domain mutations	5% - 8%	2% - 2.5%
IDH1/IDH2 mutations	17% - 33%	3% -12%
Inv(16)/t(16;16) / *CBFβ-MYH11*	4% - 6%	1% - 8%
Inv(3)/t(3;3) / EVI1	1% - 2%	0.2% - 1%
JAK2 mutations	Rare	Rare
MLL partial tandem duplications	6%	2% - 4%
NPM1 mutations	19% - 35%	12% - 16%
NRAS mutations	6% - 10%	11% - 12%
PTPN11 mutations	3% - 5%	4.%
RUNX1 mutations	5% - 10%	4% - 9%
t(15;17) / *PML-RARα*	4% - 11%	2% - 3%
t(8;21) / *RUNX1-ETO*	5% - 9%	2% - 5%
t(9;11) / *MLLT3-MLL*	1% - 2%	6% - 11%
t(v;11)(v;q23) / *MLL* rearrangements	2% - 4%	4% - 12%
TET2 mutations	8% - 13%	9%
TP53 mutations	10-15%	18% - 25%
WT1 mutations	4% - 7%	17%

References: Abbas et al., 2010; Ahmad et al., 2009; Bacher et al., 2011; Bacher et al., 2007; Christiansen et al., 2005; Christiansen et al., 2004; Christiansen et al.,2007; Fried et al., 2012; Gaidzik et al., 2011; Green et al., 2010; Kayser et al., 2011; Kosmider et al., 2011; Lee et al., 2004; Lin et al., 2005; Marcucci et al., 2010; Mauritzson et al., 2002; Paschka et al., 2010; Pedersen-Bjergaard et al., 2008; Preudhomme et al., 2002; Shen et al., 2011; Takahashi et al., 2000; Thiede et al., 2002; Westman et al., 2011.

Table 4. Chromosome and molecular abnornalities in t-AML compared to de novo AML.

The critical genetic consequences of unbalanced chromosome aberrations in MDS and AML have remained unknown (Pedersen-Bjergaard et al., 2007). The genetic consequences of a deletion may be a reduction in the level of one or more critical gene products (haploinsufficiency), or complete loss of function. The latter model, known as the "two-hit model", predicts that loss of function of both alleles of the target gene would occur, in one instance through a detectable chromosomal loss or deletion and, in the other, as a result of a subtle inactivating mutation, or other mechanisms, such as transcriptional silencing. However, the respective genes on the "intact copy" seem to be not affected, since no submicroscopic deletions or mutations of the remaining allele in any of the genes within the commonly deleted segment (CDS) were detected (reviewed in Le Beau & Olney, 2009). Therefore, most probably loss of only a single copy of a relevant gene (haploinsufficiency) perturbs cell fate. Deletions of putative tumor suppressor genes at chromosomes 5q and 7q are believed to underlie the molecular pathogenesis of alkylating agent- related leukemias. Since similar aberrations occur in de novo MDS/AML, knowledge on potential regions of involvement at chromosomes 5q and 7q derives from de novo and treatment-related cases, but the specific genes in these regions that are important in leukemia pathogenesis continue to remain elusive (Jerez et al., 2011).

On chromosome 5q, two CDSs were identified in 5q31.2 (de novo and t-MDS/t-AML) and 5q33.1 (in 5q− syndrome). The 970 kb CDS within 5q31.2 comprises 20 genes that encoded proteins that take part in regulation of mitosis and G2 checkpoint, transcriptional control, and translational regulation. The second 1.5 Mb CDS is located within 5q33.1, distal to the CDS in 5q31.2 and contains 40 genes, 33 of which are expressed within the CD34+ hematopoietic stem/progenitor cell compartment cells and, therefore, represent candidate genes (Boultwood et al., 2002).The genes that might be involved in leukemogenesis due to gene dosage effect include *RPS14, EGR1, NPM1, APC,* and *CTNNA1* (reviewed in Qian et al., 2010).

Monosomy 7 and del(7q) occur in a variety of clinical contexts including de novo MDS and AML, leukemias associated with a constitutional predisposition, and therapy-related MDS or AML (Luna-Fineman et al., 1995). Several regions with allelic loss were identified in patients with 7q deletions, including entire regions from chromosome 7q22 to 7q31, 7q32-7q35, etc. (Kratz et al., 2001; Le Beau et al., 1996; Dohner et al.,1998). Besides, case analysis of allelic loss at 7q31 and 7q22 loci revealed retention of sequences between these loci or submicroscopic allele imbalance for a different distal locus, suggesting that multiple distinct critical chromosme7q genes are involved in MDS and AML.

Critical genes affected by monosomy 7 and del(7q) are still unknown. Several candidate genes have been suggested as involved in leukemogenesis. *hDMP1* (cyclin D-binding Myb-like protein) gene, that negatively regulates cell proliferation is considered as possible as a tumor suppressor in acute leukemias with deletions of the long arm of chromosome 7 (Bodner et al., 1999). *MLL5* is a candidate tumor suppressor gene located within a 2.5-Mb interval of chromosome band 7q22, that seems to be a key regulator of normal hematopoiesis and which is frequently deleted in human myeloid malignancies. Since no inactivating mutations and decreased *MLL5* mRNA expression were detected, the most probable mechanism of gene inactivation is haploinsufficiency (Heuser et al., 2009; Zhang et al., 2009; Emerling et al., 2002).

PIK3CG, which encodes the catalytic subunit p110 gamma of phosphoinositide 3-OH-kinase-gamma (PI3K gamma), has been assigned to the same frequently deleted in myeloid malignancies chromosome band 7q22. Although that missense variations affecting residue 859 in the N-terminal catalytic domain of the protein were found, this fact probably represents a polymorphism and it is unlikely that the gene acts as a recessive TSG in myeloid leukemias with monosomy 7 (Kratz et al., 2002).

Deletions of chromosome band 17p13 or loss of a whole chromosome 17 harboring the *p53* gene were shown to be associated with point mutations of *p53*. Patients with *p53* mutations characteristically present complex karyotypes and complicated chromosome rearrangements with duplication or amplification of chromosome bands 11q23 and 21q22 encompassing the *MLL* and the *AML1* genes, resulting in "sandwich-like" marker chromosomes made of material from at least three different chromosomes.

Application of multicolor fluorescence in situ hybridization (M-FISH) allows better identification of chromosome abnormalities compared to G-banding. A clustering of breakpoints was observed in the centromeric or pericentromeric region of chromosomes 1, 5, 7, 13, 17, 21, and 22 in almost 50% of patients with t-MDS and t-AML and an abnormal karyotype. In most of the patients with chromosome derivatives containing material from 3 or more chromosomes or having "sandwich-like" chromosomes, those made up of several small interchanging layers of material from two chromosomes, showed mutations of *TP53* (Andersen et al., 2005).

In some patients treated with alkylating agents an amplification or duplication of *AML1* gene (21q22) or *MLL* gene (11q23) can be found. Generally, no point mutations in *AML1* gene or *MLL* gene rearrangements were seen in these cases. Interestingly, almost all these patients presented with acquired point mutations of the *TP53* gene, which supports the pivotal role of the impaired *TP53* function in the development of gene amplification or duplication in t-MDS and t-AML (Andersen MK, et al.,2001; Andersen MK, et al. 2005).

6.2. Balanced chromosome aberrations

Balanced chromosome translocations and inversions have been found in 10.6% of t-AML. These types of aberrations are observed most commonly in patients treated with agents targeting topoisomerase II. Other typical features of t-AML with balances chromosome abnormalities comprise presentation of the disease as an overt leukemia without a myelodysplastic phase and a short latency period (6–36 months). The formation of these chromosome abnormalities is considered as a result of multiple DNA strand breaks following the topoisomerase II inhibitors. Generally, chromosomal breakpoints have been found to be preferential sites of topoisomerase II cleavage that seems to be repaired by the nonhomologous end-joining DNA repair pathway to generate chimaeric oncoproteins that underlie the resultant leukaemias (Joannides & Grimwade, 2010).

http://dx.doi.org/10.5772/52459

Most often, chromosome translocations involve chromosome bands 11q23 or 21q22 with rearrangement of the *MLL* and the *AML1* genes, but also less frequently other balanced rearrangements such as the inv(16)(p13q22), and the t(15;17)(q22;q11) (Dissing et al., 1998; Andersen MK et al.,1998), etc. Translocations are often present as the sole abnormality.

It seems, that an association between the nature of the applied drug and the type of translocation exists, since translocations involving 11q23 are more frequent after treatment with epipodophyllotoxins, whereas translocations affecting 21q22, inv(16), and t(15;17) are more common after anthracyclines (Andersen et al., 1998). Other less common, recurrent, balanced cytogenetic abnormalities occurring in myeloid neoplasms associated with previous therapy include 3q21q26, 11p15, t(9;22)(q34;q11), 12p13, and t(8;16)(p11;p13) (Czader et al., 2009).

Recently, translocations involving the *NUP98* gene on chromosome 11p15.5 have been cloned from patients with hematological malignancies. To date, at least 8 different chromosomal rearrangements involving *NUP98* have been identified. The resultant chimeric transcripts encode fusion proteins that juxtapose the N-terminal GLFG repeats of *NUP98* to the C-terminus of the partner gene. Of note, several of these translocations have been found in patients with t-AML, suggesting that genotoxic chemotherapeutic agents may play an important role in generating chromosomal rearrangements involving *NUP98* (Lam & Aplan, 2001).

Generally, the recurrent balanced chromosome aberrations lead to the formation of fusion genes, with the participation of hematopoietic transcription factors genes, that encode himeric oncoproteins playing a crtical role in leukemogenesis.

6.2.1. Translocations involving chromosome 11q23/ MLL gene

MLL encodes a histone methyltransferase that play a key role in the regulation of gene expression. In leukemia, this function is subverted due to replacement of the C-terminal functional domains of *MLL* with those of a fusion partner, yielding a newly formed chimeric protein with an altered function that endows hematopoietic progenitors with self-renewing and leukemogenic activity (Eguchi M, 2005). Although the molecular basis for the oncogenic activity of MLL chimeric proteins is not completely understood, it seems to be derived, at least in part, through activation of clustered homeobox (HOX) genes (Harper & Aplan, 2008).

Translocations involving chromosome 11q23, where the *MLL* gene is located, are typical aberrations observed in adults with t-AML, where the frequency is significantly higher compared to de novo AML cases – 9.4% vs. 2.6% (Schoch et al., 2003). Frequent partners are chromosomes 9, 19 and 4 in the t(9;11), t(19;11) and t(4;11) translocations. Particularly higher frequency in t-AML was reported in regard to t(9;11), compared to de novo AML - 11% versus 1% respectively (Kayser et al., 2011). Besides, some structural differences between de novo AML and t-AML exist, although their clinical significance is still unclear. Typical examples of such differences are the t-AML with *MLL* rearrangements that, similarly to infant leukemias, have genomic breakpoints in *MLL* tending to cluster in the 3' portion, in contrast to adults with de novo AML, in whom the breakpoint is located in the 5' portion of the

8.3 kb breakpoint cluster region (BCR) (Zhang & Rowley,2006). Younger age, a mean period of latency of 2 years and monocytic subtypes are characteristic features of this type of leukaemia (Leone et al., 2001).

6.2.2. Translocations involving chromosome 21q22 / AML1 (CBFA2/RUNX1) gene

T-AML with balanced 21q22 aberrations has been associated with prior exposure to radiation, epipodophyllotoxins, and anthracyclines. Translocations involving chromosome 21q22 comprise multiple abnormalities, presented as t(8;21) (56%), t(3;21) (20%), and t(16;21) (5%) (Slovak et al., 2002), t(1;21)/*RUNX1-PRDM16* (Sakai et al., 2005) and other partner chromosomes (Slovak et al., 2002). The median latency for 21q22 patients is 39 months, compared to 26 months for 11q23 patients, 22 months for inv(16), 69 months for rare recurring aberrations, and 59 months for Unique (nonrecurring) balanced aberration (Slovak et al., 2002).

6.2.3. Translocations involving chromosome 11p15/ NUP98 gene

The *NUP98* gene has been reported to be fused with at least 15 partner genes in leukemias with 11p15 translocations, including *PRRX1* (*PMX1*), *HOXD13*, *RAP1GDS1*, *HOXC13*, *TOP1*, etc. (Kobzev et al., 2004). The resultant chimeric transcripts encode fusion proteins that juxtapose the N-terminal GLFG repeats of *NUP98* to the C-terminus of the partner gene. Of note, several of these translocations have been found in patients with t-AML, suggesting that genotoxic chemotherapan important role in generating chromosomal rearrangements involving *NUP98* (Lam & Aplan, 2001).In a survey of childhood t-AML/t-MDS, 11p15 translocations were found in 6% of the cases, including t(11;17)(p15;q21), t(11;12)(p15;q13), t(7;11) (p15;p15), inv(11)(p15q22), and add(11)(p15) and it has been suggested that *NUP98* may be a target gene for t-AML/MDS, and that t-AML/MDS with a fusion of *NUP98* and *HOX* or *DDX10* genes may be more frequent in children than in patients of other age groups (Nishiyama et al.,1999).

6.2.4. Translocations associated with "favorable" prognosis

A relatively distinct subgroup of t-AML comprises patients bearing "favorable" cytogenetic abnormalities, such as inv(16) and t(15;17) (Andersen MK et al. 2002), and more rarely – t(8;21) (Gustafson et al., 2009). These aberrations have been observed after alkylating agents and/or topoisomerase II inhibitors. High frequency of t(15;17), inv(16) and t(8;21) (18-29%, 21%, and 15% respectively) has also been reported in patients treated with radiotherapy only (Andersen et al., 2002; Yin et al., 2005).

The median latency period after the treatment is 22 months in patients with inv(16), 29 months in patients with t(15;17) and 37 months in patients with t(8;21). More than half of the cases in each group had additional cytogenetic abnormalities. Trisomy of chromosomes 8, 21, 22 and del(7q) are the most frequent additional abnormalities in the inv(16) subgroup, whereas trisomy 8, monosomy 5, and del(16q) are most frequent in the t(15;17) subgroup. Additional abnormalities commonly associated with t(8;21) include loss of a sex chromosome and Trisomy 4 (Andersen et al., 2002; Gustafson et al., 2009; Yin et al., 2005).

Interestingly, some structural differences were observed between patients positive for these aberrations with de novo AML and t-AML.In t-AML with inv(16)/t(16;16), the unusual rare types of fusion *CBFB-MYH11* transcripts were found to be significantly more frequent compared to de novo AML (Schnittger et al., 2007).

In therapy related t(15;17) APL, a prevalence of short form of *PML-RARa* transcripts (bcr3) was reported (62% of cases), while in de novo APL, the frequency of cases with a short form varied from 15% to 40-47% (Lin et al., 2004; Douer et al., 2003). On the other hand, in 39% of t-APL exposed to mitoxantrone (a topoisomerase II poison) and in none of the cases arising de novo, the translocation breakpoints are tightly clustered in an 8-bp region within *PML* intron 6, associated with the synthesis of long (bcr1) (Mistry et al., 2005; Hasan et al., 2010). In functional assays, this "hot spot" and the corresponding RARA breakpoints were common sites of mitoxantrone-induced cleavage by topoisomerase II (Mistry et al.,2005).

As to *RARA* breakpoints, significant clustering of *RARA* breakpoints in a 3' region of intron 2 (region B) was found in 65% of t-APL as compared to 28% de novo APLs. Furthermore, approximately 300 bp downstream of *RARA* region B contained a sequence highly homologous to a topoisomerase II consensus sequence. Biased distribution of DNA breakpoints at both *PML* and *RARA* loci suggests the existence of different pathogenetic mechanisms in t-APL as compared with de novo APL (Hasan et al., 2010). Furthermore, a significant breakpoint clustering has been also observed in *PML* and *RARA* loci, with *PML* breakpoints lying outside the mitoxantrone-associated hotspot region in epirubicin-related t-APL, that were shown to be preferential sites of topo II-induced DNA damage, enhanced by epirubicin (Mays et al., 2010).

On the other hand, almost all chromosome translocations in leukemia that have been analyzed to date show no consistent homologous sequences at the breakpoint with small deletions and duplications in each breakpoint, and micro-homologies and non-template insertions at genomic junctions of each chromosome translocation. The size of these deletions and duplications in the same translocation is much larger in de novo leukemia than in therapy-related leukemia (Zhang & Rowley, 2006).

6.3. Molecular abnormalities, unrelated to chromosome aberrations

Several molecular abnormalities were identified in both de novo AML and t-AML that are not a result of chromosome abnormalities, including mainly point mutations and gene tandem duplications. Significant differences in frequency of some of them were reported in t-AML.

Internal tandem duplications (ITD) and point mutations within the tyrosine kinase domain (TKD) of the FMS-like tyrosine kinase 3 (*FLT3*) gene are among the most frequent molecular abnormalities in de novo AML, accounting for more than 22% - 35% of the cases, and showing significant associations with the presence of a normal karyotype. In contrast, these mutations are only rarely seen in t-AML (Qian et al., 2010). Interestingly, in a small study of t-APL, *FLT3* mutations were detected in 42% of the patients, an incidence similar to that found in de novo APL cases (30%) (Chillón et al., 2010). These results and the preferential use of S-form of *PML-RARA* transcripts suggest that different molecular mechanisms are involved in t-APL compared with de novo APL (Yin et al., 2005). *NPM1* and *CEBPA* mutations, that are generally associated with favorable prognosis, are also detected with a significantly lower frequency – 30% to 40-50% and 15-20%, respectively, in de novo AML compared to 4-5% and less in t-AML (Pedersen-Bjergaard et al., 2007; Kayser et al., 2011).

In contrast, higher incidence in t-AML was reported for *TP53* mutations – 20% to 30% versus 10-15% in de novo AML. The spectrum of mutations includes missense mutations in exons 4–8, as well as loss of the wild type allele, typically as a result of a cytogenetic abnormality of 17p. In t-MDS/t-AML, *TP53* mutations are associated with −5/del(5q) and a complex karyotype (Pedersen-Bjergaard et al., 2007; Qian et al., 2010).

Point mutations in the *RUNX1* gene are another mode of genetic alteration in development of leukemia, in addition to gene rearrangements associated with chromosomal translocation. Sporadic point mutations are frequently found in three leukemia entities: AML M0 subtype, MDS-AML, and secondary (therapy-related) MDS/AML. In t-MDS/t-AML, as well as after atomic bomb radiation exposure, the reported incidence for point mutations was higher (15–30%), frequently with an association with activating mutations of the RAS pathway, compared to de novo disease (2-3%). Mutations are commonly located in the N-terminal Runt homology domain (RHD) or in the C-terminal region including the transactivation domain (TAD) and could be found in patients treated in alkylating agents (Osato M., 2004). Cases with *RUNX1* mutations usually present as t-MDS, with deletion or loss of chromosome arm 7q and with subsequent transformation to overt t-AML (Christiansen et al., 2004). In contrast, in de novo AML, *RUNX1* mutations are most frequent in cases with +13, whereas frequencies are similar in other cytogenetic groups (26%-36%) (Schnittger et al.,2007). No significant differences have been reported in regard to *NRAS, KRAS, MLL-PTD, PTPN11, JAK2.*

To study the frequency and spectrum of molecular abnormalities with a proven or suggestive role in leukemic transformation in patients with t-AML we analysed 407 consecutive adult AML patients, diagnosed and treated in our institution, for a 12-years period. Among them, 26 cases had history for a previous malignancy treated with chemotherapy and/or radiotherapy which accounts for 6,1% of the cases – 12 (46%) males and 14 (54%) females, at a mean age of 53.5 years (ranging 22-83 years).AML was diagnosed after radio and/or chemotherapy for solid tumours in 16 (61.5%) of the patients and haematopoietic neoplasms – in 10 (38.5%). Qualitative, semi-quantitative or quantitative real-time Reverse transcription polymerase chain reaction (RT-PCR) was applied in all patients for screening of molecular abnormalities, as follows: (i) fusion transcripts *BCR-ABL* (P210; P190), *PML-RARA, AML1-ETO, CBFb-MYH11, MLL-AF9, MLL-AF6, DEK-CAN,* (ii) internal or partial tandem duplication of *FLT3* (*FLT3*-ITD) and *MLL* (*MLL*-ITD) genes respectively, (iii) aberrant over-expression of *Survivin, EVI1, BAALC, MLF1, PRAME, MDR1* and *AID* genes, and type A mutation of *NPM1* gene. At least one molecular marker was detected in all patients. The most frequent type of molecular abnormalities were the aberrant gene over-expression. Among the overexpressed genes, *MDR1* over-expression was the most common finding. The established frequency (61.5%) was significantly higher compared to that in patients with de novo AML (25.0%) (Schaich et al., 2004). Molecular equivalents of recurrent translocations according to the WHO classification (2008) were found in 34.6% of the cases [9/26]. The "favourable" fusion transcripts *PML-RARA, CBFb-MYH11, AML1-ETO* were detected in 30.8% of t-AML, and their frequency was similar to that reported in de novo AML (Grimwade et al., 2010). In contrast, the *MLL*-PTD was significantly more frequent (11.5%) compared to de novo AML (5.0%) (Patel et al., 2012), while the incidence of *FLT3*-ITD was significantly lower (7.7% vs 25-25%) (Kindler et al., 2010). Despite the remarkable heterogeneity of detected molecular abnormalities, three groups of t-AML could be defined including: patients with "favourable" fusion transcripts,patients with overexpression of multiple "unfavourable" genes, and patients without a specific pattern (Data presented on Table 5.).

Eight of the patients (30.8%) beared "favourable" fusion transcripts *PML-RARA, CBFb-MYH11,* or *AML1-ETO* mRNA. In addition, *PRAME*(+) was observed in 3/7 evaluable cases, as well as *FLT3*-ITD, *Survivin*(+) and *NPM1* mutation – found in 1 case each. *MDR1*overexpression was found in 5/8 (62.5%) patients. Interestingly, the patients in this group were significantly younger compared to the remaining patients (41.9 yrs vs 57.8 yrs, respectively). The analysis identified 7 (26.7%) patients with with multiple "unfavourable" abnormalities - *BAALC* and *Survivin* genes were overexpressed in 7/7 cases, in combination with *EVI1* gene overexpression in 5/7 patients or *MLF1* – in 4/7, *MLL*-PTD – in 2/7, *FLT3*-ITD - in 1/7. Interestingly ≥3 concomitant arerrations were detected in 6/7 cases. *MDR1* overexpression was found in all patients. The remaining 11 (42.3%) patients did not show any specific pattern. Single molecular abnormalities such as *MLL*-PTD; *MLL-AF9; EVI1* gene overexpression, associated with *Survivin*(+) in half of the cases were observed, while *MDR1* overexpression was found in 5/11 (45.4%) patients. Clinical observation revealed 6 cases of early deaths. The OS was significantly different in the three groups (log rank test p=0.006) being the worst in patients with with multiple "unfavourable" abnormalities and the best – in the "favourable"fusion transcripts group (Balatzenko & Guenova, 2012).

6.4. Cooperating mutations in MDS and AML

According to the model proposed by Deguchi & Gilliland (2002), development of AML is the consequence of collaboration between at least two broad classes of mutations: (i) class I mutations which result in constitutively activated tyrosine kinases (gain of function) and confer a proliferative and/or survival advantage without affecting differentiation - *c-KIT* D816, *FLT3*-ITD; *FLT3* D835Y; N- or K-*RAS* mutations; *PTPN11; JAK3;* and (ii) class II mutations that affect genes encoding hematopoietic transcription factors (loss of function) and serve primarily to impair hematopoietic differentiation - *RUNX1-EVI1; RUNX1-ETO; CBFb-MYH11; MLL* fusions; *NUP98-HOXA9; C/EBPa; PU.1; NPM1* (Deguchi & Gilliland, 2002; Stavropoulou et al., 2010). In a recent study of 140 cases of t-AML, 33 (26%) showed evidence of Class I mutations, 47 (34%) - of Class II mutations, and only 18 (13%) demonstrated both Class I and Class II mutations (Pedersen-Bjergaardet al., 2006). Several studies confirm the applicability of the model of collaboration between the classes of mutations in t-AML.

At least 14 different genes have been identified as mutated in t-MDS and t-AML, clustering differently and characteristically in the eight genetic pathways. Class I and Class II mutations are significantly associated, indicating their cooperation in leukemogenesis (Pedersen-Bjergaard et al., 2007). Several examples of such cooperative genetic alterations were reported.

Group	Patient's age and gender	*BCR-ABL*	*PML-RARA*	*AML-ETO*	*CBFb-MYH11*	*MLL-AF9*	*MLL-AF6*	*MLL-PTD*	*FLT3-ITD*	*DEK-CAN*	*EVI1*	*BAACL*	*MLF1*	*PRAME*	*MDR1*	*Survivin*	*AID*	*NPM1 Mut A*
I n=8 30.8%	52/m	0	1	0	0	0	0	0	0	0	0	0	0	0	0	0	0	0
	62/f	0	1	0	0	0	0	0	0	0	0	0	0	0	0	0	0	0
	49/f	0	1	0	0	0	0	0	1	0	0	0	0	1	1	0	0	0
	23/f	0	0	0	1	0	0	0	0	0	0	0	0	0	1	1	0	1
	27/f	0	0	0	1	0	0	0	0	0	0	0	0	0	0	0	0	0
	72/m	0	0	1	0	0	0	0	0	0	0	0	0	0	1	0	0	0
	28/m	0	0	1	0	0	0	0	0	0	0	0	0	1	1	0	0	0
	22/m	0	0	1	0	0	0	0	0	0	0	0	0	1	1	0	0	0
II n=7 26.9%	67/f	0	0	0	0	0	0	0	1	0	0	1	1	0	1	1	0	0
	48/f	0	0	0	0	0	0	0	0	0	1	1	1	0	1	1	0	1
	65/f	0	0	0	0	0	0	0	0	0	1	1	0	0	1	1	0	0
	50/f	0	0	0	0	0	0	1	0	0	1	1	1	1	1	1	0	0
	30/m	0	0	0	0	0	0	1	0	0	1	1	0	0	1	1	0	1
	57/m	0	0	0	0	0	0	0	0	0	1	1	1	0	1	1	0	0
	82/m	0	0	0	0	0	0	0	0	0	0	1	0	0	1	1	0	0
III n=11 42.3%	57/f	0	0	0	0	0	0	0	0	0	1	0	1	0	1	N	0	0
	83/m	0	0	0	0	0	0	1	0	0	0	0	0	0	0	0	0	0
	74/m	0	0	0	0	0	0	0	0	0	0	0	0	0	1	1	0	N
	44/f	0	0	0	0	0	0	0	0	0	0	0	0	0	0	1	0	0
	67/f	0	0	0	0	0	0	0	0	0	0	0	0	0	1	1	0	1
	47/f	0	0	0	0	0	0	0	0	0	0	0	1	0	0	0	0	1
	56/m	0	0	0	0	0	0	0	0	0	0	0	0	0	0	1	0	0
	55/f	0	0	0	0	0	0	0	0	0	0	0	0	0	1	0	0	0
	68/m	0	0	0	0	0	0	0	0	0	0	0	N	0	0	0	0	0
	49/m	0	0	0	0	0	0	0	0	0	0	0	0	0	1	0	0	0
	41/f	0	0	0	0	1	0	0	0	0	0	0	0	0	0	0	0	0
Total		0%	11.5%	11.5%	7.7%	3.8%	0%	11.5%	7.7%	0%	23.1%	26.9%	24.0%	15.4%	61.5%	48.0%	0%	16%

Table 5. Molecular alterations in therapy-related acute myeloid leukemias. Group I - patients with "favourable" fusion transcripts, Group II - patients with overexpression of multiple "unfavourable" genes, Group III - patients without a specific pattern. Abreviations: f – female, m – male, N – not done.

Mutations of *RUNX1* are common in therapy-related myelodysplasia following therapy with alkylating agents and are significantly associated with deletion or loss of chromosome arm 7q and with a subsequent leukemic transformation. *FLT3* mutation and trisomy 21 are thought to be second hits in AML with *RUNX1* Mutations (Osato M., 2004; Christiansen et al., 2004). Another example that supported cooperation between Class I and Class II mutations in leukemogenesis is the report of 4 cases with mutations of the *PTPN11* gene; 3 of which had -7/7q-, 2 cases had rare balanced translocations to chromosome band 21q22 with rearrangement of the *RUNX1* gene and the other two patients had rare balanced translocations to chromosome band 3q26 with a rearrangement of the *EVI1* gene (Christiansen et al., 2007). Significant association had also been reported between –5/5q– and *p53* mutations and complex chromosome rearrangements; *MLL* rearrangements and mutations of *NRAS, KRAS* or *BRAF*; *PML-RARA* and *FLT3*-ITD; *RUNX1* mutations (Class II) and *N-RAS* mutation (Class I); *MLL-CBP* (Class II) and *FLT3*-ITD (Class I), etc. (Imagawa et al., 2010). Many of the associations observed in t-AML, such as the *NPM1-FLT3, AML1-cKIT* and *RARA-FLT3* combinations, have previously been emphasized in de novo AML. According to Pedersen-Bjergaard et al., 2007, in t-AML, at least 8 alternative genetic pathways have been defined based on characteristic recurrent chromosome abnormalities: (i) patients with 7q–/–7 but normal chromosomes 5 and without balanced aberrations, (ii) patients with 5q–/–5, but without balanced aberrations; (iii) patients with t-AML and balanced translocations involving the chromosomal band 11q23, resulting in chimeric rearrangements between the MLL gene and one of its numerous alternative partner genes; (iv) patients with balanced translocations to chromosome band 21q22 or inv(16); (v) patients with promyelocytic leukemia and chimeric rearrangement of the PML and RARA genes; (vi) patients with chimeric rearrangement of the NUP98 gene on 11p15; (vii) patients with a normal karyotype; (viii) patients with other, often unique chromosome aberrations.

7. Prognostic factors

The diagnosis of therapy-related myeloid leukemia (t-MDS/t-AML) identifies a group of high-risk patients with multiple and varied poor prognostic features (Larson, 2007), such as overrepresentation of 11q23 translocations, adverse cytogenetics, including complex and monosomal karyotypes, and *MDR1* gene overexpression, as well as reduced frequency of "favorable" *NPM1*, and *CEBPA* mutations. Besides, frequent comorbidities and cummulative toxicities, related to previous cytotoxic treatments also contribute to a worse prognosis compared to de novo AML (D'Alò et al., 2011; Kayser S, et al., 2011). In a recent study, the outcome of patients with t-AML was significantly inferior in comparison to de novo AML: the 4-year relapse-free survival (RFS) was 24.5% versus 39.5%; and the 4-year overall survival (OS) was of 25.5% versus and 37.9%, respectively (Kayser et al., 2011). During the follow-up of 109 t-AML patients after treatment for epithelial ovarian carcinoma, a median survival of 3 months from the time of secondary leukemia diagnosis was found compared to 6 month in patients with de novo AML (Vay et al., 2011). Schoch et al., 2004 found significantly shorter median OS in t-AML than in de novo AML (10 vs 15 months). Within patients with t-

AML, there were significant correlations between OS and both unfavorable and favorable cytogenetics, while age and WBC count had no impact on OS (Schoch et al., 2004). The critical impact of karyotype on the prognosis was reported by Kern et al., clearly demonstrated significant differences in the median survival between t-AML patients groups with favorable karyotype (26.7 months) and unfavorable karyotype (5.6 months) (Kern et al., 2004).

Encouraging results were reported after allogeneic hematopoietic stem cells transplantation (allo-HSCT). The follow-up of 461 patients with t-MDS or t-AML who underwent allo-HSCT detected 3-year RFS and OS rates of 33% and 35%, respectively. In a multivariate analysis, the following risk factors were identified: (1) not being in complete remission at the time of transplantation, (2) abnormal cytogenetics, (3) higher patients' age and (4) therapy-related MDS. Using age (<40 years), abnormal cytogenetics and not being in complete remission at the time of transplantation as risk factors, three different risk groups with OS of 62%, 33% and 24% could be easily distinguished (Kröger et al., 2009). Similar results were observed by Litzow et al., 2010. The analysis of outcomes in a total of 868 patients, including t-AML (n=545) or t-MDS (n=323), revealed disease-free (DFS) and OS of 32% and 37% at 1 year and 21% and 22% at 5 years, respectively. In a multivariate analysis, 4 risk factors with adverse impacts on DFS and OS were identified: (1) age older than 35 years; (2) poor-risk cytogenetics; (3) t-AML not in remission or advanced t-MDS; and (4) donor other than an HLA-identical sibling or a partially or well-matched unrelated donor. The 5-years survival for subjects with none, 1, 2, 3, or 4 of these risk factors was 50%, 26%, 21%, 10%, and 4%, respectively [Litzow et al.,2010].

T-AMLs with "favorable" genetic abnormalities involving CBF-transcription complex - t(8;21)/*RUNX1-ETO* and inv(16)/t(16;16)/*CBFβ-MYH1* and APL with t(15;17)/*PML-RARα* are of particular interest since the reported results concerning the prognostic significance of these aberrations are contradictory and vary from study to study.

According to some studies these patients have treatment outcome comparable with primary AML patients (de Witte et al., 2002). Complete remission can be obtained in 85% of intensively treated patients with inv(16), and in 69% with t(15;17), with a median OS of 29 months in both cytogenetic subgroups, thus the response rates to intensive chemotherapy are comparable to those of de novo disease (Andersen et al., 2002). Similarly, t-AML with t(15;17) and t(8;21), treated according to standard protocols, had an outcome similar to de novo cases, indicating the dominant prognostic role of good karyotypes (D'Alò et al., 2011). The comparison of clinical and pathologic findings in therapy-related APL and de novo APL cases revealed abnormal promyelocytes with similar morphologic and immunophenotypic features, comparable cytogenetic findings, comparable rates of FMS-like tyrosine kinase mutations, and similar rates of recurrent disease and death, suggesting that secondary APL is similar to de novo APL and, thus, should be considered distinct from other secondary acute myeloid neoplasms (Duffield et al., 2012).

In contrast, matched analysis (by age, Eastern Cooperative Oncology Group performance status, and additional cytogenetic abnormalities) indicated worse OS and event-free survival (EFS) in patients with therapy-related CBF AML carrying the recurrent chromosomal aberrations inv(16) or t(8;21) – a median OS of 100 weeks compared to 376 weeks in de novo CBF AMLs (Borthakuret al., 2009). In patients with t-AML and t(8;21), the OS is significantly inferior to that of patients with de novo t(8;21) AMLs (19 months vs not reached). These findings suggest that t(8;21) t-AMLs share many features with de novo AML with t(8;21)(q22;q22), but the affected patients have a worse outcome (Gustafson et al., 2009). Interstingly, it has been reported recently that despite that fewer complete remissions are achieved in t-APL (63.6%) compared to de novo APL (92.5%), this was a result of the higher induction mortality rate of 36.4% vs. 7.5%, respectively. No cases of leukemic resistance were seen in either group. However, OS was also inferior in t-APL compared to de novo APL (51% vs. 84%, respectively) (Elliott et al., 2012).

8. Treatment

The survival of patients with t-AML is often poor despite prompt diagnosis and treatment. There is a paucity of prospective treatment data since these patients are often excluded from frontline chemotherapy trials and turned to best supportive care. However, despite that the CR rate of t-AML patients (28% up to 50%) has been demonstrated to be inferior to patients with de novo AML (65-80%), this difference can be attributed to the higher number of patients with unfavourable karyotypes. Within cytogenetically defined subgroups, the prognosis of t-AML patients does not differ significantly from patients with de novo AML. Treatment recommendations should be further based on the patient's performance status, which likely reflects age, comorbidities, the status of the primary disease, and the presence of complications from primary therapy, as well as the clonal abnormalities detected in the t-AML cells. Standard chemotherapy, haematopoietic stem cell transplantation, as well as experimental trials are applied.

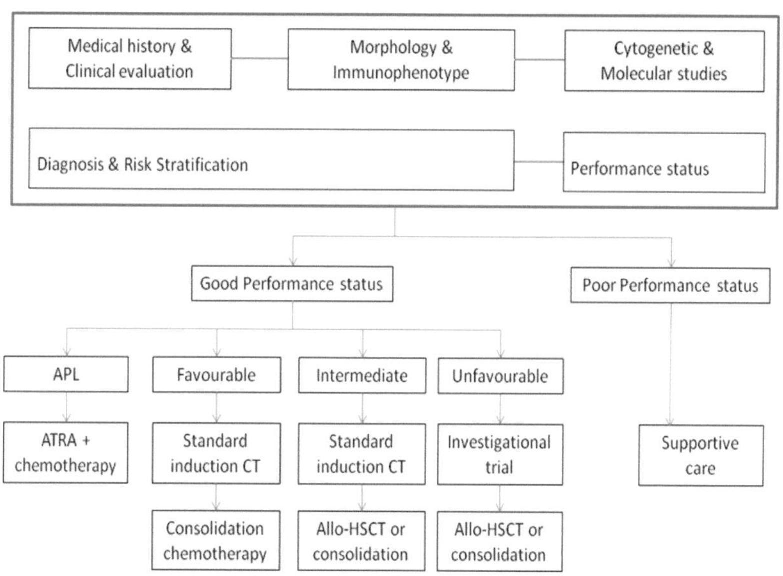

Figure 1. Clinical algorythm in the management of t-AML patients.

Intriguingly, several studies found that results after induction therapy were not different between t-AML and de novo AML patients. Furthermore, analyses of CR-rates, OS and DFS, when corrected for the influence of age, cytogenetic abnormalities, performance status and leucocyte count, showed that the presence of a t-AML may even lose prognostic significance and patients with secondary AML should be offered the chance of benefiting from treatment according to current frontline AML protocols (Ostgård et al., 2010). The dosage and modality of treatment during postremission therapy however have a marked impact on the cumulative toxicity of cancer therapy. Therefore, intensive induction therapy should not be withheld for t-AML patients, and dose-reduced regimes for allogeneic HSCT should be considered. In contrast, t-AML patients >60 years show a significantly greater relapse rates probably due to the lower dosage of applied chemotherapy during postremission therapy compared with younger patients (Kayser et al., 2011). Encouraging results are reported after allogeneic transplantation. The identification of relevant risk factors allows for a more precise prediction of outcome and identification of subjects most likely to benefit from allogeneic transplantation.Allogeneic transplantation should be proposed timely to these patients after an accurate analysis of patient history (Litzow et al., 2010; Spina et al., 2012). Novel transplantation strategies using reduced intensity conditioning regimens as well as novel drugs – demethylating agents and targeted therapies, await clinical testing and may improve outcome (de Witte et al., 2002).

9. Conclusion

As the number of patients with t-AMLs is expected to rise, safety issues of cytotoxic therapies are becoming increasingly important in order to develop strategies to reduce the risk for therapy-related malignancies without compromising success rates for the respective primary disorders. Besides, there is clinical and biological overlap between therapy related and high-risk de novo leukaemias suggesting similar mechanisms of leukaemogenesis. Deeper insights into pathogenetic mechanisms will eventually help to establish a more differentiated clinical approach to successfully treat, but hopefully also prevent, these often fatal consequences of cytotoxic therapies.

Acknowledgements

The reported own data on therapy-related AML were generated in the Center of Excellence "Translational Research in Haematology" of the National Specialised Hospital for Active Treatment of Hematological Diseases, supported by National Science Fund (grant CVP01-119/D02-35/2009), as follows: morphology and immunophenotype were evaluated at the Laboratory of Haematopathology and Immunology, cytogenetic and molecular studies were performed at the Laboratory of Cytogenetics and Molecular Biology, clinical management was performed at the Haematology Clinic. MG and GB contributed equally to the development of the manuscript. GM was responsible for the treatment section. MG and GB

http://dx.doi.org/10.5772/52459

have been supported by EuGESMA COST Action BM0801: European Genetic and Epigenetic Study on AML and MDS.

Author details

Margarita Guenova[1,4*], Gueorgui Balatzenko[2,4] and Georgi Mihaylov[3,4]

*Address all correspondence to: margenova@gmail.com

1 Laboratory of Haematopathology and Immunology, National Specialized Hospital for Active Treatment of Haematological Diseases, Sofia, Bulgaria

2 Laboratory of Cytogenetics and Molecular Biology, National Specialized Hospital for Active Treatment of Haematological Diseases, Sofia, Bulgaria

3 Haematology Clinic, National Specialized Hospital for Active Treatment of Haematological Diseases, Sofia, Bulgaria

4 Center of Excellence – Translational Research in Haematology, National Specialized Hospital for Active Treatment of Haematological Diseases, Sofia, Bulgaria

References

[1] Abbas, S., Lugthart, S., Kavelaars, F. G., Schelen, A., Koenders, J. E., Zeilemaker, A., van Putten, W. J., Rijneveld, A. W., Löwenberg, B., & Valk, P. J. Acquired mutations in the genes encoding IDH1 and IDH2 both are recurrent aberrations in acute myeloid leukemia: prevalence and prognostic value. Blood. (2010). , 116(12), 2122-6.

[2] Ahmad F, Mandava S, Das BR. Mutations of NPM1 gene in de novo acute myeloid leukaemia: determination of incidence, distribution pattern and identification of two novel mutations in Indian population. Hematol Oncol. 2009;27(2):90-7.

[3] Allan, J. M., Wild, Rollinson. S., Willett, E. V., Moorman, A. V., Dovey, G. J., Roddam, P. L., Roman, E., Cartwright, R. A., & Morgan, G. J. Polymorphism in glutathione S-transferase is associated with susceptibility to chemotherapy-induced leukemia. Proc Natl Acad Sci U S A. (2001). , 1.

[4] Andersen, M. K., Johansson, B., Larsen, S. O., & Pedersen-Bjergaard, J. Chromosomal abnormalities in secondary MDS and AML.Relationship to drugs and radiation with specific emphasis on the balanced rearrangements.Haematologica. (1998). Jun;, 83(6), 483-8.

[5] Andersen, M. K., Christiansen, D. H., Kirchhoff, M., & Pedersen-Bjergaard, J. Duplication or amplification of chromosome band 11q23, including the unrearranged MLL

gene, is a recurrent abnormality in therapy-related MDS an dAML, and is closely related to mutation of the TP53 gene and to previous therapy with alkylating agents. Genes Chromosomes Cancer. (2001)., 31(1), 33-41.

[6] Andersen, M. K., Larson, R. A., Mauritzson, N., Schnittger, S., Jhanwar, S. C., & Pedersen-Bjergaard, J. Balanced chromosome abnormalities inv(16) and t(15;17) in therapy-related myelodysplastic syndromes and acute leukemia: report from an international workshop. Genes Chromosomes Cancer. (2002)., 33(4), 395-400.

[7] Andersen, M. K., Christiansen, D. H., & Pedersen-Bjergaard, J. Centromeric breakage and highly rearranged chromosome derivatives associated with mutations of TP53 are common in therapy-related MDS and AML after therapy with alkylating agents: an M-FISH study. Genes Chromosomes Cancer. (2005)., 42(4), 358-71.

[8] Anderson, L. A., Pfeiffer, R. M., Landgren, O., Gadalla, S., Berndt, S. I., & Engels, E. A. Risks of myeloid malignancies in patients with autoimmune conditions. Br J Cancer. (2009)., 100(5), 822-8.

[9] Arber, D. A., Slovak, M. L., Popplewell, L., Bedell, V., Ikle, D., Rowley, , International, Workshop., on, Leukemia., Karyotype, , & Prior, Therapy. Therapy-related acute myeloid leukemia/myelodysplasia with balanced 21q22 translocations.Am J Clin Pathol. (2002)., 117(2), 306-13.

[10] Askling, J., Fored, C. M., Baecklund, E., Brandt, L., Backlin, C., Ekbom, A., et al. Haematopoietic malignancies in rheumatoid arthritis: lymphoma risk and characteristics after exposure to tumour necrosis factor antagonists. Ann Rheum Dis. (2005)., 64(10), 1414-20.

[11] Au, W. Y., Wan, S. K., Man, T. S., Kwong, C., & , Y. L. Pentasomy 8q in therapy-related myelodysplastic syndrome due to cyclophosphamide therapy for fibrosing alveolitis. Cancer Genet Cytogenet. (2003)., 141(1), 79-82.

[12] Bacher, U., Haferlach, C., Schnittger, D., Alpermann, T., Kern, W., & Haferlach, T. Patients with Therapy-Related Myeloid Disorders Share Genetic Features but Can Be Separated by Blast Counts and Cytogenetic Risk Groups Into Prognostically Relevant Subgroups, Blood (ASH Annual Meeting Abstracts), (2011). Abstract 3583

[13] Bacher U, Haferlach T, Kern W, Haferlach C, Schnittger S.A comparative study of molecular mutations in 381 patients with myelodysplastic syndrome and in 4130 patients with acute myeloid leukemia.Haematologica. 2007;92(6):744-52.

[14] Balatzenko, G., & Guenova, M. Spectrum of molecular alterations in therapy-related acute myeloid leukemias. COST Action:BM0801: 8th MC meeting & 6th WG meeting. April (2012). Beldrade, Serbia, 23-24.

[15] Barlogie, B., Tricot, G., Haessler, J., van Rhee, F., Cottler-Fox, M., Anaissie, E., Waldron, J., Pineda-Roman, M., Thertulien, R., Zangari, M., Hollmig, K., Mohiuddin, A., Alsayed, Y., Hoering, A., Crowley, J., & Sawyer, J. Cytogenetically defined myelodysplasia after melphalan-based autotransplantation for multiple myeloma linked to

poor hematopoietic stem-cell mobilization: the Arkansas experience in more than 3,000 patients treated since 1989. Blood. (2008)., 111(1), 94-100.

[16] Barnard DR, Woods WG.Treatment-related myelodysplastic syndrome/acute myeloid leukemia in survivors of childhood cancer--an update. Leuk Lymphoma. (2005)., 46(5), 651-63.

[17] Beekman R, Touw IP. G-CSF and its receptor in myeloid malignancy.Blood. 2010;115(25):5131-6.

[18] Bennett, J. M., Troxel, A. B., Gelman, R., Falkson, G., Coccia-Portugal, Dreicer. R., Tormey, D. C., & Rushing, D. Myelodysplastic syndrome and acute myeloid leukemia secondary to mitolactol treatment in patients with breast cancer. J Clin Oncol. (1994)., 12(4), 874-5.

[19] Bhatia, S., Robison, L. L., Oberlin, O., Greenberg, M., Bunin, G., Fossati-Bellani, F., & Meadows, A. T. Breast cancer and other second neoplasms after childhood Hodgkin's disease. N Engl J Med. (1996)., 334(12), 745-51.

[20] Bhavnani M, Azzawi SA, Yin JA, Lucas GS.Therapy-related acute promyelocytic leukaemia.Br J Haematol. 1994;86(1):231-2.

[21] Blanco, J. G., Dervieux, T., Edick, Mehta. P. K., Rubnitz, J. E., Shurtleff, S., Raimondi, S. C., Behm, F. G., Pui, C. H., & Relling, M. V. Molecular emergence of acute myeloid leukemia during treatment for acute lymphoblastic leukemia. Proc Natl Acad Sci U S A. (2001)., 98(18), 10338-43.

[22] Bo, J., Schrøder, H., Kristinsson, J., Madsen, B., Szumlanski, C., Weinshilboum, R., Andersen, J. B., & Schmiegelow, K. Possible carcinogenic effect of 6-mercaptopurine on bone marrow stem cells: relation to thiopurine metabolism. Cancer.(1999)., 86(6), 1080-6.

[23] Bodner SM, Naeve CW, Rakestraw KM, Jones BG, Valentine VA, Valentine MB, Luthardt FW, Willman CL, Raimondi SC, Downing JR, Roussel MF, Sherr CJ, Look AT.Cloning and chromosomal localization of the gene encoding human cyclin Dbinding Myb-like protein (hDMP1). Gene. (1999).,229(1-2), 223-8.

[24] Bogni, A., Cheng, C., Liu, W., Yang, W., Pfeffer, J., Mukatira, S., French, D., Downing, J. R., Pui, C. H., & Relling, M. V. Genome-wide approach to identify risk factors for therapy-related myeloid leukemia.Leukemia. (2006)., 20(2), 239-46.

[25] Boice Jr, Greene. M. H., Killen, J. Y., Jr Ellenberg, S. S., Keehn, R. J., Mc Fadden, E., Chen, T. T., Fraumeni, J. F., & Jr , . Leukemia and preleukemia after adjuvant treatment of gastrointestinal cancer with semustine (methyl-CCNU). N Engl J Med. (1983)., 309(18), 1079-84.

[26] Bolufer, P., Collado, M., Barragan, E., Calasanz, Colomer. D., Tormo, M., González, M., Brunet, S., Batlle, M., Cervera, J., & Sanz, . Profile of polymorphisms of drug-metabolising enzymes and the risk of therapy-related leukaemia.Br J Haematol. (2007)., 136(4), 590-6.

[27] Borthakur, G., Lin, E., Jain, N., Estey, Cortes. J. E., O'Brien, S., Faderl, S., Ravandi, F., Pierce, S., & Kantarjian, H. Survival is poorer in patients with secondary core-binding factor acute myelogenous leukemia compared with de novo core-binding factor leukemia. Cancer. (2009). , 115(14), 3217-21.

[28] Boultwood, J., Fidler, C., Strickson, A. J., Watkins, F., Gama, S., Kearney, L., Tosi, S., Kasprzyk, A., Cheng, J. F., Jaju, R. J., & Wainscoat, J. S. Narrowing and genomic annotation of the commonly deleted region of the 5q- syndrome.Blood. (2002). , 99(12), 4638-41.

[29] Carli, P. M., Sgro, C., Parchin-Geneste, N., Isambert, N., Mugneret, F., Girodon, F., & Maynadié, M. Increase therapy-related leukemia secondary to breast cancer. Leukemia. (2000). , 14(6), 1014-7.

[30] Chak LY, Sikic BI, Tucker MA, Horns RC Jr, Cox RS.Increased incidence of acute nonlymphocytic leukemia following therapy in patients with small cell carcinoma of the lung.J Clin Oncol. (1984). , 2(5), 385-90.

[31] Chakraborty, S., Sun, C. L., Francisco, L., Sabado, M., Li, L., Chang, K. L., Forman, S., Bhatia, S., & Bhatia, R. Accelerated telomere shortening precedes development of therapy-related myelodysplasia or acute myelogenous leukemia after autologous transplantation for lymphoma. J Clin Oncol. (2009). , 27(5), 791-8.

[32] Chandra, P., Luthra, R., Zuo, Z., Yao, H., Ravandi, F., Reddy, N., Garcia-Manero, G., Kantarjian, H., & Jones, D. Acute myeloid leukemia with t(9;11)(q23): common properties of dysregulated ras pathway signaling and genomic progression characterize de novo and therapy-related cases. Am J Clin Pathol. (2010)., 133(5), 21-22.

[33] Chillón, M. C., Santamaría, C., García-Sanz, R., Balanzategui, A., Sarasquete, Alcoceba. M., Marín, L., Caballero, Vidriales. M. B., Ramos, F., Bernal, T., Díaz-Mediavilla, J., García de, Coca. A., Peñarrubia, Queizán. J. A., Giraldo, P., San, Miguel. J. F., & González, M. Long FLT3 internal tandem duplications and reduced PML-RARα expression at diagnosis characterize a high-risk subgroup of acute promyelocytic leukemia patients. Haematologica. (2010). , 95(5), 745-51.

[34] Christiansen, D. H., Andersen, M. K., Desta, F., & Pedersen-Bjergaard, J. Mutations of genes in the receptor tyrosine kinase (RTK)/RAS-BRAF signal transduction pathway in therapy-related myelodysplasia and acute myeloid leukemia. Leukemia. (2005). , 19(12), 2232-40.

[35] Christiansen DH, Andersen MK, Desta F, Pedersen-Bjergaard J. Mutations of genes in the receptor tyrosine kinase (RTK)/RAS-BRAF signal transduction pathway in therapy-related myelodysplasia and acute myeloid leukemia. Leukemia. 2005;19(12): 2232-40.

[36] Christiansen, D. H., Desta, F., Andersen, M. K., & Pedersen-Bjergaard, J. Mutations of the PTPN11 gene in therapy-related MDS and AML with rare balanced chromosome translocations. Genes Chromosomes Cancer. (2007). , 46(6), 517-21.

[37] Cimino, G., Papa, G., Tura, S., Mazza, P., Rossi, Ferrini. P. L., Bosi, A., Amadori, S., Lo, Coco. F., D'Arcangelo, E., Giannarelli, D., et al. Second primary cancer following Hodgkin's disease: updated results of an Italian multicentric study. J Clin Oncol. (1991). , 9(3), 432-7.

[38] Collins, C. M., Morgan, Mosse. C., & Sosman, J. Dacarbazine induced acute myeloid leukemia in melanoma. Melanoma Res. (2009). , 19(5), 337-40.

[39] Colovic, N., Suvajdzic, N., Kraguljac, Kurtovic. N., Djordjevic, V., Dencic, Fekete. M., Drulovic, J., Vidovic, A., & Tomin, D. Therapy-related acute leukemia in two patients with multiple sclerosis treated with Mitoxantrone. Biomed Pharmacother. (2012). , 66(3), 173-4.

[40] Cowell IG, Sondka Z, Smith K, Lee KC, Manville CM, Sidorczuk-Lesthuruge M, Rance HA, Padget K, Jackson GH, Adachi N, Austin CA. Model for MLL translocations in therapy-related leukemia involving topoisomerase IIβ-mediated DNA strand breaks and gene proximity. Proc Natl Acad Sci U S A. 2012;109(23):8989-94.

[41] Curtis, R. E., Boice, Stovall. M., et al. Risk of leukemia after chemotherapy and radiation treatment for breast cancer. N Engl J Med (1992). , 326, 1754-1.

[42] Czader M, Orazi A. Therapy-related myeloid neoplasms. Am J Clin Pathol. 2009;132(3):410-25.

[43] D'Alò, F., Fianchi, L., Fabiani, E., Criscuolo, M., Greco, M., Guidi, F., Pagano, L., Leone, G., & Voso, M. T. Similarities and differences between therapy-related and elderly acute myeloid leukemia.Mediterr J Hematol Infect Dis. (2011). e2011052

[44] Dann EJ, Rowe JM.Biology and therapy of secondary leukaemias. Best Pract Res Clin Haematol. (2001). , 14(1), 119-37.

[45] Dastugue N, Pris J, Colombies P. Translocation t(3;21)(q26;q22) in acute myeloblastic leukemia secondary to polycythemia vera. Cancer Genet Cytogenet.1990;44(2):275-6.

[46] de Witte, T., Oosterveld, M., Span, B., Muus, P., & Schattenberg, A. Stem cell transplantation for leukemias following myelodysplastic syndromes or secondary to cytotoxic therapy. Rev Clin Exp Hematol. (2002). , 6(1), 72-85.

[47] Deguchi, K., & Gilliland, D. G. Cooperativity between mutations in tyrosine kinases and in hematopoietic transcription factors in AML. Leukemia. (2002). , 16(4), 740-4.

[48] Devereux, S., Selassie, T. G., Vaughan, Hudson. G., Vaughan, Hudson. B., & Linch, D. C. Leukaemia complicating treatment for Hodgkin's disease: the experience of the British National Lymphoma Investigation. BMJ. (1990). , 301(6760), 1077-80.

[49] Diamandidou, E., Buzdar, A. U., Smith, T. L., Frye, D., Witjaksono, M., & Hortobagyi, G. N. Treatment-related leukemia in breast cancer patients treated with fluorouracil-doxorubicin-cyclophosphamide combination adjuvant chemotherapy: theUniversity of Texas M.D. Anderson Cancer Center experience. J Clin Oncol. (1996). , 14(10), 2722-30.

[50] Dissing, M., Le Beau-Bjergaard, Pedersen., & , J. Inversion of chromosome 16 and uncommon rearrangements of the CBFB and MYH11 genes in therapy-related acute myeloid leukemia: rare events related to DNA-topoisomerase II inhibitors? J Clin Oncol. (1998). , 16(5), 1890-6.

[51] Döhner, K., Brown, J., Hehmann, U., Hetzel, C., Stewart, J., Lowther, G., Scholl, C., Fröhling, S., Cuneo, A., Tsui, L. C., Lichter, P., Scherer, S. W., & Döhner, H. Molecular cytogenetic characterization of a critical region in bands 7q35-q36 commonly deleted in malignant myeloid disorders. Blood. (1998). , 92(11), 4031-5.

[52] Dores, G. M., Metayer, C., Curtis, R. E., Lynch, C. F., Clarke, E. A., Glimelius, B., Storm, H., Pukkala, E., van Leeuwen, F. E., Holowaty, E. J., Andersson, M., Wiklund, T., Joensuu, T., van't, Veer. M. B., Stovall, M., Gospodarowicz, M., & Travis, L. B. Second malignant neoplasms amonglong-term survivors of Hodgkin's disease: a population-based evaluation over 25 years. J Clin Oncol. (2002). , 20(16), 3484-94.

[53] Douer, D., Santillana, S., Ramezani, L., Samanez, C., Slovak, M. L., Lee, Watkins. K., Williams, T., & Vallejos, C. Acute promyelocytic leukaemia in patients originating in Latin America is associated with an increased frequency of the bcr1 subtype of the PML/RARalpha fusion gene. Br J Haematol. (2003). , 122(4), 563-70.

[54] Drabløs, F., Feyzi, E., Vaagbø, P. A., Kavli, C. B., Bratlie, B., Peña-Diaz, J., Otterlei, M., Slupphaug, G., & Krokan, H. E. Alkylation damage in DNA and RNA--repair mechanisms and medical significance. DNA Repair (Amst). (2004). , 3(11), 1389-407.

[55] Duffield, Aoki. J., Levis, M., Cowan, K., Gocke, C. D., Burns, K. H., Borowitz-Ross, Vuica., & , M. Clinical and pathologic features of secondary acute promyelocytic leukemia. Am J Clin Pathol. (2012). , 137(3), 395-402.

[56] Eguchi, M., Eguchi-Ishimae, M., & Greaves, M. Molecular pathogenesis of MLL-associated leukemias. Int J Hematol. (2005). , 82(1), 9-20.

[57] Elliott, Letendre. L., Tefferi, A., Hogan, W. J., Hook, C., Kaufmann, S. H., Pruthi, R. K., Pardanani, A., Begna, K. H., Ashrani, Wolanskyj. A. P., Al-Kali, A., & Litzow, M. R. Therapy-related acute promyelocytic leukemia: observations relating to APL pathogenesis and therapy. Eur J Haematol. (2012). , 88(3), 237-43.

[58] Ellis NA, Huo D, Yildiz O, Worrillow LJ, Banerjee M, Le Beau MM, Larson RA,Allan JM, Onel K. MDM2 SNP309 and TP53 Arg72Pro interact to alter therapy-related acute myeloid leukemia susceptibility. Blood. 2008;112(3):741-9.

[59] Emerling BM, Bonifas J, Kratz CP, Donovan S, Taylor BR, Green ED, Le Beau MM, Shannon KM. MLL5, a homolog of Drosophila trithorax located within a segment of chromosome band 7q22 implicated in myeloid leukemia. Oncogene. 2002;21(31): 4849-54.

[60] Ezoe, S. Secondary Leukemia Associated with the Anti-Cancer Agent, Etoposide, a Topoisomerase II Inhibitor. Int J Environ Res Public Health. (2012). , 9(7), 2444-53.

[61] Faurschou, M., Sorensen, I. J., Mellemkjaer, L., Loft, A. G., Thomsen, Tvede. N., & Baslund, B. Malignancies in Wegener's granulomatosis: incidence and relation to cyclophosphamide therapy in a cohort of 293 patients. J Rheumatol. (2008). , 35(1), 100-5.

[62] Felix CA.Secondary leukemias induced by topoisomerase-targeted drugs. Biochim Biophys Acta. (1998).

[63] Felix CA, Hosler MR, Provisor D, Salhany K, Sexsmith EA, Slater DJ, Cheung NK,Winick NJ, Strauss EA, Heyn R, Lange BJ, Malkin D. The p53 gene in pediatric therapy-related leukemia and myelodysplasia.Blood. 1996;87(10):4376-81.

[64] Fisher, B., Rockette, H., Fisher, E. R., et al. Leukemia in breast cancer patients following adjuvant chemotherapy, or postoperative radiation: the NSABP experience. J Clin Oncol (1985)., 3, 1640-58.

[65] Flaig, T. W., Tangen, C. M., Hussain, M. H., Stadler, W. M., Raghavan, D., Crawford, E. D., Glodé, L. M., Southwest, Oncology., & Group, . Randomization reveals unexpected acute leukemias in Southwest Oncology Group prostate cancer trial. J Clin Oncol. (2008)., 26(9), 1532-6.

[66] Fried I, Bodner C, Pichler MM, Lind K, Beham-Schmid C, Quehenberger F, Sperr WR, Linkesch W, Sill H, Wölfler A. Frequency, onset and clinical impact of somatic DNMT3A mutations in therapy-related and secondary acute myeloid leukemia. Haematologica. 2012;97(2):246-50.

[67] Gaidzik VI, Bullinger L, Schlenk RF, Zimmermann AS, Röck J, Paschka P, Corbacioglu A, Krauter J, Schlegelberger B, Ganser A, Späth D, Kündgen A,Schmidt-Wolf IG, Götze K, Nachbaur D, Pfreundschuh M, Horst HA, Döhner H, Döhner K. RUNX1 mutations in acute myeloid leukemia: results from a comprehensive genetic and clinical analysis from the AML study group. J Clin Oncol. 2011;29(10):1364-72

[68] Godley LA, Larson RA.Therapy-related myeloid leukemia.Semin Oncol. (2008). , 35(4), 418-29.

[69] Godley LA, Le Beau MM. Therapy-Related AML. In: Acute Myelogenous Leukemia, Ed. Karp JE, Humana Press Inc.,. (2007). 71-96.

[70] Greco, M., D'Alò, F., Scardocci, A., Criscuolo, M., Fabiani, E., Guidi, F., Di Ruscio, A., Migliara, G., Pagano, L., Fianchi, L., Chiusolo, P., Hohaus, S., Leone, G., & Voso, M. T. Promoter methylation of DAPK1, E-cadherin and thrombospondin-1 in de novo and therapy-related myeloid neoplasms.Blood Cells Mol Dis. (2010)., 45(3), 181-5.

[71] Green CL, Koo KK, Hills RK, Burnett AK, Linch DC, Gale RE.Prognostic significance of CEBPA mutations in a large cohort of younger adult patients with acute myeloid leukemia: impact of double CEBPA mutations and the interaction with FLT3 and NPM1 mutations. J Clin Oncol. (2010)., 28(16), 2739-47.

[72] Griesinger, F., Metz, M., Trümper, L., Schulz, T., & Haase, D. Secondary leukaemia after cure for locally advanced NSCLC: alkylating type secondary leukaemia after in-

duction therapy with docetaxel and carboplatin for NSCLC IIIB. Lung Cancer. (2004)., 44(2), 261-5.

[73] Grimwade, D., Hills, R. K., Moorman, A. V., Walker, H., Chatters, S., Goldstone, A. H., Wheatley, K., Harrison, C. J., Burnett, A. K., National, Cancer., Research, Institute., Adult, Leukaemia., & Working, Group. Refinement of cytogenetic classification in acute myeloid leukemia: determination of prognostic significance of rare recurring chromosomal abnormalities among 5876 younger adult patients treated in the United Kingdom Medical Research Council trials. Blood. (2010)., 116(3), 354-65.

[74] Guidelines for CarcinogenRisk Assessment.EPA/630/F. Risk Assessment Forum U.S. Environmental Protection Agency, Washington, DC, (2005)., 03.

[75] Guillem VM, Collado M, Terol MJ, Calasanz MJ, Esteve J, Gonzalez M, Sanzo C,Nomdedeu J, Bolufer P, Lluch A, Tormo M. Role of MTHFR (677, 1298) haplotype in the risk of developing secondary leukemia after treatment of breast cancer and hematological malignancies. Leukemia. 2007;21(7):1413-22.

[76] Gustafson, S. A., Lin, P., Chen, S. S., Chen, L., Abruzzo, L. V., Luthra, R., Medeiros, L. J., & Wang, S. A. Therapy-related acute myeloid leukemia with t(8;21) (q22;q22) shares many features with de novo acute myeloid leukemia with t(8;21)(q22;q22) but does not have a favorable outcome. Am J Clin Pathol. (2009)., 131(5), 647-55.

[77] Harada, Y., & Harada, H. Molecular mechanisms that produce secondary MDS/AML by RUNX1/AML1 point mutations. J Cell Biochem.(2011)., 112(2), 425-32.

[78] Harper DP, Aplan PD.Chromosomal rearrangements leading to MLL gene fusions: clinical and biological aspects. Cancer Res. (2008)., 68(24), 10024-7.

[79] Hasan SK, Ottone T, Schlenk RF, Xiao Y, Wiemels JL, Mitra ME, Bernasconi P, Di Raimondo F, Stanghellini MT, Marco P, Mays AN, Döhner H, Sanz MA, Amadori S,Grimwade D, Lo-Coco F. Analysis of t(15;17) chromosomal breakpoint sequences in therapy-related versus de novo acute promyelocytic leukemia: association of DNA breaks with specific DNA motifs at PML and RARA loci. Genes Chromosomes Cancer.2010;49(8):726-32.

[80] Haupt, R., Fears, T. R., Rosso, P., Colella, R., Loiacono, G., de Terlizzi, M., Mancini, A., Comelli, A., Indolfi, P., Donfrancesco, A., et al. Increased risk of secondary leukemia after single-agent treatment with etoposide for Langerhans' cell histiocytosis. Pediatr Hematol Oncol. (1994)., 11(5), 499-507.

[81] Helleday T, Petermann E, Lundin C, Hodgson B, Sharma RA.DNA repair pathways as targets for cancer therapy.Nat Rev Cancer. 2008;8(3):193-204.

[82] Hershman, D., Neugut, A. I., Jacobson, J. S., Wang, J., Tsai, W. Y., Mc Bride, R., Bennett, C. L., & Grann, V. R. Acute myeloid leukemia or myelodysplastic syndrome following use of granulocyte colony-stimulating factors during breast cancer adjuvant chemotherapy. J Natl Cancer Inst. (2007)., 99(3), 196-205.

[83] Heuser M, Yap DB, Leung M, de Algara TR, Tafech A, McKinney S, Dixon J,Thresher R, Colledge B, Carlton M, Humphries RK, Aparicio SA. Loss of MLL5 results in pleiotropic hematopoietic defects, reduced neutrophil immune function, and extreme sensitivity to DNA demethylation. Blood. 2009;113(7):1432-43.

[84] Hijiya N, Hudson MM, Lensing S, Zacher M, Onciu M, Behm FG, Razzouk BI, Ribeiro RC, Rubnitz JE, Sandlund JT, Rivera GK, Evans WE, Relling MV, Pui CH.Cumulative incidence of secondary neoplasms as a first event after childhood acute lymphoblastic leukemia. JAMA. 2007;297(11):1207-15.

[85] Howe, R., Micallef, I. N., Inwards, D. J., Ansell, S. M., Dewald, G. W., Dispenzieri, A., Gastineau, D. A., Gertz, Geyer. S. M., Hanson, Lacy. M. Q., Tefferi, A., & Litzow, M. R. Secondary myelodysplastic syndrome and acute myelogenous leukemia are significant complications following autologous stem cell transplantation for lymphoma. Bone Marrow Transplant. (2003)., 32(3), 317-24.

[86] Imagawa, J., Harada, Y., Shimomura, T., Tanaka, H., Okikawa, Y., Hyodo, H., Kimura, A., & Harada, H. Clinical and genetic features of therapy-related myeloid neoplasms after chemotherapy for acute promyelocytic leukemia. Blood. (2010)., 116(26), 6018-22.

[87] Itzhar, N., Dessen, P., Toujani, S., Auger, N., Preudhomme, C., Richon, C., Lazar, V., Saada, V., Bennaceur, A., Bourhis, J. H., de Botton, S., & Bernheim, A. Chromosomal minimal critical regions in therapy-related leukemia appear different from those of de novo leukemia by high-resolution aCGH. PLoS One. (2011). e16623.

[88] Jawad, M., Seedhouse, C. H., Russell, N., & Plumb, M. Polymorphisms in human homeobox HLX1 and DNA repair RAD51 genes increase the risk of therapy-related acute myeloid leukemia. Blood. (2006)., 108(12), 3916-8.

[89] Jerez A, Yuka Sugimoto, Hideki Makishima, Amit Verma, Christine L O'Keefe, Ramon V Tiu, Azim M Mohamedali, Michael A McDevitt, Ghulam J. Mufti, Jacqueline Boultwood, and Jaroslaw P Maciejewski, Clinical and Genomic Characterization of Chromosome 7 Lesions in Myeloid Malignancies, Blood (ASH Annual Meeting Abstracts), 2011; 118: 3549.

[90] Joannides, M., & Grimwade, D. Molecular biology of therapy-related leukaemias. Clin Transl Oncol. (2010)., 12(1), 8-14.

[91] Johnson KJ, Blair CM, Fink JM, Cerhan JR, Roesler MA, Hirsch BA, Nguyen PL, Ross JA.Medical conditions and risk of adult myeloid leukemia.Cancer Causes Control. (2012)., 23(7), 1083-9.

[92] Josting, A., Wiedenmann, S., Franklin, J., May, M., Sieber, M., Wolf, J., Engert, A., Diehl, V., German, Hodgkin's., Lymphoma, Study., & Group, . Secondary myeloid leukemia and myelodysplastic syndromes in patients treated for Hodgkin's disease: a report from the German Hodgkin's Lymphoma Study Group. J Clin Oncol. (2003)., 21(18), 3440-6.

[93] Libura, J., Slater, D. J., & Felix, Richardson. C. Therapy-related acute myeloid leukemia-like MLL rearrangements are induced by etoposide in primary human CD34+ cells and remain stable after clonal expansion. Blood. (2005). Mar 1;, 105(5), 2124-31.

[94] Kaldor, J. M., Day, N. E., Clarke, E. A., Van Leeuwen, F. E., Henry-Amar, M., Fiorentino, M. V., Bell, J., Pedersen, D., Band, P., Assouline, D., et al. Leukemia following Hodgkin's disease. N Engl J Med. (1990)., 322(1), 7-13.

[95] Kaldor, J. M., Day, N. E., Pettersson, F., Clarke, E. A., Pedersen, D., Mehnert, W., Bell, J., Høst, H., Prior, P., Karjalainen, S., et al. Leukemia following chemotherapy for ovarian cancer. N Engl J Med. (1990)., 322(1), 1-6.

[96] Kayser S, Döhner K, Krauter J, Köhne CH, Horst HA, Held G, von Lilienfeld-Toal M, Wilhelm S, Kündgen A, Götze K, Rummel M, Nachbaur D, Schlegelberger B, Göhring G, Späth D, Morlok C, Zucknick M, Ganser A, Döhner H, Schlenk RF; German-Austrian AMLSG. The impact of therapy-related acute myeloid leukemia (AML) on outcome in 2853 adult patients with newly diagnosed AML. Blood. 2011;117(7): 2137-45.

[97] Kern, W., Haferlach, T., Schnittger, S., Hiddemann, W., & Schoch, C. Prognosis in therapy-related acute myeloid leukemia and impact of karyotype. J Clin Oncol. (2004)., 22(12), 2510-1.

[98] Kindler T, Lipka DB, Fischer T. FLT3 as a therapeutic target in AML: still challenging after all these years. Blood. 2010;116(24):5089-102.

[99] Klymenko S, Trott K, Atkinson M, Bink K, Bebeshko V, Bazyka D, Dmytrenko I, Abramenko I, Bilous N, Misurin A, Zitzelsberger H, Rosemann M. Aml1 gene rearrangements and mutations in radiation-associated acute myeloid leukemia and myelodysplastic syndromes. J Radiat Res. 2005;46(2):249-55.

[100] Knight, J. A., Skol, A. D., Shinde, A., Hastings, D., Walgren, R. A., Shao, J., Tennant, T. R., Banerjee, M., Allan, J. M., Le Beau, Larson. R. A., Graubert, T. A., Cox, N. J., & Onel, K. Genome-wide association study to identify novel loci associated with therapy-related myeloid leukemia susceptibility. Blood. (2009)., 113(22), 5575-82.

[101] Knoche, E., Mc Leod, H. L., & Graubert, T. A. Pharmacogenetics of alkylator-associated acute myeloid leukemia. Pharmacogenomics. (2006)., 7(5), 719-29.

[102] Kobzev, Y. N., Martinez-Climent, J., Lee, S., Chen, J., & Rowley, . Analysis of translocations that involve the NUP98 gene in patients with 11chromosomal rearrangements. Genes Chromosomes Cancer. (2004)., 41(4), 339-52.

[103] Kolte, B., Baer, A. N., Sait, S. N., O'Loughlin, K. L., Stewart, C. C., Barcos, M., Wetzler, M., & Baer, M. R. Acute myeloid leukemia in the setting of low dose weekly methotrexate therapy for rheumatoid arthritis. Leuk Lymphoma. (2001)., 42(3), 371-8.

[104] Kosmider O, Delabesse E, de Mas VM, Cornillet-Lefebvre P, Blanchet O, Delmer A, Recher C, Raynaud S, Bouscary D, Viguié F, Lacombe C, Bernard OA, Ifrah N, Drey-

fus F, Fontenay M; GOELAMS Investigators. TET2 mutations in secondary acute myeloid leukemias: a French retrospective study. Haematologica. 2011;96(7):1059-63.

[105] Kristinsson SY, Björkholm M, Hultcrantz M, Derolf ÅR, Landgren O, Goldin LR.Chronic immune stimulation might act as a trigger for the development of acute myeloid leukemia or myelodysplastic syndromes. J Clin Oncol. 2011;29(21):2897-903.

[106] Kratz CP, Emerling BM, Donovan S, Laig-Webster M, Taylor BR, Thompson P, Jensen S, Banerjee A, Bonifas J, Makalowski W, Green ED, Le Beau MM, Shannon KM.Candidate gene isolation and comparative analysis of a commonly deleted segment of 7q22 implicated in myeloid malignancies. Genomics. 2001;77(3):171-80.

[107] Kröger N, Brand R, van Biezen A, Zander A, Dierlamm J, Niederwieser D, Devergie A, Ruutu T, Cornish J, Ljungman P, Gratwohl A, Cordonnier C, Beelen D, Deconinck E, Symeonidis A, de Witte T; Myelodysplastic Syndromes Subcommittee of The Chronic Leukaemia Working Party of European Group for Blood and Marrow Transplantation (EBMT). Risk factors for therapy-related myelodysplastic syndrome and acute myeloid leukemia treated with allogeneic stem cell transplantation.Haematologica. 2009;94(4):542-9.

[108] Kuptsova-Clarkson N, Ambrosone CB, Weiss J, Baer MR, Sucheston LE, Zirpoli G, Kopecky KJ, Ford L, Blanco J, Wetzler M, Moysich KB. XPD DNA nucleotide excision repair gene polymorphisms associated with DNA repair deficiency predict better treatment outcomes in secondary acute myeloid leukemia. Int J Mol Epidemiol Genet. 2010;1(4):278-94.

[109] Kwong YL. Azathioprine: association with therapy-related myelodysplastic syndrome and acute myeloid leukemia.J Rheumatol. (2010). , 37(3), 485-90.

[110] Kyle RA, Pierre RV, Bayrd ED.Multiple myeloma and acute myelomonocytic leukemia. N Engl J Med. (1970). , 283(21), 1121-5.

[111] Lam DH, Aplan PD. NUP98 gene fusions in hematologic malignancies. Leukemia. 2001;15(11):1689-95.

[112] Larson RA, Le Beau MM.Prognosis and therapy when acute promyelocytic leukemia and other "good risk" acute myeloid leukemias occur as a therapy-related myeloid neoplasm. Mediterr J Hematol Infect Dis. (2011). e2011032.

[113] Larson RA. Therapy-related myeloid leukemia: stochastic or idiosyncratic? Blood,. (2004). 104, 602-603.

[114] Larson RA.Etiology and management of therapy-related myeloid leukemia. Hematology Am Soc Hematol Educ Program. (2007). , 2007, 453-9.

[115] Latagliata, R., Petti, M. C., Fenu, S., Mancini, M., Spiriti, Breccia. M., Brunetti, G. A., Avvisati, G., Lo, Coco. F., & Mandelli, F. Therapy-related myelodysplastic syndrome-acute myelogenous leukemia in patients treated for acute promyelocytic leukemia: an emerging problem. Blood. (2002). , 99(3), 822-4.

[116] Le Beau, Espinosa. R., 3rd Davis, E. M., Eisenbart, Larson. R. A., & Green, E. D. Cytogenetic and molecular delineation of a region of chromosome 7 commonly deleted in malignant myeloid diseases. Blood. (1996). Sep 15;, 88(6), 1930-5.

[117] Le Beau MM, Olney HJ. Myelodysplastic Syndroms. In: Cancer Cytogenetics: Chromosomal and Molecular Genetic Abberations of Tumor Cells.Eds. Heim S, Mitelman F. 3rd ed.- Oxford : Wiley-Blackwell, (2009). , 141-178.

[118] Le Deley, M. C., Leblanc, T., Shamsaldin, A., Raquin, Lacour. B., Sommelet, D., Chompret, A., Cayuela, J. M., Bayle, C., Bernheim, A., de Vathaire, F., Vassal, G., Hill, C., Société, Française., & d'Oncologie, Pédiatrique. Risk of secondary leukemia after a solid tumor in childhood according to the dose of epipodophyllotoxins and anthracyclines: a case-control study by the Société Française d'Oncologie Pédiatrique. J Clin Oncol. (2003). , 21(6), 1074-81.

[119] Lee JW, Soung YH, Park WS, Kim SY, Nam SW, Min WS, Lee JY, Yoo NJ, Lee SH.BRAF mutations in acute leukemias.Leukemia. (2004). , 18(1), 170-2.

[120] Leone, G., Pagano, L., Ben-Yehuda, D., & Voso, M. T. Therapy-related leukemia and myelodysplasia: susceptibility and incidence. Haematologica. (2007). , 92(10), 1389-98.

[121] Lenz, G., Dreyling, M., Schiegnitz, E., Haferlach, T., Hasford, J., Unterhalt, M., & Hiddemann, W. Moderate increase of secondary hematologic malignancies after myeloablative radiochemotherapy and autologous stem-cell transplantation in patients with indolent lymphoma: results of a prospective randomized trial of the German Low Grade Lymphoma Study Group. J Clin Oncol. (2004). , 22(24), 4926-33.

[122] Leone, G., Pagano, L., Ben-Yehuda, D., & Voso, M. T. Therapy-related leukemia and myelodysplasia: susceptibility and incidence. Haematologica. (2007). , 92(10), 1389-98.

[123] Leone G, Pagano L, Ben-Yehuda D, Voso MT. Therapy-related leukemia and myelodysplasia: susceptibility and incidence. Haematologica. 2007;92(10):1389-98.

[124] Li, L., Li, M., Sun, C., Francisco, L., Chakraborty, S., Sabado, M., Mc Donald, T., Gyorffy, J., Chang, K., Wang, S., Fan, W., Li, J., Zhao, L. P., Radich, J., Forman, S., Bhatia, S., & Bhatia, R. Altered hematopoietic cell gene expression precedes development of therapy-related myelodysplasia/acute myeloid leukemia and identifies patients at risk. Cancer Cell. (2011). , 20(5), 591-605.

[125] Lichtman MA.Is there an entity of chemically induced BCR-ABL-positive chronic myelogenous leukemia? Oncologist. (2008)., 13(6), 645-54.

[126] Lin LI, Chen CY, Lin DT, Tsay W, Tang JL, Yeh YC, Shen HL, Su FH, Yao M, Huang SY, Tien HF. Characterization of CEBPA mutations in acute myeloid leukemia: most patients with CEBPA mutations have biallelic mutations and show a distinct immunophenotype of the leukemic cells. Clin Cancer Res. 2005;11(4):1372-9.

[127] Litzow, M. R., Tarima, S., Pérez, W. S., Bolwell, B. J., Cairo, Camitta., Cutler, C. S., de Lima, M., Dipersio, J. F., Gale, R. P., Keating, A., Lazarus, H. M., Luger, S., Marks, D. I., Maziarz, R. T., Mc Carthy, P. L., Pasquini, M. C., Phillips, G. L., Rizzo, Sierra. J., & Tallman, Weisdorf. D. J. Allogeneic transplantation for therapy-related myelodysplastic syndrome and acute myeloid leukemia.Blood.(2010). , 115(9), 1850-7.

[128] Lofstrom, B., Backlin, C., Sundstrom, C., Hellstrom-Lindberg, E., Ekbom, A., & Lundberg, I. E. Myeloid leukaemia in systemic lupus erythematosus--a nested case-control study based on Swedish registers.Rheumatology (Oxford) (2009). , 48(10), 1222-6.

[129] Lyman, G. H., Dale, D. C., Wolff, D. A., Culakova, E., Poniewierski, Kuderer. N. M., & Crawford, J. Acute myeloid leukemia or myelodysplastic syndrome in randomized controlled clinical trials of cancer chemotherapy with granulocyte colony-stimulating factor: a systematic review. J Clin Oncol. (2010). Jun 10;, 28(17), 2914-24.

[130] Luna-Fineman S, Shannon KM, Lange BJ. Childhood monosomy 7: epidemiology,biology, and mechanistic implications. Blood. 1995;85(8):1985-99.

[131] Mailankody, S., Pfeiffer, R. M., Kristinsson, S. Y., Korde, N., Bjorkholm, M., Goldin, L. R., Turesson, I., & Landgren, O. Risk of acute myeloid leukemia and myelodysplastic syndromes after multiple myeloma and its precursor disease (MGUS). Blood. (2011). , 118(15), 4086-92.

[132] Marcucci G, Maharry K, Wu YZ, Radmacher MD, Mrózek K, Margeson D, Holland KB, Whitman SP, Becker H, Schwind S, Metzeler KH, Powell BL, Carter TH, Kolitz JE, Wetzler M, Carroll AJ, Baer MR, Caligiuri MA, Larson RA, Bloomfield CD. IDH1 and IDH2 gene mutations identify novel molecular subsets within de novo cytogenetically normal acute myeloid leukemia: a Cancer and Leukemia Group B study. J Clin Oncol. 2010;28(14):2348-55.

[133] Maris JM, Wiersma SR, Mahgoub N, Thompson P, Geyer RJ, Hurwitz CG, Lange BJ,Shannon KM. Monosomy 7 myelodysplastic syndrome and other second malignant neoplasms in children with neurofibromatosis type 1. Cancer. 1997;79(7): 1438-46.

[134] Martin, M. G., Welch, J. S., Luo, J., Ellis, Graubert. T. A., & Walter, . Therapy related acute myeloid leukemia in breast cancer survivors, a population-based study. Breast Cancer Res Treat. (2009). , 118(3), 593-8.

[135] Martinelli V, Radaelli M, Straffi L, Rodegher M, Comi G. Mitoxantrone: benefits and risks in multiple sclerosis patients. Neurol Sci. 2009;30(Suppl 2):S167–70

[136] Mauch, P. M., Kalish, L. A., Marcus, K. C., Coleman, C. N., Shulman, L. N., Krill, E., Come, S., Silver, B., Canellos, G. P., & Tarbell, N. J. Second malignancies after treatment for laparotomy staged IA-IIIB Hodgkin's disease: long-term analysis of risk factors and outcome. Blood. (1996). , 87(9), 3625-32.

[137] Mauritzson, N., Albin, M., Rylander, L., et al. Pooled analysis of clinical and cytogenetic features in treatment-related and de novo adult acute myeloid leukemia and

myelodysplastic syndromes based on a consecutive series of 761 patients analyzed 1976-1993 and on 5098 unselected cases reported in the literature 1974-2001. Leukemia. (2002). , 16(12), 2366-78.

[138] Mays, A. N., Osheroff, N., Xiao, Y., Wiemels, J. L., Felix, Byl. J. A., Saravanamuttu, K., Peniket, A., Corser, R., Chang, C., Hoyle, C., Parker, A. N., Hasan, S. K., Lo-Coco, F., Solomon, E., & Grimwade, D. Evidence for direct involvement of epirubicin in the formation of chromosomal translocations in t(15;17) therapy-related acute promyelocytic leukemia. Blood. (2010). , 115(2), 326-30.

[139] Metayer, C., Curtis, R. E., Vose, J., Sobocinski, K. A., Horowitz, Bhatia. S., Fay, J. W., Freytes, C. O., Goldstein, S. C., Herzig, R. H., Keating, A., Miller, C. B., Nevill, T. J., Pecora, A. L., Rizzo, Williams. S. F., Li, C. Y., Travis, L. B., & Weisdorf, D. J. Myelodysplastic syndrome and acute myeloid leukemia after autotransplantation for lymphoma: a multicenter case-control study. Blood. (2003). , 101(5), 2015-23.

[140] Micallef, I. N., Lillington, D. M., Apostolidis, J., Amess, J. A., Neat, M., Matthews, J., Clark, T., Foran, J. M., Salam, A., Lister, T. A., & Rohatiner, A. Z. Therapy-related myelodysplasia and secondary acute myelogenous leukemia after high-dose therapy with autologous hematopoietic progenitor-cell support for lymphoid malignancies. J Clin Oncol. (2000). , 18(5), 947-55.

[141] Mistry AR, Felix CA, Whitmarsh RJ, Mason A, Reiter A, Cassinat B, Parry A, Walz C, Wiemels JL, Segal MR, Adès L, Blair IA, Osheroff N, Peniket AJ,Lafage-Pochitaloff M, Cross NC, Chomienne C, Solomon E, Fenaux P, Grimwade D. DNA topoisomerase II in therapy-related acute promyelocytic leukemia. N Engl J Med. 2005;352(15): 1529-38.

[142] Miyata A, Deguchi S, Fujita M, Kikuchi T, Honda K. [Therapy-related AML(M2) with t(8;21) that developed three years after chemo-therapy for hepatocellular carcinoma]. Rinsho Ketsueki. 1996;37(5):448-51.

[143] Morrison, V. A., Rai, K. R., Peterson, B. L., Kolitz, J. E., Elias, L., Appelbaum, F. R., Hines, Shepherd. L., Larson, R. A., & Schiffer, . Therapy-related myeloid leukemias are observed in patients with chronic lymphocytic leukemia after treatment with fludarabine and chlorambucil: results of an intergroup study, cancer and leukemia group B 9011. J Clin Oncol. (2002). , 20(18), 3878-84.

[144] Mudie, N. Y., Swerdlow, A. J., Higgins, C. D., Smith, P., Qiao, Z., Hancock, B. W., Hoskin, P. J., & Linch, D. C. Risk of second malignancy after non-Hodgkin's lymphoma: a British Cohort Study. J Clin Oncol. (2006). , 24(10), 1568-74.

[145] Nakamori, Y., Miyazaki, M., Tominaga, T., Taguchi, A., & Shinohara, K. Therapy-related erythroleukemia caused by the administration of UFT and mitomycin C in a patient with colon cancer. Int J Clin Oncol. (2003). , 8(1), 56-9.

[146] Nardi, V., Winkfield, K. M., Ok, C. Y., Niemierko, A., Kluk, Attar. E. C., Garcia-Manero, G., Wang, S. A., & Hasserjian, R. P. Acute myeloid leukemia and myelodysplas-

tic syndromes after radiation therapy are similar to de novo disease and differ from other therapy-related myeloid neoplasms. J Clin Oncol. (2012). , 30(19), 2340-7.

[147] Nishiyama M, Arai Y, Tsunematsu Y, Kobayashi H, Asami K, Yabe M, Kato S, Oda M, Eguchi H, Ohki M, Kaneko Y. 11p15 translocations involving the NUP98 gene in childhood therapy-related acute myeloid leukemia/myelodysplastic syndrome. Genes Chromosomes Cancer. 1999;26(3):215-20.

[148] Noronha V, Berliner N, Ballen KK, Lacy J, Kracher J, Baehring J, Henson JW. Treatment-related myelodysplasia/AML in a patient with a history of breast cancer and an oligodendroglioma treated with temozolomide: case study and review of the literature. Neuro Oncol. 2006;8(3):280-3.

[149] Offman J, Opelz G, Doehler B, Cummins D, Halil O, Banner NR, Burke MM, Sullivan D, Macpherson P, Karran P. Defective DNA mismatch repair in acute myeloid leukemia/myelodysplastic syndrome after organ transplantation. Blood. 2004;104(3):822-8.

[150] Ojha, R. P., Fischbach, L. A., Zhou, Y., Felini, Singh. K. P., & Thertulien, R. Acute myeloid leukemia incidence following radiation therapy for localized or locally advanced prostate adenocarcinoma.Cancer Epidemiol. (2010). , 34(3), 274-8.

[151] Osato, M. Point mutations in the RUNX1/AML1 gene: another actor in RUNX leukemia. Oncogene. (2004). , 23(24), 4284-96.

[152] Ostgård, L. S., Kjeldsen, E., Holm, Brown., Pde, N., Pedersen, B. B., Bendix, K., Johansen, P., Kristensen, J. S., & Nørgaard, J. M. Reasons for treating secondary AML as de novo AML. Eur J Haematol. (2010). , 85(3), 217-26.

[153] Pagano, L., Pulsoni, A., Tosti, Avvisati. G., Mele, L., Mele, M., Martino, B., Visani, G., Cerri, R., Di Bona, E., Invernizzi, R., Nosari, A., Clavio, M., Allione, B., Coser, P., Candoni, A., Levis, A., Camera, A., Melillo, L., Leone, G., Mandelli, F., Gruppo, Italiano., Malattie, Ematologiche., & Maligne, dell'Adulto. Clinical and biological features of acute myeloid leukaemia occurring as second malignancy: GIMEMA archive of adult acute leukaemia. Br J Haematol. (2001). , 112(1), 109-17.

[154] Paschka P, Schlenk RF, Gaidzik VI, Habdank M, Krönke J, Bullinger L, Späth D, Kayser S, Zucknick M, Götze K, Horst HA, Germing U, Döhner H, Döhner K. IDH1 and IDH2 mutations are frequent genetic alterations in acute myeloid leukemia and confer adverse prognosis in cytogenetically normal acute myeloid leukemia with NPM1 mutation without FLT3 internal tandem duplication. J Clin Oncol. 2010;28(22): 3636-43.

[155] Patel, J. P., Gönen, M., Figueroa, Fernandez. H., Sun, Z., Racevskis, J., Van Vlierberghe, P., Dolgalev, I., Thomas, S., Aminova, O., Huberman, K., Cheng, J., Viale, A., Socci, N. D., Heguy, A., Cherry, A., Vance, G., Higgins, R. R., Ketterling, R. P., Gallagher, R. E., Litzow, M., van den, Brink. M. R., Lazarus, H. M., Rowe, J. M., Luger, S., Ferrando, A., Paietta, E., Tallman, Melnick. A., Abdel-Wahab, O., & Levine, R. L. Prognostic relevance of integrated genetic profiling in acute myeloid leukemia. N Engl J Med. (2012). , 366(12), 1079-89.

[156] Pedersen-Bjergaard, J. Insights into leukemogenesis from therapy-related leukemia. N Engl J Med. (2005). , 352(15), 1591-4.

[157] Pedersen-Bjergaard, J., Andersen, M. K., Andersen, M. T., & Christiansen, D. H. Genetics of therapy-related myelodysplasia and acute myeloid leukemia.Leukemia. (2008). , 22(2), 240-8.

[158] Pedersen-Bjergaard, J., Andersen, M. T., & Andersen, M. K. Genetic pathways in the pathogenesis of therapy-related myelodysplasia and acute myeloid leukemia.Hematology Am Soc Hematol Educ Program.(2007). , 2007, 392-7.

[159] Pedersen-Bjergaard, J., Christiansen, D. H., Desta, F., & Andersen, M. K. Alternative genetic pathways and cooperating genetic abnormalities in the pathogenesis of therapy-related myelodysplasia and acute myeloid leukemia. Leukemia. (2006). , 20(11), 1943-9.

[160] Pedersen-Bjergaard, J., Daugaard, G., Hansen, S. W., Philip, P., Larsen, S. O., & Rørth, M. Increased risk of myelodysplasia and leukaemia after etoposide, cisplatin, and bleomycin for germ-cell tumours. Lancet. (1991). , 338(8763), 359-63.

[161] Pedersen-Bjergaard, J., Nissen, N. I., Sørensen, H. M., Hou-Jensen, K., Larsen, Ernst. P., Ersbøl, J., Knudtzon, S., & Rose, C. Acute non-lymphocytic leukemia in patients with ovarian carcinoma following long-term treatment with Treosulfan (=dihydroxybusulfan). Cancer. (1980). , 45(1), 19-29.

[162] Pedersen-Bjergaard, J. Molecular cytogenetics in cancer.Lancet. (2001). , 357(9255), 491-2.

[163] Perentesis JP.Genetic predisposition and treatment-related leukemia.Med Pediatr Oncol. (2001). , 36(5), 541-8.

[164] Perry JR, Brown MT, Gockerman JP.Acute leukemia following treatment of malignant glioma.J Neurooncol. 1998;40(1):39-46.

[165] Praga, C., Bergh, J., Bliss, J., Bonneterre, J., Cesana, B., Coombes, R. C., Fargeot, P., Folin, A., Fumoleau, P., Giuliani, R., Kerbrat, P., Hery, M., Nilsson, J., Onida, F., Piccart, M., Shepherd, L., Therasse, P., Wils, J., & Rogers, D. Risk of acute myeloid leukemia and myelodysplastic syndrome in trials of adjuvant epirubicin for early breast cancer: correlation with doses of epirubicin and cyclophosphamide. J Clin Oncol. (2005). , 23(18), 4179-91.

[166] Preudhomme, C., Sagot, C., Boissel, N., Cayuela, J. M., Tigaud, I., de Botton, S., Thomas, X., Raffoux, E., Lamandin, C., Castaigne, S., Fenaux, P., Dombret, H., & Group, A. L. F. A. Favorable prognostic significance of CEBPA mutations in patients with de novo acute myeloid leukemia: a study from the Acute Leukemia French Association (ALFA). Blood. (2002). , 100(8), 2717-23.

[167] Pui-H, C., Behm, F. G., Raimondi, S. C., Dodge, R. K., George, S. L., Rivera, G. K., Mirro, J., Kalwinsky, D. K., Dahl, G. V., Murphy, S. B., Crist, W. M., & Williams, D. L.

Secondary Acute Myeloid Leukemia in Children Treated for Acute Lymphoid Leukemia. N Engl J Med (1989)., 321(3), 136-142.

[168] Pyatt DW, Aylward LL, Hays SM.Is age an independent risk factor for chemically induced acute myelogenous leukemia in children?J Toxicol Environ Health B Crit Rev. 2007;10(5):379-400

[169] Qian, Z., Fernald, Godley. L. A., Larson, R. A., & Le Beau, . Expression profiling of CD34+ hematopoietic stem/ progenitor cells reveals distinct subtypes of therapy-related acute myeloid leukemia. Proc Natl Acad Sci U S A. (2002). , 99(23), 14925-30.

[170] Qian, Z., Joslin, J. M., Tennant, T. R., Reshmi, S. C., Young, D. J., Stoddart, A., Larson, R. A., & Le Beau, . Cytogenetic and genetic pathways in therapy-related acute myeloid leukemia.Chem Biol Interact. (2010)., 184(1-2), 50-7.

[171] Quesnel, B., Kantarjian, H., Bjergaard, J. P., Brault, P., Estey, E., Lai, J. L., Tilly, H., Stoppa, A. M., Archimbaud, E., Harousseau, J. L., et al. Therapy-related acute myeloid leukemia with t(8;21), inv(16), and t(8;16): a report on 25 cases and review of the literature. J Clin Oncol. (1993). , 11(12), 2370-9.

[172] Ramadan, S. M., Fouad, T. M., Summa, V., Hasan, S., Kh-Coco, Lo., & , F. Acute myeloid leukemia developing in patients with autoimmune diseases. Haematologica. (2012). , 97(6), 805-17.

[173] Rassool FV, Gaymes TJ, Omidvar N, Brady N, Beurlet S, Pla M, Reboul M, Lea N, Chomienne C, Thomas NS, Mufti GJ, Padua RA. Reactive oxygen species, DNA damage, and error-prone repair: a model for genomic instability with progression in myeloid leukemia? Cancer Res. 2007;67(18):8762-71.

[174] Relling, M. V., Boyett, J. M., Blanco, J. G., Raimondi, S., Behm, F. G., Sandlund, J. T., Rivera, G. K., Kun, L. E., Evans, W. E., & Pui, C. H. Granulocyte colony-stimulating factor and the risk of secondary myeloid malignancy after etoposide treatment. Blood. (2003). , 101(10), 3862-7.

[175] Ries LAG, Harkins D, Krapcho M, et al. SEER cancer statistics review, 1975-2003. Based on November 2005 SEER data submission. Bethesda, Md: National Cancer Institute; 2006. Available at: http://seer.cancer.gov/csr/1975_2003 Accessed October 7, 2008.

[176] Riggi M, Riva A. Therapy-related leukemia: what is the role of 4-epidoxorubicin? J Clin Oncol. 1993;11(7):1430-1.

[177] Rosenthal NS, Farhi DC.Myelodys-plastic syndromes and acute myeloid leukemia in connective tissue disease after single-agent chemotherapy.Am J Clin Pathol. 1996;106(5):676-9.

[178] Rund, D., & Ben-Yehuda, D. Therapy-related leukemia and myelodysplasia: evolving concepts of pathogenesis and treatment. Hematology. (2004). , 9(3), 179-87.

[179] Rund D, Krichevsky S, Bar-Cohen S, Goldschmidt N, Kedmi M, Malik E, Gural A,Shafran-Tikva S, Ben-Neriah S, Ben-Yehuda D. Therapy-related leukemia: clinical

characteristics and analysis of new molecular risk factors in 96 adult patients. Leukemia. 2005;19(11):1919-28.

[180] Sakai I, Tamura T, Narumi H, Uchida N, Yakushijin Y, Hato T, Fujita S,Yasukawa M. Novel RUNX1-PRDM16 fusion transcripts in a patient with acute myeloid leukemia showing t(1;21)(p36;q22). Genes Chromosomes Cancer. 2005;44(3):265-70.

[181] Salas, C., Pérez-Vera, P., & Frías, S. Genetic abnormalities in leukemia secondary to treatment in patients with Hodgkin's disease. Rev Invest Clin. (2011)., 63(1), 53-63.

[182] Sala-Torra, O., Hanna, C., Loken, M. R., Flowers, Maris. M., Ladne, P. A., Mason, J. R., Senitzer, D., Rodriguez, R., Forman, S. J., Deeg, H. J., & Radich, J. P. Evidence of donor-derived hematologic malignancies after hematopoietic stem cell transplantation.Biol Blood Marrow Transplant. (2006)., 12(5), 511-7.

[183] Samanta, D. R., Senapati, S. N., Sharma, P. K., Mohanty, A., & Samantaray, S. Acute myelogenous leukemia following treatment of invasive cervix carcinoma: a case report and a review of the literature. J Cancer Res Ther. (2009)., 5(4), 302-4.

[184] Sandoval C, Head DR, Mirro J Jr, Behm FG, Ayers GD, Raimondi SC. Translocation (9;11)(p21;q23) in pediatric de novo and secondary acute myeloblastic leukemia. Leukemia. 1992;6(6):513-9

[185] Scaradavou, A., Heller, G., Sklar, Ren. L., & Ghavimi, F. Second malignant neoplasms in long-term survivors of childhood rhabdomyosarcoma. Cancer. (1995). , 76(10), 1860-7.

[186] Schaich, M., Ritter, M., Illmer, T., Lisske, P., Thiede, C., Schäkel, U., Mohr, B., Ehninger, G., & Neubauer, A. Mutations in ras proto-oncogenes are associated with lower mdr1 gene expression in adult acute myeloid leukaemia. Br J Haematol. (2001). , 112(2), 300-7.

[187] Schneider, D. T., Hilgenfeld, E., Schwabe, D., Behnisch, W., Zoubek, A., Wessalowski, R., & Göbel, U. Acute myelogenous leukemia after treatment for malignant germ cell tumors in children. J Clin Oncol. (1999)., 17(10), 3226-33.

[188] Schnittger S, Bacher U, Haferlach C, Kern W, Haferlach T. Rare CBFB-MYH11 fusion transcripts in AML with inv(16)/t(16;16) are associated with therapy-related AML M4eo, atypical cytomorphology, atypical immunophenotype, atypical additional chromosomal rearrangements and low white blood cell count: a study on 162 patients. Leukemia. 2007;21(4):725-31.

[189] Schoch C, Schnittger S, Klaus M, Kern W, Hiddemann W, Haferlach T. AML with 11q23/MLL abnormalities as defined by the WHO classification: incidence, partner chromosomes, FAB subtype, age distribution, and prognostic impact in an unselected series of 1897 cytogenetically analyzed AML cases. Blood. 2003;102(7):2395-40

[190] Schoch, C., Kern, W., Schnittger, S., Hiddemann, W., & Haferlach, T. Karyotype is an independent prognostic parameter in therapy-related acute myeloid leukemia (t-

AML): an analysis of 93 patients with t-AML in comparison to 1091 patients with de novo AML. Leukemia.(2004). , 18(1), 120-5.

[191] See, H. T., Thomas, D. A., Bueso-Ramos, C., & Kavanagh, J. Secondary leukemia after treatment with paclitaxel and carboplatin in a patient with recurrent ovarian cancer. Int J Gynecol Cancer. (2006)., 16(Suppl 1), 236-40.

[192] Seedhouse, C., Bainton, R., Lewis, M., Harding, A., Russell, N., & Das-Gupta, E. The genotype distribution of the XRCC1 gene indicates a role for base excision repair in the development of therapy-related acute myeloblastic leukemia. Blood. (2002). , 100(10), 3761-6.

[193] Seedhouse, C., Faulkner, R., Ashraf, N., Das-Gupta, E., & Russell, N. Polymorphisms in genes involved in homologous recombination repair interact to increase the risk of developing acute myeloid leukemia. Clin Cancer Res. (2004). , 10(8), 2675-80.

[194] Seedhouse, C., & Russell, N. Advances in the understanding of susceptibility to treatment-related acute myeloid leukaemia. Br J Haematol. (2007). , 137(6), 513-29.

[195] Shen, Y., Zhu, Y. M., Fan, X., Shi, J. Y., Wang, Q. R., Yan, X. J., Gu, Z. H., Wang, Y. Y., Chen, B., Jiang, C. L., Yan, H., Chen, F. F., Chen, H. M., Chen, Z., Jin, J., & Chen, S. J. Gene mutation patterns and their prognostic impact in a cohort of 1185 patients with acute myeloid leukemia.Blood. (2011). , 118(20), 5593-603.

[196] Sill, H., Olipitz, W., Zebisch, A., Schulz, E., Wölfler, A., Therapy-related, myeloid., neoplasms, pathobiology., & clinical, characteristics. Br J Pharmacol. (2011). , 162(4), 792-805.

[197] Slovak ML, Bedell V, Popplewell L, Arber DA, Schoch C, Slater R. 21q22 balanced chromosome aberrations in therapy-related hematopoietic disorders: report from an international workshop. Genes Chromosomes Cancer. 2002;33(4):379-94.

[198] Smit, C. G., & Meyler, L. Acute myeloid leukaemia after treatment with cytostatic agents. Lancet. (1970). , 2(7674), 671-2.

[199] Smith, M. R., Neuberg, D., Flinn, I. W., Grever, M. R., Lazarus, H. M., Rowe, J. M., Dewald, G., Bennett, J. M., Paietta, E. M., Byrd, J. C., Hussein, Appelbaum. F. R., Larson, R. A., Litzow, M. R., & Tallman, . Incidence of therapy-related myeloid neoplasia after initial therapy for chronic lymphocytic leukemia with fludarabine-cyclophosphamide versus fludarabine: long-term follow-up of US Intergroup Study E2997. Blood. (2011). , 118(13), 3525-7.

[200] Smith, S. M., Le Beau, Huo. D., Karrison, T., Sobecks, R. M., Anastasi, J., Vardiman, J. W., & Rowley, Larson. R. A. Clinical-cytogenetic associations in 306 patients with therapy-related myelodysplasia and myeloid leukemia: the University of Chicago series. Blood. (2003). , 102(1), 43-52.

[201] Spina, F., Alessandrino, P. E., Milani, R., Bonifazi, F., Bernardi, M., Luksch, R., Fagioli, F., Formica, C., & Farina, L. Allogeneic stem cell transplantation in therapy-related

acute myeloid leukemia and myelodysplastic syndromes: impact of patient characteristics and timing of transplant. Leuk Lymphoma. (2012). , 53(1), 96-102.

[202] Stavropoulou, V., Brault, L., & Schwaller, J. Insights into molecular pathways for targeted therapeutics in acute leukemia. Swiss Med Wkly. (2010). w13068.

[203] Suvajdžić, N., Cvetković, Z., Dorđević, V., Kraguljac-Kurtović, N., Stanisavljević, D., Bogdanović, A., Djunić, I., Colović, N., Vidović, A., Elezović, I., & Tomin, D. Prognostic factors for therapy-related acute myeloid leukaemia (t-AML)- A single centre experience. Biomed Pharmacother. (2012). , 66(4), 285-92.

[204] Takahashi, T., Yamamoto, R., Tanaka, K., Kamada, N., & Miyagawa, K. Mutation analysis of the WT1 gene in secondary leukemia. Leukemia. (2000). , 14(7), 1316-7.

[205] Talwalkar SS, Yin CC, Naeem RC, Hicks MJ, Strong LC, Abruzzo LV.Myelodysplastic syndromes arising in patients with germline TP53 mutation and Li-Fraumeni syndrome. Arch Pathol Lab Med. (2010). , 134(7), 1010-5.

[206] Tarella, C., Passera, R., Magni, M., Benedetti, F., Rossi, A., Gueli, A., Patti, C., Parvis, G., Ciceri, F., Gallamini, A., Cortelazzo, S., Zoli, V., Corradini, P., Carobbio, A., Mulé, A., Bosa, M., Barbui, A., Di Nicola, M., Sorio, M., Caracciolo, D., Gianni, A. M., & Rambaldi, A. Risk factors for the development of secondary malignancy after high-dose chemotherapyand autograft, with or without rituximab: a 20-year retrospective follow-up study in patients with lymphoma. J Clin Oncol. (2011). , 29(7), 814-24.

[207] Tavernier, E., Le de Botton, Q. H., Dhédin, S., Bulabois, N., Reman, O., Vey, N., Lhéritier, V., Dombret, H., & Thomas, X. Secondary or concomitant neoplasms among adults diagnosed with acute lymphoblastic leukemia and treated according to the LALA-87 and LALA-94 trials. Cancer. (2007). , 110(12), 2747-55.

[208] Thiede, C., Steudel, C., Mohr, B., Schaich, M., Schäkel, U., Platzbecker, U., Wermke, M., Bornhäuser, M., Ritter, M., Neubauer, A., Ehninger, G., & Illmer, T. Analysis of FLT3-activating mutations in 979 patients with acute myelogenous leukemia: association with FAB subtypes and identification of subgroups with poor prognosis. Blood. (2002). , 99(12), 4326-35.

[209] Touw IP, Bontenbal M. Granulocyte colony-stimulating factor: key (f)actor or innocent bystander in the development of secondary myeloid malignancy?J Natl Cancer Inst. 2007;99(3):183-6.

[210] Travis, L. B., Andersson, M., Gospodarowicz, M., van Leeuwen, F. E., Bergfeldt, K., Lynch, C. F., Curtis, R. E., Kohler, Wiklund. T., Storm, H., Holowaty, E., Hall, P., Pukkala, E., Sleijfer, D. T., Clarke, E. A., Boice Jr, Stovall. M., & Gilbert, E. Treatment-associated leukemia following testicular cancer. J Natl Cancer Inst. (2000). , 92(14), 1165-71.

[211] Travis LB, Curtis RE, Boice JD Jr, Hankey BF, Fraumeni JF Jr.Second cancers following non-Hodgkin's lymphoma.Cancer. (1991). , 67(7), 2002-9.

[212] Travis, L. B., Curtis, R. E., Storm, H., Hall, P., Holowaty, E., Van Leeuwen, F. E., Kohler, Pukkala. E., Lynch, C. F., Andersson, M., Bergfeldt, K., Clarke, E. A., Wiklund, T., Stoter, G., Gospodarowicz, M., Sturgeon, J., Fraumeni, J. F., & Jr Boice Jr, . Risk of second malignant neoplasms among long-term survivors of testicular cancer. J Natl Cancer Inst. (1997). , 89(19), 1429-39.

[213] Travis, L. B., Curtis, R. E., Stovall, M., Holowaty, E. J., van Leeuwen, F. E., Glimelius, B., Lynch, C. F., Hagenbeek, A., Li, C. Y., Banks, P. M., et al. Risk of leukemia following treatment for non-Hodgkin's lymphoma. J Natl Cancer Inst. (1994). , 86(19), 1450-7.

[214] Travis, L. B., Holowaty, E. J., Bergfeldt, K., Lynch, C. F., Kohler, Wiklund. T., Curtis, R. E., Hall, P., Andersson, M., Pukkala, E., Sturgeon, J., & Stovall, M. Risk of leukemia after platinum-based chemotherapy for ovarian cancer. N Engl J Med. (1999). , 340(5), 351-7.

[215] Travis, L. B., Weeks, J., Curtis, R. E., Chaffey, J. T., Stovall, M., Banks, P. M., & Boice Jr, . Leukemia following low-dose total body irradiation and chemotherapy for non-Hodgkin's lymphoma. J Clin Oncol. (1996). , 14(2), 565-71.

[216] Travis LB.The epidemiology of second primary cancers. Cancer Epidemiol Biomarkers Prev (2006). , 15(11), 2020-6.

[217] Trumpp, A., Essers, M., & Wilson, A. Awakening dormant haematopoietic stem cells.Nat Rev Immunol. (2010). , 10(3), 201-9.

[218] Turker, A., & Güler, N. Therapy related acute myeloid leukemia after exposure to 5-fluorouracil: a case report. Hematol Cell Ther. (1999). , 41(5), 195-6.

[219] United National Scientific Committee on the Effects of Atomic Radiation (UNSCEAR). UNSCEAR 2000 Report to General Assembly, with scientific annexes, sources, and effects of ionizing radiation. New York: United Nations; (2000).

[220] van Leeuwen, F. E., Stiggelbout, A. M., van den-Dusebout, Belt., Noyon, A. W., Eliel, R., R,van, M., Kerkhoff, E. H., Delemarre, J. F., & Somers, R. Second cancer risk following testicular cancer: a follow-up study of 1,909 patients. J Clin Oncol. (1993). , 11(3), 415-24.

[221] Vardiman J, Arber DA, Brunning RD, et al. Therapy-related myeloid neoplasms. In: WHO Classification of Tumours of Haematopoietic and Lymphoid Tissues (eds S.H. Swerdlow, E. Campo, N.L. Harris, E.S. Jaffe, S.a. Pileri, H. Stein, J. thiele & J.W. Vardiman), 2008, pp. 127-129.IARC, Lyon.

[222] Vardiman JW, Thiele J, Arber DA, Brunning RD, Borowitz MJ, Porwit A, Harris NL, Le Beau MM, Hellström-Lindberg E, Tefferi A, Bloomfield CD. The 2008 revision of the World Health Organization (WHO) classification of myeloid neoplasms and acute leukemia: rationale and important changes. Blood. 2009;114(5):937-51.

[223] Vay, A., Kumar, S., Seward, S., Semaan, A., Schiffer, Munkarah. A. R., & Morris, R. T. Therapy-related myeloid leukemia after treatment for epithelial ovarian carcinoma: an epidemiological analysis. Gynecol Oncol. (2011). , 123(3), 456-60.

[224] Verma, D., O'Brien, S., Thomas, D., Faderl, S., Koller, C., Pierce, S., Kebriaei, P., Garcia-Manero, G., Cortes, J., Kantarjian, H., & Ravandi, F. Therapy-related acute myelogenous leukemia and myelodysplastic syndrome in patients with acute lymphoblastic leukemia treated with the hyperfractionated cyclophosphamide, vincristine, doxorubicin, and dexamethasone regimens. Cancer. (2009). , 115(1), 101-6.

[225] Voso, M. T., D'Alò, F., Greco, M., Fabiani, E., Criscuolo, M., Migliara, G., Pagano, L., Fianchi, L., Guidi, F., Hohaus, S., & Leone, G. Epigenetic changes in therapy-related MDS/AML. Chem Biol Interact. (2010).

[226] Wang, E., Hutchinson, C. B., Huang, Q., Lu, C. M., Crow, J., Wang, F. F., Sebastian, S., Rehder, C., Lagoo, A., Horwitz, M., Rizzieri, D., Yu, J., Goodman, B., Datto, M., & Buckley, P. Donor cell-derived leukemias/myelodysplastic neoplasms in allogeneic hematopoietic stem cell transplant recipients: a clinicopathologic study of 10 cases and a comprehensive review of the literature. Am J Clin Pathol. (2011). , 135(4), 525-40.

[227] Westman MK, Andersen MT, Pedersen-Bjergaard J, Andersen MK. IDH1 and IDH2 Mutations in Therapy-Related Acute Myeloid Leukemia Are Associated with a Normal Karyotype or Der(1;7)(q10;p10) Combined with RUNX1 Mutations. Blood (ASH Annual Meeting Abstracts), 2011, abstact 3514

[228] Wood BL. Myeloid malignancies: myelodysplastic syndromes, myeloproliferative disorders, and acute myeloid leukemia.Clin Lab Med. (2007). , 27(3), 551-75.

[229] Xue Y, Guo Y, Xie X. Translocation t(7;11)(P15;P15) in a patient with therapy-related acute myeloid leukemia following bimolane and ICRF-154 treatment for psoriasis. Leuk Res. 1997;21(2):107-9.

[230] Yang, J., Terebelo, H. R., & Zonder, J. A. Secondary Primary Malignancies in Multiple Myeloma: An Old Nemesis Revisited. Adv Hematol. (2012)., 2012:801495.

[231] Yin CC, Glassman AB, Lin P, Valbuena JR, Jones D, Luthra R, Medeiros LJ. Morphologic, cytogenetic, and molecular abnormalities in therapy-related acute promyelocytic leukemia.Am J Clin Pathol. 2005;123(6):840-8.

[232] Yonal, I., Hindilerden, F., Ozcan, E., Palanduz, S., & Aktan, M. The co-presence of deletion 7q, 20q and inversion 16 in therapy-related acute myeloid leukemia developed secondary to treatment of breast cancer with cyclophosphamide, doxorubicin, and radiotherapy: a case report. J Med Case Rep. (2012)., 6:67.

[233] Zhang, Y., & Rowley, . Chromatin structural elements and chromosomal translocations in leukemia. DNA Repair (Amst). (2006)., 5(9-10), 1282-97.

[234] Zhang Y, Wong J, Klinger M, Tran MT, Shannon KM, Killeen N. MLL5 contributes to hematopoietic stem cell fitness and homeostasis. Blood. 2009;113(7):1455-63.

[235] Zebisch A, Haller M, Hiden K, Goebel T, Hoefler G, Troppmair J, Sill H. Loss of RAF kinase inhibitor protein is a somatic event in the pathogenesis of therapy-related acute myeloid leukemias with C-RAF germline mutations. Leukemia. 2009;23(6): 1049-53.

Chapter 5

Treatment of Myelodysplastic Syndrome and Acute Myeloid Leukemia by Immunomodulatory and Epigenetic Drugs

Ota Fuchs

Additional information is available at the end of the chapter

http://dx.doi.org/10.5772/52099

1. Introduction

Acute myeloid leukemia (AML) is associated with poor prognosis in elderly patients. More effective, less toxic therapies for older patients with AML who are not eligible for standard intensive induction therapy or have refractory or relapsed disease after chemotherapy are urgently needed. Epigenetic approaches with hypomethylating agents and histone deacetylase inhibitors and immunomodulatory drugs used in advance in the treatment of patients with myelodysplastic syndrome (MDS) have been also studied in patients with AML [1-15].

MDS is a diverse goup of clonal hematopoietic stem cell disorders manifested by ineffective production of blood cells with varying need for transfusions, risk of infection, and risk of transformation to AML. Epigenetic changes, such as DNA methylation, histone acetylation, and RNA interference alter gene expression impacting disease biology and play an important role in the pathogenesis of both, MDS and AML. Hypermethylation of CpG islands in the promoters of key genes involved in cell cycle regulation, apoptosis, tumor suppressor control and in response to chemotherapy and the consequent silencing of their expression is well documented in MDS. Hypermethylated DNA sequences of key cellular machinery provide an attractive potential therapeutic target for the treatment of MDS. DNA methylation and histone modification not only regulate the expression of protein-encoding genes but also microRNAs (miRs), such as let-7a, miR-9, miR-34a, miR-124, miR-137, miR-148, miR-203 and miR-223 [16-22]. The only approved way to inhibit DNA methylation is to use clinically available inhibitors of enzymes- DNA methyltransferases (DNMTs). Treatment with DNMT inhibitors is a rational strategy with the aim to reinduce the expression of epigenetically silenced genes for tumor suppressors and other targeted genes, often connected with response to chemotherapy. It can induce a broad spektrum of apoptotic pathways. This strategy is valid not only for MDS but for human cancer generally, including AML. 5-Aza-cytidine (azacidine, Vidaza) and 5-aza-2′-deoxycytidine (5-azaCdR decitabine) have become the standard in the treatment of patients with higher-risk MDS, in particular older individuals, where intensive chemotherapy and allogeneic stem cell transplantation is not possible.

Azacitidine (Vidaza, Celgene Corporation, Summit, NJ, USA or Celgene Europe Ltd., Winsdor, UK) was the first drug approved for the treatment of MDS in the United States and in the European Union. Decitabine (Dacogen, Eisai Inc., Woodcliff Lake, NJ, USA under license from Astex Pharmaceuticals, Inc., Dublin, CA, USA) received initial regulatory approval from the US Food and Drug Administration (FDA) in May 2006 for the treatment of patients with all MDS subtypes [23-25]. Since then, decitabine has also gained regulatory approval in Russia, Malaysia, South Korea, the Philippines, Uruguay, Chile, Argentina, Peru, Colombia, and Brazil, and is considered for approval in other countries. European Organisation for Research and Treatment of Cancer (EORTC) conducted study, which failed to reveal a significant improvement in overall survival, time to AML transformation and death, for low-dose decitabine compared to the best supportive care [26-31].

About 80-90% of 5-aza-cytidine is incorporated into RNA which disrupts nucleic acid and protein metabolism leading to apoptosis. The rest of 5-azacytidine (10-20%) inhibits DNA synthesis through conversion to decitabine triphosphate and subsequent DNA incorporation. Recently, precise mechanism of azacitidine action has been described. Azacitidine inhibits ribonucleotide reductase subunit and causes perturbation of the pool of deoxyribonucleotide triphosphates.

The median survival for azacitidine-treated patients with AML (75mg/m^2/day for 7 days) in a phase III randomized trial was 24.5 months, compared with 16 months for AML patients receiving conventional care regimens [4]. Complete remisson rates were 18% for patients receiving azacitidine, 15% for patients receiving low-dose cytarabine, and 55% for patients receiving intensive induction therapy [4, 5]. Multicenter, phase II study of decitabine (20 mg/m^2/day for 5 days) for the first-line treatment of older patients with AML found remissions in 25% of patients, with a median overall survival of 7.7 months and a 30-day mortality rate of 7% [5]. Another study in older AML patients treated with a 10-day schedule of decitabine showed that 47% of patients achieved complete remission without added toxicity [32]. Despite these encouraging results, in a randomized phase III trial, decitabine produced complete remission in 18% older patients with AML but without the significant improvement in overall survival in comparison with patients receiving supportive care or low-dose cytarabine [25]. Several new studies show a little better results [33, 34]. New randomized studies evaluating single-agent decitabine versus conventional treatment are warranted. A low incidence of treatment-related toxicity has been reported for both these agents, azacitidine and decitabine, supports their use for older AML patients, mainly for those unable or unwilling to receive standard intensive chemotherapy.

Decitabine maintains normal hematopoietic stem cell (HSC) self-renewal but induces terminal differentiation in AML cells. AML cells express low levels of the key late differentiation factor CEBPE (CCAAT/enhancer binding protein epsilon). *CEBPE* promoter CpGs are usually hypomethylated during granulocyte maturation but are significantly hypermethylated in AML cells [35]. Decitabine-induced hypomethylation is greatest at these and other promoter CpGs that are usually hypomethylated with myeloid maturation, accompanied by cellular differentiation of AML cells. In contrast, decitabine-treated normal HSC retained immature morphology. High expression of lineage-specifying factor and aberrant epigenetic repression of some late differentiation factors distinguishes AML cells from normal HSCs and could explain the contrasting differentiation and methylation responses to decitabine. Decitabine induced upregulation of several apoptosis-related genes, in particular of *DAP-kinase 1* and *BCL2L10*. *BCL2L10* was hypermethylated in 45% of AML but not in healthy controls [36].

Another inhibitors of DNMTs (5,6-dihydro-5-azacytidine, 2′-deoxy-5,6-dihydro-5-azacytidine, a second-generation hypo-methylating agent SGI-110 /a dinucleotide of decitabine and deoxyguanosine linked with a natural phosphodiester linkage/, zebularine, procaine, epigallocatechin-3-gallate, and N-phthalyl-L-tryptophan) are in preclinical studies or in clinical trials [37, 38].

The second epigenetic target for which drugs are available is histone deacetylation. There are several histone deacetylases (HDAC) inhibitors (romidepsin, vorinostat, belinostat, sodium phenylbutyrate, valproic acid, entinostat, and mocetinostat) in preclinical studies or in clinical trials [6, 10, 11]. Vorinostat and valproic acid received approval from the US FDA and are available for clinical use in the USA.

Clinical studies with dual pharmacologic targeting of DNMT and HDAC enzymes (azacitidine and phenylbutyrate or decitabine plus vorinostat) reported overall response rate of 22% in MDS/AML patients and supported preclinical results where synergistic anticancer activity was found [12, 39, 40].

Clinical benefit from the immunomodulatory agent lenalidomide (CC5013, Revlimid®) in patients with lower-risk MDS associated with deletion of the long arm of chromosome 5 (del(5q)) led to its 2005 FDA approval for red blood cell transfusion-dependent anemia due to low or intermediate-1 risk MDS associated with a chromosome 5q deletion with or without additional cytogenetic abnormalities. Lenalidomide functions through immunomodulatory, anti-inflammatory, anti-angiogenic and direct neoplastic cells inhibitory mechanisms [41-43]. The highly encouraging results with lenalidomide in del(5q) lower-risk MDS were not repeated in del(5q) AML. The cause of this difference is in many cases deletion of another commonly deleted region 5q31 and not of the 5q32-33 including *RPS14*. However, there is the clear activity of lenalidomide in a subset of patients with AML [8, 9]. Safety, efficacy and biological predictors of response to sequential azacitidine and lenalidomide for elderly patients with acute myeloid leukemia were also studied [14]. This therapy was well tolerated with encouraging clinical and biological activity.

The regulation of gene expression by DNA methylation

DNA methylation is a covalent modification at position C5 of the cytidine ring in the context of a CpG dinucleotide. This methylation is catalysed by a family of DNMTs including DNMT1, DNMT3A and DNMT3B. DNMT1 is required for maintenance methylation during DNA replication. DNMT3A and DNMT3B function in *de* novo methylation [44-47]. CpG rich regions called CpG islands are present in about half of human gene promoters. Methylation of these CpG islands is associated with transcriptional silencing from the involved promoters. When the CpG islands are highly methylated, they bind specific proteins which recruit transcriptional co-repressors such as histone deacetylases (HDACs). Epigenetic silencing is also associated with histone H3 lysine 9 (H3K9) methylation. This modification is associated with closed chromatin and results also in transcriptional suppression. Alterations in DNA methylation are important in the pathogenesis of MDS [48]. Increasing evidence shows aberrant hypermethylation of genes occurring in and potentially contributing to pathogenesis of MDS. The tumor suppressor and cell cycle regulatory gene *CDKN2B* (cyclin-dependent kinase inhibitor 2B) is an example of hypermethylated gene in MDS resulting in silenced expression of this cell cycle inhibitor $p15^{INK4B}$ (cyclin-dependent kinase 4 inhibitor B) and in uncontrolled cell cycle progression and cellular proliferation. *CDKN2B* methylation is frequent in refractory anemia with excess blasts in transformation, therapy-related MDS, and in chronic myelomonocytic leukemia [49-52]. Increased methylation of *CDKN2B* gene is connected with disease progression. Methylation level of *CDKN2B* gene might be used as a marker of leukemic transformation in MDS [53].

Reversal of aberrant methylation by the treatment with hypomethylating agents leads to re-expression of silenced tumor suppressor genes and some other genes, often connected with response to chemotherapy (*CDKN2B*, cyclin-dependent kinase inhibitor 2A /*CDKN2A*/ coding for $p16^{INK4A}$, the cell-adhesion genes /cadherin-1 /*CDH-1*/, cadherin-13 /*CDH-13*/, and immunoglobulin superfamily member 4 /*IGSF4*/, the pro-apoptotic death-associated protein serine/threonine kinase gene /*DAP-kinase*/, the suppressor of cytokine signaling-1 /*SOCS1*/, the reversion-induced LIM homeodomain containing gene /RIL/, a ligand-dependent suppressor deleted in colorectal cancer /*DCC*/, a growth regulatory and tumor suppressor gene hypermethylated in cancer /*HIC1*/, dinucleosidetriphosphatase-fragile histidine triad gene / *FHIT*/ involved in purine metabolism, calcitonin, arachidonate 12- lipoxygenase /ALOX12/ involved in the production and metabolism of fatty acid hydroperoxidases, glutathione S-transferase Mu1 /GSTM1/, testes-specific serine protease 50 /*TSP50*/, O-6-methylguanine-DNA methyltransferase /*MGMT*/, Krüppel like factor 11 /*KLF11*/, oligodendrocyte lineage transcription factor 2 /*OLIG2*/, estrogen receptor alpha /*ESR1*/, progesterone receptors *PGRA* and *PGRB*, RAS association domain family1A /*RASSF1*/, functioning in the control of microtubule polymerization and potentially in the maintenance of genomic stability, and *BLU*, both tumor suppressors genes located at 3p21.3, retinoic acid receptor beta /*RARB*/, a nuclear transcription factor which mediates cellular signaling, cell growth and differentiation, and neutrophic tyrosine kinase receptor, type 1 /*NTRK1*/), which is needed to transmit signals for cell growth and survival [54-57].

In the recent years, the discovery of a series of mutations in patients with MDS has provided insight into the pathogenesis of MDS. Among these alternations have been mutations in genes, such as *IDH1*, *IDH2*, *TET2*, and *DNMT3A*, which affect DNA methylation [58-61]. These mutations are discussed in the special chapter.

http://dx.doi.org/10.5772/52099

2. Types of histone methylation modification and their regulatory mechanisms

Histone methylation is carried out by several histone methyltransferases that methylate lysine (HKMTs) or arginines (PRMTs) in histone tails [62-65]. The four core histones, H2A, H2B, H3, and H4, make up the nucleosome, the main structural unit of chromatin. Some specific histone tail modification, such as methylation of histone 3 lysine tail residue 4 (H3K4), are associated with activation of gene expression, while others, such as methylation of histone 3 lysine 27 (H3K27), are associated with gene repression [66]. These marks are normally carefully controlled by the interplay of sequence-specific DNA binding transcription factors and transcriptional cofactors, many of which are histone-modifying enzymes. The end amino group of lysine can be mono-, di- or tri-methylated. Dependent on this methylation state, the binding affinity of chromatin-associated proteins varies greatly. Methylation of histone 3 lysines 4 and 27 is catalyzed by trithorax and polycomb family of proteins. H3K27 is di- and trimethylated by enhancer of zeste homolog 2 (EZH2), a polycomb family protein [67]. The enzyme that reverses H3K27 methylation was not known until the discovery of two demethylases, ubiquitously transcribed tetratricopeptide repeat, X chromosome (UTX) and Jumonji domain containing 3 (JMJD3), both of which are members of the Jmje domain-containing protein family [68]. EZH2 has been reported to be mutated and inactivated in MDS [69], but is also overexpressed in other subsets of MDS [70]. *UTX* mutations and/or deletions have also been observed in patients with MDS and chronic myelomonocytic leukemia [61, 71-73].

3. Histone acetylation status

Acetylation of nucleosomal histones in part regulates gene transcription in most cells. Differential acetylation of nucleosomal histones results in either transcriptional activation (hyperacetylation and an open chromatin configuration) or repression (hypoacetylation and compacted chromatin) [74, 75]. The role of chromatin remodeling in carcinogenesis was studied with the help of inhibitors of HDACs (HDIs). HDIs induce the hyperacetylation of nucleosomal histones in cells resulting in the expression of aberrantly repressed genes (e.g., tumor suppressor genes) that produce growth arrest, terminal differentiation, and/or apoptosis in carcinoma cells, depending on the HDI and dose used, and the cell type [76-79]. The inappropriate recruitment of HDACs provides at least one mechanism by which oncogenes could alter gene expression in favor of excessive proliferation. Thus, orally active HDIs with low toxicity towards normal cells and tissues, which would effectively inhibit tumor growth are needed for epigenetic anticancer therapy. In October 2006, the US Food and Drug Administration (FDA) approved the first drug of this new class, vorinostat (SAHA, Zolinza) for treatment of cutaneous T-cell lymphoma. Several further HDIs (romidepsin, belinostat, sodium phenylbutyrate, valproic acid, entinostat, and mocetinostat) are in clinical trials. HDIs have shown significant activity against a variety of hematological and solid tumors at doses that are well tolerated by patients, both in monotherapy as well as in combination therapy with other drugs. Combined DNA methyltransferase and histone deacetylase inhibition are used in experiments *in vitro* but also in clinical trials in MDS and AML patients [6, 39].

4. MicroRNAs and epigenetic machinery

MicroRNAs (miRs) belong to a class of small non-coding regulatory RNA that act through binding to the 3′ -UTR of target mRNA and leading to translational repression or degradation of target mRNA at post-transcriptional level. MiRs can directly target epigenetic effectors such as DNMTs, HDACs and polycomb repressive complexes. On the other hand, some miRs (miR-9, 34b/c, 124, 127, 137, 145, 146a, 148, -203, let-7a-3, and others) are epigenetically regulated [80, 81].

MiR-29b targets DNMT3A mRNA [18, 82, 83]. In addition, some isoforms of DNMT3B are targeted by miR-148 [84]. MiR-26a, 101, 205 and -214 regulates EZH2 [85-90].

Dostalova Merkerova et al. found nine upregulated genes for miRs located at chromosome 14q32 in CD34+ cells separated from mononuclear cells of bone marrow obtained from MDS patients [91]. 14q32 region contains 40 miR genes with imprinted expression controlled by a distant differentially methylated region. For example miR-127, a member of the 14q32 region, is involved in B-cell differentiation process through posttranscriptional regulation of *BLIMP1, XBP1,* and *BCL6* genes [91]. BLIMP1 (B lymphocyte induced maturation protein 1) is a zinc finger transcriptional repressor which functions as a master regulátor of terminal differentiation of B cells into plasma cells. XBP1 (X-box binding protein 1) is transcription factor that regulates MHC class II genes by binding to a promoter element referred to as an X box. BCL6 (B-cell lymphoma 6 protein) is a transcriptional represor which regulates germinal center B cell differentiation and inflammation.

5. Protein EVI1 and epigenetic machinery

EVI1 (the ecotropic viral integration site 1) is encoded by gene on chromosome 3q26 [92-95]. The oncoprotein EVI1 and the DNMT3 co-operate in bindig and de novo methylation of target DNA [96]. EVI1 forms a bridge between the epigenetic machinery and signaling pathway [97, 98]. EVI1 represses PTEN (phosphatase and tensin homolog) expression and activates PI3K/AKT (Protein kinase B)/mTOR via interaction with polycomb proteins [97, 98]. Overexpression of EVI1 predicts poor survival in MDS and AML [99]. MDS patients with inversion of chromosome 3 and with *EVI1* transcriptional activation achieved morphological and cytogenetic response to azacitidine [100].

6. Epigenetic therapy in MDS and AML

Treatment with DNMT inhibitors is a rational strategy with the aim to reinduce the expression of epigenetically silenced genes for tumor suppressors and other targeted genes, often

http://dx.doi.org/10.5772/52099

connected with response to chemotherapy. Responses to therapy with DNMT inhibitors are up to now not fully elucidated. We have no clear evidence for DNMT overexpression in MDS and the decrease in global methylation after treatment with demethylating agents has not correlated with disease response. Changes in differentiation and/or apoptosis, and induction of a immune response can be also involved [28-38, 101].

DNA methylation of upstream regulatory element (URE) plays an important role in downregulation of transcription of *PU.1* gene. PU.1 is the transcription factor and tumor suppressor necessary for myeloid differentiation. Azacitidine treatment demethylated *in vitro* URE leading to upregulation of PU.1 followed by derepression of its transcriptonal targets and onset of myeloid differentiation [102]. DNA demethylation and a shift from a repressive histone profile to a more active profile that includes the reassociation of RNA polymerase II (Pol II) with the targeted promoters are necessary for tumor suppressor gene reactivation [103].

Even if a complete understanding of the mechanism of action of azanucleotides remains to be elucidated, their pharmacodynamic effects promote enhanced survival independently of any ability to eliminate the MDS clone. The MDS clone persists in many patients treated by DNMT inhibitors but this clone is modulated and hematologic function is improved together with survival of patients.

It has been almost 50 years since the synthesis and antitumor activity of azacitidine (AC) was described [104, 105]. AC is a pyrimidine nucleoside analog of cytidine and is characterized by a presence of an extra nitrogen atom at position C5 of pyrimidine ring. This modification leads to a blockade of cytosine methylation via a covalent trapping of DNMT. AC is believed to utilize a dual mechanism of action following its phosphorylation: 1) hypomethylation of DNA at low doses and 2) cytotoxicity due to the incorporation into RNA and apparent interaction with protein biosynthesis at high doses. To overcome cytotoxicity, a deoxy analog of AC, 5-aza-2′-deoxycytidine (decitabine, DAC) was synthesized, which is incorporated only into the DNA following its phosphorylation. DAC significantly inhibits DNA methylation at lower concentrations and with less cytotoxicity in comparison with AC [106]. Both, AC and DAC, possess high cytotoxicity at their maximal tolerated doses and are unstable in aqueous solution.

7. Azacitidine clinical studies

Patients with MDS were randomly treated with either azacitidine or best supportive care in the CALGB 9221 study [107]. A total of 191 patients with a median age of 68 years were used. Azacitidine (75 mg/m^2/day) was injected subcutaneously in 7-day cycles beginning on days 1, 29, 57, and 85 (every 28 days). If a beneficial effect was not demonstrated by day 57 and no significant toxicity other than nausea or vomiting had occured, the dose of AC was increased by 33%. Once benefit occured on a particular dosage, AC was continued unless toxicity developed. Patients were assessed after the fourth cycle. Those who achieved complete response (CR) continued on AC until either CR or relapse occured. After 4 months of supportive care, any patients with worsening dinase were permitted to cross over to treatment with AC. Overall, 59% of patients had either refractory anemia with excess blasts (RAEB) or RAEB in transformation (RAEB-T) according to French-American-British (FAB)-defined criteria, and 65% of patients were red blood cell transfusion dependent. Sixty percent of patients in the azacitidine arm (including 7% of patients with CR, 16% with a partial response /PR/, and 37% with hematologic improvement /HI/), compared with 5% of patients in the control arm, responded to treatment ($p<0.001$). The median time to leukemic transformation or death was 21 months in patients treated with AC compared with 12 months in the best supportive care ($p=0.007$). The median overall survival was 20 months for AC-treated patients compared with 14 months for patients assigned to best supportive care. 53% of patients on best supportive care received azacitidine after crossover. A further benefit of AC over supportive care was a significant improvement in quality of life (physical functioning, fatigue, dyspnea) in patients treated with AC compared with patients in the control arm. AC did not increase the rate of infection or gastrointestinal bleeding above the rate associated with underlying disease.

The AZA-001 trial was an international, randomized phase III study designed to test the hypothesis that AC significantly extends overall survival in patients with MDS compared with standard care regimens including best supportive care, low-dose cytarabine (ara-C, 20 mg/m^2 for 14 days every 28 days for at least 4 cycles), or intensive chemotherapy consisting of induction with higher dose of ara-C (100-200 mg/m^2/day for 7 days plus 3 days of daunorubicin 45-60 mg/m^2/day, idarubicin 9-12 mg/m^2/day, or mitoxantrone 8-12 mg/m^2/day) [108]. A total of 358 patients with higher-risk MDS were randomly assigned to either azacitidine as in CALGB 9221 or to standard of care. Median age of patients was 69 years. After a median follow-up of 21.1 months, the median survival time was significantly better in azacitidine patients compared with standard of care options (24.5 versus 15.0 months, respectively $p=0.001$) irrespective of age, percentage of marrow blasts or karyotype. In particular, overall survival was prolonged for azacitidine in patients with -7 / del(7q) cytogenetic abnormality, median overall survival was 13.1 months in the azacitidine group compared with 4.6 months in the standard of care group ($p=0.00017$). Progression to AML was significantly delayed in patients treated with AC (17.8 months in the AC group versus 11.5 months in the standard of care group $p<0.001$). Transfusion requirements and rate of infections were also significantly improved in azacitidine patients.

Continued azacitidine therapy beyond time of first response improves quality of response in patients with higher-risk myelodysplastic syndromes in 48% of patients [109]. This secondary analysis of the AZA-001 phase III study evaluated the time to first response and the potential benefit of continued AC treatment beyond first response in responders. Overal, 91 of 179 patients achieved a response to azacitidine; responding patients received a median of 14 treatment cycles (range, 2-30). Median time to first response was 2 cycles (range, 1-16). Although 91% of first responses occured by 6 cycles, continued azacitidine improved response in 48% of patients. Best response was achieved by 92% of responders by 12 cycles. Median time from first response to best response was 3.5 cycles (95% confidence interval

(CI), 3.0-6.0) in 30 patients who ultimately achieved a complete response, and 3.0 cycles (95% CI, 1.0-3.0) in 21 patients who achieved a partial response.

French group studied a retrospective cohort of 282 higher-risk MDS treated with azacitidine, including 32 patients who concomitantly received erythropoiesis stimulating agents (ESA) for a median of 5.8 months after azacitidine onset [110]. Hematologic improvement was reached in 44% of the ESA and 29% of the no-ESA patients. Transfusion independence was achieved in 48% of the ESA and 20% of the no-ESA groups. Median overall survival was 19.6 months in the ESA and 11.9 months in the no-ESA patients.

Platelet doubling after the first azacitidine cycle is a promising independent predictor for response and overall survival in MDS, chronic myelomonocytic leukemia (CMML) and AML patients in the Dutch azacitidine patients [111].

8. Decitabine clinical studies

Two studies used 3-day, 9-dose regimens requiring inpatient hospitalization and two studies used 5-10 day decitabine regimens intended for outpatient administration [23, 25].

The US D-0007 phase III study compared decitabine (15 mg/m^2 continuous 3-hour intravenous infusion every 8 hours for 3 days) with supportive care in 170 patients with a confirmed diagnosisof de novo or secondary MDS. The median age of enrolled patients was 70 years (range, 30-85 years). Most patients (69%) had intermediate (Int)-2- or high- risk diseaseas defined by the International Prognostic Scoring System criteria, and were red blood cell transfusion dependent (71%) [23]. No significant difference was seen in median overall survival (OS) between patients treated with decitabine and those receiving supportive care (14.0 versus 14.9 months, respectively; p=0.636). The median duration of response to decitabine treatment was 10.3 months (range, 4.1-13.9 months). Patients received a median of 3 courses of decitabine treatment (range, 0-9).

EORTC 06011 phase III study compared decitabine given on a 3-day inpatient regimen (15 mg/m^2 intravenously over 4 hours three times a day for 3 days, every 6 weeks, for a maximum of 8 cycles) with supportive care. A total of 233 patients with primary or secondary MDS, or CMML defined by FAB classification (median age, 70 years; range, 60 to 90 years) were enrolled [25]. 53% had poor-risk cytogenetics, and the median MDS duration at random assignment was 3 months. The median OS prolongation with decitabine versus best supportive care was not statistically significant (median OS, 10.1 versus 8.5 months; p=0.38).

M.D. Anderson Cancer Center ID03-0180 randomized phase II study compared three outpatient decitabine schedules. In this single-institution study, 95 patients (77 with MDS, and 18 with CMML) were randomized to receive 20 mg/m^2/day intravenously for 5 days, 20 mg/m^2/day subcutaneously for 5 days, or 10 mg/m^2/day intravenously for 10 days. Thus, all patients received the same 100 mg/m^2 total decitabine dose in each treatment cycle. Overall, 32 patients (34%) achieved CR and 69 patients (73%) had an objective response. The 5-day intravenous schedule, which had the highest dose-intensity, was selected as optimal. The

CR rate in that arm was 39% compared with 21% in the 5-day subcutaneous arm and 24% in the 10-day intravenous arm (P<0.05). The high dose-intensity arm (the 5-day intravenous schedule) was also superior at inducing hypomethylation at day 5 and at activating the expression of the cell cycle inhibitor $p15^{INK4B}$ at days 12 or 28 after therapy. The 5-day intravenous schedule of decitabine optimizes epigenetic modulation and clinical responses in MDS.

North American multicenter DACO-020 ADOPT phase II study started on the results of the study of M.D. Anderson Cancer Center dealing with efficacy and safety of decitabine in the 5-day intravenous schedule, every 4 weeks in 99 patients with MDS (de novo or secondary). The primary end point was the overall response rate (ORR) by International Working Group criteria. Secondary end points included cytogenetic responses, hematological improvement, response duration, survival and safety. The ORR was 32% (17 complete responses plus 15 marrow complete responses and the overall improvement rate was 51%, which included 18% of hematologic improvement. Decitabine can be administered in an outpatient petting with comparable efficiacy and safety to the US FDA- approved impatient regimen.

9. Comparison of azacitidine and decitabine

Azacitidine and decitabine appear to have similar administration costs. As far as adverse events azacitidine is well tolerated. Grade 3 and 4 neutropenia was observed for 91% patients in the azacitidine treated group, and 76% in the best conventional care group. Grade 3 and 4 thrombocytopenia occurred among 85% of patients in the azacitidine treated group and 80% in the best conventional care group. Higher risk of febrile neutropenia (23%) was described in the US D-0007 phase III decitabine study. In this study 87 % of neutropenia and 85% of thrombocytopenia in response to decitabine were reported. In AZA-001 study the median OS was 24.5 months for azacitidine compared with 15.0 month for the best conventional care [108]. Decitabine has not demonstrated a survival advantage compared with the best conventional care (14.0 versus 14.9 months) [23]. In the EORTC 06011 study, the median OS was 10.1 months for decitabine and 8.5 months for supportive care [25]. Comparing results from different studies suggests similar median number of cycles to first response for azicitidine (2.3 cycles /64 days/ in CALGB 9221 study) and decitabine (2 cycles /3.3 months/ in the D-0007 study and 2 cycles /2 months/ in DACO-020 ADOPT trial) [23, 106]. For azacitidine treated patients, the median duration of response was 15 months in CALGB 9221 study [107] and 13.6 months in AZA-001 trial [108]. For decitabine treated patients, the median duration of response ranged from 8.6 months for EORTC 06011 study [25], 10 months in the DACO-020 ADOPT trial, to 10.3 months in the D-0007 study [23].

10. Biomarkers of sensitivity to hypomethylating agents

A number of research groups have focused on the identification of methylation patterns that would predict for response in MDS. No such profile exists. Baseline methylation pat-

http://dx.doi.org/10.5772/52099

terns were not associated with response to hypomethylating agents. The significant correlation was observed between reduced methylation over time and clinical outcome. Further studies of methylation dynamics both before and after treatment with hypomethylating agents will be useful to determine the ability of these markers to direct treatment. DNA methylation of upstream regulatory element (URE) controlling the transcription of *PU.1* gene may be a new biomarker for the prediction which patiens will bendit from therapy by hypomethylating agents [102].

Several other biomarkers, such as mutations in *TET2* gene and levels of miR-29b have been reported to be associated with responses to azacitidine and decitabine, respectively. TET2 is a protein involved in the conversion of 5-methylcytosine to 5-hydroxymethylcytosine and could therefore result in passive induction of DNA methylation. TET2 mutations were recently reported to be associated with clinical response to azacitidine but not with survival. Contradictory results were obtained by another research group [112]. TET2 mutations were described in 15% of 86 patients. The response rate to AC was 82% in the mutated patients and 45% in the nonmutated patients with wild *TET2* gene. Mutated TET2 ($p=0.04$) and favorable cytogenetic risk (intermediate risk: $p=0.04$, poor risk: $p=0.048$ compared with good risk) independently predicted a higher response rate. TET2 status may be a genetic predictor of response to AC, independently of karyotype. Expression levels of DNMT1, an enzyme involved in maintenance of methylation patterns, are regulated by miR-29b. Higher levels of miR-29b were associated with clinical response to decitabine.

Circulating cell-free DNAs from plasma and serum of patients with MDS can be used to detect genetic and epigenetic abnormalities. The plasma DNA concentration was found to be relatively high in patients with higher blast cell counts in bone marrow.

11. Resistance to hypomethylating agents

There is a subgroup of patients with MDS who do not respond to therapy with hypomethylating agents and a large, growing cohort of patients that lose progress while on azacidine or decitabine therapy. Since the mechanism of resistance to hypomethylating agents are not known, selection of therapy is largely empiric but must take into account the age, comorbidities, and performance status of the patient, as well as the characteristics of the disease at the time of treatment failure. Higher intensity approaches and allogeneic stem cell transplantation can yield improved response rates and long-term disease control but should be limited to a selected cohort of patients who can tolerate the treatment-related morbidities. For the majority of patients who likely will be better candidates for lower intensity therapy, several novel, investigational approaches are becoming available. Among these are newer nucleoside analogues, inhibitors of protein tyrosine kinases, molecules that interact with redox signaling within the cell, immunotherapy approaches, and others.

In clinical trials, some patients do not respond to hypomethylating agents initially (primary resistance) and most patients who initially respond to treatment, eventually relapse (secondary resistance) despite continued therapy with hypomethylating agents. Most primary mechanisms of resistance are based on metabolic pathways. The primary resistance is caused by the insufficient intracellular concentration of nucleoside triphosphates resulting from deoxycytidine kinase deficiency (DCK mutations or aberrant gene expression), increased deamination by cytidine deaminase (CDA), or high dNTP pools. Higher ratio of CDA/DCK in a subset of patients means that decitabine is less activated through mono-phosphorylation by DCK and more inactivated through deamination by CDA in non-responders. Secondary resistance is likely due alternate progression pathways as a less aberrant DNA methylation was found during the treatment with hypomethylating agent than at diagnosis, and there were no significant changes in decitabine metabolism gene expression.

12. New hypomethylating agents

Current hypomethylating agents are limited due to route of administration and potency as inducers of DNA hypomethylation. An oral compound or an agent with a better pharmacodynamic profile could improve hypomethylating therapy of MDS patients. Initial results with an oral formulation of 5-azacytidine have been reported.

2′, 3′, 5′-triacetyl-5-azacytidine demonstrates significant pharmacokinetic improvements in bioavailability, solubility, and stability over the parent compound 5-azacytidine. *In vivo* analyses indicated a lack of general toxicity coupled with significantly improved survival. Pharmacodynamic analyses confirmed its ability to suppress global methylation *in vivo.* Esterified nucleoside derivatives may be effective prodrugs for azacitidine and encourages further investigation and possible clinical evaluation.

A new salt derivative, oral decitabine mesylate, is used in ongoing trials. A barrier to efficacious and accessible DNMT1-targeted therapy is cytidine deaminase, an enzyme highly expressed in the intestine and liver that rapidly metabolizes decitabine int into inactive uridine counterparts, severely limiting exposure time and oral bioavailability. Oral administration of 3,4,5,6-tetrahydrouridine (THU), a competitive inhibitor of cytidine deaminase, before oral decitabine extended decitabine absorption time in mice and nonhuman primates and widened the concentration-time profile. Therefore, the exposure time for S-phase-specific depletion of DNMT1 is increased without the high peak of decitabine levels that can cause DNA damage and cytotoxicity. On the other hand, decreased DNA methylation in intermediate and high risk AML patients with DNMT3A mutation was linked with higher relapse rates and an inferior overall survival [113].

5,6-dihydro-5-azacytidine (DHAC) and 2′-deoxy-5,6-dihydro-5-azacytidine (DHDAC) are hydrolytically stable. There is no evidence of significant genotoxicity and/or mitochondrial toxicity on mammalian cells. Both compounds are a less toxic alternative of azacitidine and decitabine and may also be of therapeutic interest.

Another compounds actively being studied in clinical trials are SGI-110 and CP-4200, a second generation hypomethylating agents [38]. One of the limitations of the nucleoside analogues in the clinical trials has been the side effects, such as thrombocytopenia and neutropenia, which are probably caused by cytotoxic effects associated with the drug′s incorporation into the DNA or RNA independently of their DNA hypomethylation value. This has encouraged the search for inhibitors of DNA methylation that are not incorporated into DNA or RNA.

Zebularine is a cytidine deaminase inhibitor that also displays antitumor and DNA demethylating properties. Zebularine is a cytidine analog that contains a 2-(1*H*)-pyrimidinone ring.

The drug procainamide, approved by the FDA for the treatment of cardiac arrythmias, and procaine, a drug approved by the FDA for use as a local anesthetic, were proposed as non-nucleoside inhibitors of DNA methylation. This action is thought to be mediated by their binding to GC-rich DNA sequences. Both, procaine and procainamide, are derivatives of 4-amino-benzoic acid.

Dietary phytochemicals, tea catechins, polyphenols, particularly (-)-epigallocatechin-3-gallate decreased the levels of 5-methylcytosine, DNMTs activity, mRNA and protein levels of DNMT1, DNMT3A and DNMT3B and also decreased histone deacetylase aktivity and stimulated re-expression of the mRNA and proteins of silenced tumor suppressor genes.

N-phthalyl-L-tryptophan (RG108) and its dicyclo-hexyl-amine salt effectively blocked DNA methyltransferases *in vitro* and did not cause covalent enzyme tramping in human cell line. Incubation of cells with RG108 resulted in signifiant demethylation of genomic DNA without any detectable toxicity. RG108 caused demethylation and reactivation of tumor suppressor genes.

13. Combinations of hypomethylating agents with histone deacetylase inhibitors or other drugs

In vitro, most of histone deacetylase inhibitors (HDACI) have been shown to have synergistic activity when combined with either azacitidine or decitabine. Therefore, phase I and II clinical trials were performed. Combination of decitabine and valproic acid was safe and active and time to response was accelerated [6,12]. A randomized phase II trial has been conducted at M.D. Anderson Cancer Center comparing decitabine versus decitabine in combination with valproic acid [6, 12, 39]. Results did not show any significant benefit with the combination of decitabine and valproic acid. Similar results were obtained with combination of azacitidine and MS-275 (Entinostat), a potent HDACI [12, 39].

Phase I trial for combination of lenalidomide with azacitidine has shown this combination to be very safe and clinically active in MDS [114]. In this study 18 patients (2 intermediate 1-, 10 intermediate 2- and 6 high- risk) were enrolled with median age 68 years (range, 52 to 78 years). Interval from diagnosis was 5 weeks (range, 2 to 106 weeks) and follow-up was 7 months (range, 1 to 26 months). Azacitidine (75 mg/m^2/day) on days 1 through 5 and lenalidomide (10 mg) on days 1 through 21 were used. The combination of lenalidomide and azacitidine is well tolerated with encouraging clinical activity.

14. Lenalidomide with potent immunomodulatory, antiangiogenic and direct neoplastic cell inhibitory activity

Interstitial deletions involving long arm of chromosome 5 are one of the common cytogenetic abnormalities in MDS patients [115-117]. MDS with isolated del(5q) in which the sole cytogenetic abnormality is del(5q) is a distinct entity with a risk of evolution into AML of approximately 10%. It is characterized by macrocytic anemia with or without other cytopenias and/or thrombocytosis. Myeloblasts comprise less than 5% of bone marrow and less than 1% of peripheral blood.

Lenalidomide [3-(4-amino-1-oxo1,3-dihydro-2H-isoindol-2-yl)piperidine-2,6-dione] is 4-amino-glutarimide analog of thalidomide with potent immunomodulatory, antiangiogenic and direct neoplastic cell inhibitory activity [118-120]. Thalidomide was synthesized in Germany, in 1954, from α-phtaloylisoglutamine, to be used as sedative and antimetic drug. In 1957, after a short period of preclinical studies, thalidomide was approved for first trimester gestational sickness in humans. The appearance of malformations such as phocomelia in the newborn banned its use three years later. The US Food and Drug Administration (FDA) approved thalidomide in 1998 for the treatment of erythema nodosum leprosum. A small but consistent fraction of transfusion-dependent MDS patients achieved transfusion independence by treatment with thalidomide.

Lenalidomide was developed in order to avoid thalidomide side effects (sedation and neuropathy), and to increase efficacy [118-120]. Lenalidomide shares a number of structural and biological properties with thalidomide but is safer and more potent than thalidomide. Lenalidomide was first studied in a single- center trial [121]. Erythroid and cytogenetic responses were achieved in a study of 43 patients with MDS, particularly in patients with isolated del(5q31-33) [28]. Lenalidomide was administered in three different dosing schedules: 25 mg daily, 10 mg daily, and 10 mg daily for 21 days of each 28-day cycle [121]. The erythroid response rates were highest in patients with the International Prognostic scoring system (IPSS) low or intermediate 1 risk MDS. Transfusion independence was achieved in 20 of 32 patients (63%), and three additional patients had reduced red blood cells transfusion needs [121]. Ten of 12 patients (83%) with del(5q31) experienced major erythroid responses, defined as sustained transfusion independence, compared with a 57% response rate in patients with a normal karyotype and a 12% response rate in patients with other cytogenetic abnormalities. Complete cytogenetic remissions were achieved in 75% of the del(5q31) patients (9 of 12 of these patients), with one additional patient achieving at least a 50% decreases in abnormal metaphases [121]. Myelosuppression (neutropenia and/or thrombocytopenia) was the most common adverse event, but it was dose-dependent, favoring the 10 mg daily dose for 21 days of each 28-day cycle.

15. Multicenter phase II trials of lenalidomide

After encouraging results of a single-center trial (MDS-001) [28], the effect of lenalidomide on the 5q31 deletion MDS syndrome was investigated in a large multicenter phase II study (MDS-003) and led to its FDA approval for red blood cell transfusion-dependent anemia due to low or intermediate-1 risk MDS associated with a chromosome 5q deletion with or without additional cytogenetic abnormalities [122]. The initial schedule was 10 mg of lenalidomide for 21 days every 4 weeks, but the treatment schedule was subsequently amended so that the 10 mg dose was given every day because of the shorter interval between initiation of treatment and a response in the pilot study. Of the 148 transfusion-dependent patients who were included in the study, 46 were treated on the 21-day schedule and 102 received continuous daily dosing. Overall, 112 (76%) patients responded to treatment with a median time to response 4.6 weeks. Among these, 99 no longer needed transfusions by week 24, while the remaining 13 patients had a reduction of 50% or greater in the number of transfusions required. There was no significant difference in response rate between the two treatment schedules. Response rate was independent of additional chromosomal aberrations. Patients with pretreatment thrombocytopenia had an inferior outcome. Almost half of the patients, including some with complex karyotypes, had a complete cytogenetic response. Neutropenia and thrombocytopenia were the most common treatment-associated adverse events. Most other adverse events were of low or moderate severity and included pruritus, rash, diarrhea, and fatigue. Adjustment of the lenalidomide dose due to intolerance was required in 124 patients, including 93 of those receiving continuous daily dosing and 31 of those receiving 21-day dosing. Thirty patients discontinued lenalidomide treatment because of adverse events including thrombocytopenia or neutropenia, rash AML, anemia, facial edema, congestive heart failure, urticaria, diarrhea, weight loss, renal insufficiency, cerebrovascular accident, dementia, dyspnea, pyrexia, and pneumonia.

However, the European Medicine Agency (EMEA) did not approve lenalidomide for this indication, raising the concern, based on the results of the MDS-003 trial, that lenalidomide may trigger progression to AML in some patients with del(5q).

Current recommendation state that treatment with lenalidomide in del(5q) MDS should be continued until disease progression [123]. The question whether interrruption of lenalidomide treatment for patients in remission would be beneficial has been also addressed [124]. It is important for several reasons: 1) it could reduce costs and side effects; 2) it could facilitate disease progression to AML. Different mechanisms have been discussed to explain AML progression. Evidence that pre-therapeutic telomere length was significantly shorter in those patients who ultimately transformed to AML than in those who did not was presented [125]. Transformation to AML is occasionally observed, paticularly in patients without a cytogenetic response to lenalidomide. Jädersten et al. [126] performed molecular studies in a patient with classical 5q- syndrome with complete erythroid and partial cytogenetic response to lenalidomide, who evolved to high-risk MDS with complex karyotype. Immunohistochemistry of pretreatment marrow biopsies revealed a small fraction of progenitors with overexpression of p53 and sequencing confirmed a *TP53* mutation. *TP53* mutated subclones have not previously been detected in 5q- syndrome and indicates heterogeneity of this disease. Subsequently, *TP53* mutations with a median clone size of 11% (range, 1% to 54%) were detected in 10 from 55 (18%) low-risk MDS or intermediate-1 risk patients with del(5q) by next-generation sequencing [127]. *TP53* mutations are associated with strong nuclear p53 protein expression. Patients with mutation had significantly worse outcome. *TP53* mutations may lead to genetic instability and disease progression. This clonal heterogeneity in low-risk MDS patients with del(5q) may be of importance when assessing the prognosis and selecting the therapy in these patients. It has been speculated that continuous administration of lenalidomide may lead to selective pressure on stem cells that induces genomic instability, resulting in acute leukemia transformation [128].

Longest transfusion-free intervals are achieved in patients low-risk MDS patients with del(5q) who are exposed to lenalidomide 6 months beyond complete cytogenetic remission [41, 124]. Lenalidomide should not be withdrawn prematurely in patients who achieve transfusion independence as partial cytogenetic remission patients seem to have a higher relapse rate than complete cytogenetic remission patients.

Treatment by lenalidomide is based on scientific knowledge because small deletions in several ribosomal genes, including *RPS14*, were found in CD34+ cells not only in patients with del(5q) but also in patients with non-del(5q) MDS [41, 42, 129-131]. This observation suggested that deregulated ribosomal biogenesis may not be limited to del(5q) MDS. Czibere et al. [132] showed that lower risk non-del(5q) MDS patients with *RPS14* haploinsufficiency tend to have prolonged survival. Defective ribosomal biogenesis has a lead role in disrupting erythropoiesis in a variety of anemias. Disruption of ribosomal biogenesis has been clearly demonstrated in multiple ribosomopathies to greatly perturb p53 signaling [130, 131].

Bone marrow aspirates of patients who responded to lenalidomide showed before treatment decreased expression of the set of the genes needed for erythroid differentiation. Lenalidomide seems to overcome differentiation block in del(5q) patients with decreased expression of these genes compared to the non-responders [131]. Thus, lenalidomide restored erythroid differentiation potential by upregulation of the suppressed erythroid gene signature (genes for α- and β-globin, ankyrin 1, band 3, band 4.2, carbonic anhydrase, ferrochelatase and glycophorin B) [133].

The "Groupe Francophone des Myélodysplasies" conducted a multicenter phase 2 trial with lenalidomide in intermediate-2 (19 patients) and high-risk MDS (28 patients) with del(5q). Forty seven patients (24 males and 23 females, with a median age of 69 years, range, 36-84 years) were treated. Forty three patients of 47 patients had transfusion-dependent anemia. Patients received 10 mg lenalidomide once daily orally during 21 days every 4 weeks. In patients without response after 8 weeks, the lenalidomide dose was increased to 15 mg/day in the same time schedule during an additional 8 weeks. If no response was found in this additional time of treatment, lenalidomide was discontinued. Thirteen of the 47 patients (27%) achieved response according to International Working Group (IWG) 2006 criteria. Median duration of overall response was 6.5 months, 11.5 months in patients who achieved the complete remission. Grade 3 and 4 neutropenia and thrombocytopenia were seen in most patients.

Möllgård et al. [7] hypothesized that increasing doses of lenalidomide may be successfully used in high-risk MDS and AML with chromosome 5 abnormalities. They tested this hypothesis in prospective phase II multicenter trial with 28 patients (12 with intermediate-risk 2 or high-risk MDS and 16 with AML). Oral lenalidomide was given at a dose of 10 mg/day in weeks 1 to 5. The dose was increased to 20 mg/day in weeks 6 to 9, and to 30 mg/day in weeks 10 to 16. In the case of suspected drug-related toxicity the dose was lowered to 5 mg/day. The overall response rate in treated patients with MDS was 36% (4/11) and that for AML patients was 20% (3/15). Seven patients stopped therapy due to progressive disease and nine because of complications, most of which were disease-related. Patients with *TP53* mutations responded less well than those without mutations. No responses were observed among 11 cases with deleterious *TP53* mutation [7].

16. Randomized phase III placebo-controlled study of lenalidomide in del(5q) patients

This study [134] examined the safety of lenalidomide in a randomized phase III trial (MDS-004) in low-/int-1-risk myelodysplastic syndromes (MDS) with a del(5q) abnormality.

The similar criteria as in the MDS-003 study were chosen. Two hundred five patients were randomized to receive treatment with either lenalidomide 10 mg orally daily for 21 days of each 28-day cycle, lenalidomide 5 mg orally daily for 28 days of each 28-day cycle, or placebo. Erythroid responses were assessed at 16 weeks. Nonresponders were then in open-label treatment and they were excluded from the efficacy analysis. Red blood cell transfusion independence was achieved in 53.6% of patients treated on 10 mg arm, 33.3% on 5 mg arm and 6% on the placebo arm. Cytogenetic response rates were also highest in the 10 mg arm (41.5% of patients), while in 5 mg arm (17.4%) and in the placebo arm (0%). The median rise in hemoglobin at the time of the best response was also higher in patients treated with the 10 mg lenalidomide. No difference in the rate of AML trandsformation among three arms was found. This study confirmed that the preferred starting dose of lenalidomide in patients with del(5q) low-/int-1-risk MDS remains 10 mg.

17. Further clinical studies of lower risk MDS patients with del(5q) treated with lenalidomide

Many of the initial clinical and laboratory observations obtained in the MDS-003 trial were confirmed in the study of Le Bras et al. [135]. Ninety five lower risk MDS patients (low and intermediate 1 risk in IPSS, 25 males and 70 females with a median age of 70.4 years) with del(5q) were treated with 10 mg of lenalidomide daily, 21 days every 28 days for at least 16 weeks. Patients with at least a minor erythroid response after 16 weeks were treated in the same way until disease progression, treatment failure or treatment-limiting toxicity.

Erythroid response was evaluated according to international working group (IWG) 2000 criteria. Sixty two of the 95 patients (65%) achieved erythroid response according to IWG 2006 criteria. In these 62 patients, 60 patients (63% from 95 patients) achieved red blood cell transfusion independence. Median time to transfusion independence was 16 weeks (range 8-33 weeks). Fifteen patients who achieved transfusion independence were analyzed for cytogenetic response (20% of complete and 40% of partial cytogenetic response). The rest of these 15 patients (40%) had no cytogenetic response. Six (6.3%) patients progressed to AML and 15 patients died, including 6 patients who had achieved transfusion independence. In the MDS-003 trial, the primary endpoint was hematological response, while in the study of Le Bras et al. transfusion independence. The cytogenetic remission rate was higher in the MDS-003 trial (73% versus 60% in the study of Le Bras et al. [135]. Neutropenia and thrombocytopenia were the most common adverse events in both studies.

A Japanese multiinstitutional study MDS-007 in MDS patients with del(5q) treated with lenalidomide has been recently performed. This study was targeted on morphologic analysis and evaluation of the relationship among erythroid response, change of morphologic findings and cytogenetic response. MDS-007 trial was a single-arm, open-label study. Eleven patients were enrolled in this study, including 5 patients with transfusion-dependent anemia and 6 patients with transfusion-independent symptomatic anemia. Nine patients showed less than 25% of bone marrow erythroblasts before therapy with lenalidomide and no patient had more than 40% of bone marrow erythroblasts at that time. Eight patients showed a rapid increase of bone marrow erythroblasts to more than 40% on day 85. All patients except one achieved a major erythroid response as defined by either transfusion independence or by rapid increase of hemoglobin level in most patients on day 169 of lenalidomide therapy. One patient without any hematologic response by day 169, achieved a major erythroid response on day 218. Erythroid response could be achieved even without a cytogenetic response. No patient in this analysis showed a hematological relapse prior to cytogenetic one. These findings suggested that lenalidomide can improve anemia by more than one mechanism of action and also through mechanism different from del(5q) elimination.

18. Therapy with lenalidomide in combination with another drug in MDS

In order to maximize the potential benefit from lenalidomide therapy combination strategies were developed. Lenalidomide in attemp to improve outcome of patients can be combined with erythropoiesis-stimulating agents (ESA), such as erythropoietin or darbepoietin alpha. This therapy is based on preclinical observations shoving that lenalidomide significantly potentiated erythropoietin receptor signaling. The addition of erythropoietin (40, 000 U/week) for an additional 8-week course had the beneficial effect in low and intermediate-1 risk MDS patients who had failed prior treatment with lenalidomide monotherapy for 16 weeks. To evaluate the potential benefit of the combination of lenalidomide and ESA, Park et al. [136] tried the association in three del5q MDS patients, who were resistant or partially responding to lenalidomide alone. Lenalidomide had two different actions, one on the disapperance of the 5q- clone and the other one on the stimulation of the erythroid production in combination with ESA.

In low to intermediate-1 risk non-del(5q) MDS, lenalidomide treatment is less effective with a lower response rate (25%) and shorter response duration than in the same risk MDS with del(5q) [41]. Combination of lenalidomide with another drug could improve outcome of patients with low to intermediate-1 risk non-del(5q) MDS. Ezatiostat hydrochloride (Telintra, TLK199), a tripeptide glutathione analog is a reversible inhibitor of the enzyme glutathione S-transferase P1-1 (GSTP1-1) inhibitor. This inhibitor was developed for the treatment of cytopenias associated with lower risk MDS. Ezatiostat activates jun-N-terminal kinase (JNK), promoting the growth and maturation of hematopoietic progenitors, while inducing apoptosis in human leukemia blasts. The ability of ezatiostat to activate the caspase-dependent pathway may help eliminate or inhibit the emergence of malignant clones. Alternatively, ezatiostat increases reactive oxygen species in dysplastic cells and contibutes by this effect also to apoptotic death. Based on these mechanisms of action, response rates, non-overlapping toxicities, and tolerability observed in a single agent ezatiostat phase 1 and 2 studies in MDS, a study of the combination of ezatiostat and lenalidomide was conducted to determine the safety and efficacy of ezatiostat with lenalidomide in non-del(5q) low to intermediate-1 risk MDS. Eighteen patients (median age 73 years; range 57-82; 72% male) were enrolled in the study. Thirteen patients (72%) were intermediate-1 risk and 5 patients (28%) were low risk. Four patients had abnormal cytogenetics. Twelve patients (67%) were red blood cell transfusion-dependent and 2 patients (11%) were were platelet transfusion-dependent. Three of 8 (38%) patients achieved transfusion independence including 1 responder who did not respond to prior lenalidomide. Ezatiostat caused clinically significant reduction in red blood cell and platelet transfusions. Since ezatiostat is non-myelosuppressive, it is a good candidate for combination with lenalidomide. The recommended doses of this combination regimen for future studies is the ezatiostat.

Lenalidomide and azacitidine combination has been already described [14, 114].

Romiplostim (AMG 531, Nplate) is an Fc-peptide fusion protein (peptibody) that acts as a thrombopoietin receptor agonist. It has no amino acid sequence homology with endogenous thrombopoietin. Romiplostim stimulates megakaryopoiesis and thrombopoiesis by binding to and activating the thrombopoietin receptor and downstream signaling. Romiplostim appeared well tolerated in patients with lower risk MDS and thrombocytopenia. Low platelet counts in patients with MDS may be due to the underlying disease or due to treatment with disease-modifying agents, and platelet transfusions are often the only treatment for clinically significant thrombocytopenia or bleeding. Randomized phase II study evaluating the efficacy and safety of romiplostim treatment of patients with low or intermediate-1 risk MDS receiving lenalidomide was performed. This was double-blind, placebo controlled, dose finding study that evaluated the effect of romiplostim on the incidence of clinically significant thrombocytopenia events (grade 3 or 4 thrombocytopenia and/or receipt of platelet transfusions) and the safety of romiplostim in patients with low or intermediate-1 risk MDS receiving lenalidomide. Thirty nine patients (median age 74 years; range, 39 to 90) were randomized into treatment groups receiving placebo, 500 μg romiplostim, or 750 μg romiplostim by weekly subcutaneous injections in combination with lenalidomide (one 10 mg capsule by mouth daily for each 28-day cycle). Fifteen patients (39%) had platelet counts◎50x10^9/L and 7 (18%) had del(5q). Treatment continued for a total of four cycles. Twelve patients (31%) discontinued the study. Disease progression to AML was reported in 1 patient in the romiplostim 500 µg group. Response was 8% for the placebo, 36% for 500 µg romiplostim, and 15% for 750 µg romiplostim groups. Romiplostim appeared to be well toll-erated in low or intermediate-1 risk MDS patients receiving lenalidomide.

It is possible that effect of lenalidomide could be augmented with the addition of another immunomodulation agent, cyclosporine A. A single-arm, open-label study of the efficacy and safety of lenalidomide in combination with cyclosporine A in red blood cell transfusion-dependent both 5q- and non 5q- MDS patients started at Weill Cornell Medical College in New York.

Other drugs are tried and will be probably used in combinations with lenalidomide in the treatment MDS patients with del(5q) in the future. Dexamethasone and lenalidomide rescue erythropoiesis, alone and in combination, in RPS14- and RPS19- (ribosomal proteins of small ribosomal subunit) deficient cells [137]. L-leucine was also studied in RPS14- and RPS19- deficient cells [138-141]. The combined use of L-leucine and lenalidomide might be considered for therapy in MDS patients with the del(5q) since there is evidence to suggest that these two drugs act through different mechanism and their effect may be synergistic.

19. Mechanisms of action of lenalidomide

Lenalidomide shares a number of structural and biological properties with thalidomide but is safer and more potent than thalidomide. Both drugs appear to function through four mechanisms: immunomodulatory, anti-inflammatory, anti-angiogenic and direct neoplastic cells inhibitory [41, 42, 142]. Lenalidomide has a direct erythropoiesis stimulating effect. Wei et al. [143] demonstrated that the haplodeficient enzymatic targets of lenalidomide within the commonly deleted region are two dual-specificity phosphatases, the cell division cycle 25C (Cdc25C) and the protein phosphatase 2A (PP2A). These phosphatases are coregulators of G2-M checkpoint in the cell cycle and thus, their inhibition by lenalidomide leads to G2 arrest and apoptosis of del(5q) specimens. The mechanism of action is different in non-del(5q), where lenalidomide restores and promotes effective erythropoiesis with no direct cytotoxic effect [144]. Lenalidomide promotes erythropoiesis and fetal hemoglobin production in human CD34+ cells [144]. The increased fetal hemoglobin expression was associated with epigenetic effect on chromatin (an increase in histone 3 acetylation on the γ-globin gene promoter).

The similar epigenetic modulation of gene for p21(CIP1/WAF1) by lenalidomide was described in both lymphoma and multiple myeloma. A potent cyclin-dependent kinase inhibitor p21(CIP1/WAF1) decreases activity of cyclinE-CDK2 or cyclinD-CDK4/6 complexes, and thus functions as a regulator of cell cycle progression. The p21 protein can mediate cellular senescence and also interact with proliferating cell nuclear antigen (PCNA), a DNA polymerase accessory factor, and plays a regulatory role in S phase DNA replication and DNA damage repair.

Most MDS patients including those with del(5q) become refractory to erythropoietin (EPO). EPO is an essential glycoprotein that facilitates red blood cell maturation from erythroid progenitors and mediates erythropoiesis. EPO acts through EPO-receptor (EPO-R) and the signal transducer and activator of transcription 5 (STAT5). Disruption of STAT5 results in a variety of cell-specific effects, one of which is the impaired erythropoiesis. Lenalidomide relieves repression of ligand-dependent activation of the EPO-R/STAT5 pathway. Ebert et al. [133] showed that target genes of this pathway are underexpressed in lenalidomide-responsive MDS patients wihout del (5q). Lenalidomide promotes erythropoiesis in MDS by CD45 protein tyrosine phosphatase inhibition. CD45 phosphatase is overactivated in MDS and may inhibit phosphorylation of STAt5 stimulated by EPO-R. Lenalidomide is able to restore EPO-R/STAT5 signaling that is essential for hematopoiesis. Lenalidomide restores and promotes effective erythropoiesis in non-del(5q) without direct cytotoxic effect.

A deregulated immune system plays the important role in pathogenesis of MDS. Deregulation is caused by the alteration of cytokines in the bone marrow microenvironment, deffective T-cell regulation and diminished natural killer (NK) cell activity. Deficiences in T cells, NK cells and interferon-γ (IFN-γ) production were described in the bone marrow and peripheral blood of MDS patients. Lenalidomide exhibits potent T-cell costimulatory properties and augmented production of IL-2 and IFN-γ [118]. Akt (proteinase B) signaling pathway and transcription factor AP1 (activator protein 1) are involved in T-cell activation. Increased numbers and activation of NK and NK T-cell populations were also observed in peripheral blood cells cultured with lenalidomide.

Anti-inflammatory effects of lenalidomide is based on the inhibition of proinflammatory cytokines and chemokines, such as TNF-α, IL-1β, IL-6, IL-12, monocyte chemotactic protein-1 and macrophage inflammatory protein-1α. On the other hand, lenalidomide elevates anti-inflammatory cytokine IL-10. Interestingly, haploinsuficiency of miR-145 and miR-146a in 5q - syndrome increases IL-6 levels by elevation of interleukin-1 receptor-associated kinase 1 (IRAK1), Toll-interleukin-1 receptor domain-containing adaptor protein (TIRAP), tumor necrosis factor receptor-associated factor-6 (TRAF6), and NF-κB [145].

Angiogenesis, the formation of new blood vessels, plays an important role in the growth and progression of MDS. Anti-angiogenic effects of lenalidomide are independent of immunomodulatory effects and are mediated through endothelial cell migration inhibition. The mechanism by which lenalidomide inhibited vascular endothelial growth factor (VEGF)-induced endothelial cell migration may be related to VEGF-induced inhibition of Akt phosphorylation. Furthermore, loss of anti-angiogenic effect of lenalidomide predicted disease progression and an increased risk of transformation to AML.

Lenalidomide does not affect DNA synthesis but inhibits cytokinesis of MDS cells. Cytokinesis occurs as the final stage of cell division after mitosis. A contractile ring, made of non-muscle myosin and actin filaments assembles in the middle of the cell adjacent to the cell membrane. Formins are Rho-GTPase effector proteins that are involved in the polymerization of actin and effects microtubule during meiosis, mitosis, the maintenance of cell polarity, vesicular trafficking and signaling to the nucleus. Diaphanous (mDia)-related formin mDia1 is encoded by *DIAPH1* located on the long arm of chromosome 5 (5q31.3) and lies between the two commonly deleted regions in MDS patients with 5q- syndrome. It is not clear whether mDia1 plays a role in lenalidomide effect on cytokinesis. Knock-out of *DIAPH1* in mice has T cell responses and myelodysplastic phenotype.

The clinical effect of lenalidomide is associated with significant increases in the numbers of erythroid, myeloid and megakaryocytic colony-forming cells and a substantial improvement in the hematopoiesis-supporting capacity of bone marrow stroma. Lenalidomide induces significant alterations in the adhesion profile of hematopoietic progenitor cells, including over-expression of membrane ligands (CXCR4/CD184, CD54/ICAM1, CD11a and CD49d where CD is cluster of differentiation) and overproduction of soluble stromal cell-derived factor-1 (SDF-1) and of ICAM1 in the bone marrow microenvironment. CXCR4 is C-X-C chemokine receptor type 4 also known as fusin or CD184. ICAM1 (intracellular adhesion molecule 1 also known as CD54) is a cell surface glycoprotein. All these effects favor the maintenance of CD34+ cells in the bone marrow. Lenalidomide-mediated induction of the SLAM antigen CD48 on patients′ CD34+ cells may be associated with the drug′s apoptosis-inducing effect through co-stimulatory interactions between CD34+ cells and cytotoxic lymphocytes in the bone marrow microenvironment.

20. Conclusion and perspectives

Despite the encouraging results with azacitidine and decitabine, it is obvious that it will be important to have access to second generation agents with the capacity to increase faster early response rates with acceptable toxicity profiles. Preliminary results with oral formulation of both azacitine and decitabine are promising and these forms could improve hypomethylating therapy of MDS patients in future. Another approach is to develop combination strategies using either azacitidine or decitabine. Several such approaches are currently studied and many are promising but not yet fully understood. Including of cytidine deaminase inhibitor in these combinations appears to be important for better results but it needs new clinical studies. Lenalidomide is currently the treatment of choice for lower risk transfusion-dependent del(5q) MDS patients, and remains a treatment alternative for the management of anemia in lower risk MDS without 5q deletion MDS patients with adequate neutrophil and platelet counts [41, 42]. Lenalidomide has also activity in higher risk MDS and AML with del(5q) and even in non(del5q) MDS.

Though the mechanism of lenalidomide action has not been definitively determined, it is clear that there is difference between mechanisms in MDS with del(5q) and MDS with non-del(5q).

In MDS with del(5q), lenalidomide acts through inhibition of phosphatase activity in the commonly deleted region of the long arm of chromosome 5. This phosphatases play a key role in in cell cycle regulation. The inhibition of these phosphatases by lenalidomide leads to G2 arrest, followed by apoptosis of del(5q) specimens. The direct cytotoxic effects of lenalidomide on the del(5q) clone are also very important. Lenalidomide inhibits the malignant clone and up-regulates the *SPARC* gene mapping to the commonly deleted region in 5q-syndrome patients. However, SPARC is dispensable for murine hematopoiesis [146]. While haploinsufficiency of the *RPS14* gene appears to be a key contributor to erythropoietic failure associated with del(5q) MDS, the critical genes responsible for clonal dominance in del(5q) high-risk MDS and AML are less well-defined. It is known that this deleted region is different in del(5q) high-risk MDS and AML [147]. The effect of lenalidomide in these cases needs to identify further biologic features accounting for response, thereby allowing rational use of this drug, both alone and in combination with another agents.

In MDS with non-del(5q), an increased expression of adhesion molecules caused by lenalidomide treatment leads to recovery and maintenance of the CD34+ cells through interactions between the hematopoietic and stromal cells. This effect of lenalidomide on the bone marrow microenvironment causes abrogation of the function of pro-apoptotic and pro-inflammatory cytokines. Lenalidomide is capable to increase red blood cell production independently of ribosome dysfunction. Lenalidomide restores and promotes effective erythropoiesis without direct cytotoxic effect. Lenalidomide activates the EPO-R/STAT5 pathway.

New cytogenetic tools such as fluorescence in situ hybridization (FISH) or single nucleotide polymorphism array (SNP-A)-based karyotyping increased the diagnostic yield over metaphase cytogenetics. Sugimoto et al. [148] have recently found with help of these new cytogenetic tools that normal karyotype and gain of chromosome 8 were predictive of response to lenalidomide in non-del(5q) patients with myeloid malignancies.

The presence of multiple cellular and genetic abnormalities in MDS and AML is common and suggests that combination therapy targeting different mechanisms of action may be beneficial particularly in higher-risk MDS disease, for which both microenvironment and cell regulatory mechanisms play a role. The optimal dose, schedule and duration of treatment is still an area of active investigation, especially in the use of lenalidomide combinations with other drugs.

Acknowledgements

This work was supported by the research grant NT/13836-4/2012 from the Ministry of Health of the Czech Republic.

Author details

Ota Fuchs*

Address all correspondence to:

Institute of Hematology and Blood Transfusion, Prague, Czech Republic

References

[1] Tone, R.M. (2009). How I treat patients with myelodysplastic syndromes. *Blood*, 113(25), 6296-6303.

[2] Fehniger, T. A., Byrd, J. C., Marcucci, G., Abboud, C. N., Kefauver, C., Payton, J. E., Vij, R., & Blum, W. (2009). Single-agent lenalidomide induces complete remission of acute leukemia in patiens with isolated trisomy 13. *Blood*, 113(5), 1002-1005.

[3] Fenaux, P., Bowen, D., Gattermann, N., Hellström-Lindberg, E., Hofmann, W. K., Pfeilstöcker, M., Sanz, G., & Santini, V. (2010). Practical use of azacitidine in higher-risk myelodysplastic syndromes: An expert panel opinion. *Leukemia Research*, 34(11), 1410-1416.

[4] Fenaux, P., Mufti, G. J., Hellström-Lindberg, E., Santini, V., Gattermann, N., Germing, U., Sanz, G., List, A. F., Gore, S., Seymour, J. F., Dombret, H., Backstrom, J., Zimmerman, L., Mc Kenzie, D., Beach, C. L., & Silverman, L. R. (2010). Azacitidine prolongs overall survival compared with conventional care regimens in elderly patients with low bone marrow blast count acute myeloid leukemia. *Journal of Clinical Oncology*, 28(4), 562-569.

[5] Cashen, A. F., Schiller, G. J., O', Donnell. M. R., & Di Persio, J. F. (2010). Multicenter, phase II study of decitabine for the first-line treatment of older patients with acute myeloid leukemia. *Journal of Clinical Oncology*, 28(4), 556-561.

[6] Abujamra, A. L., Dos, Santos. M. P., Roesler, R., Schwartsmann, G., & Brunetto, A. L. (2010). Histone deacetylase inhibitors: *A new perspective for the treatment of leukemia. Leukemia Research*, 34(6), 687-695.

[7] Möllgård, L., Saft, L., Treppendahl, M. B., Dybedal, I., Nørgaard, J. M., Astermark, J., Ejerblad, E., Garelius, H., Dufva, I. H., Jansson, M., Jädersten, M., Kjeldsen, L., Linder, O., Nilsson, L., Vestergaard, H., Porwit, A., Grønbaek, K., & Hellström-Lindberg, E. (2011). Clinical effect of increasing doses of lenalidomide in high-risk myelodysplastic syndrome and acute myeloid leukemia with chromosome 5 abnormalities. *Haematologica*, 96(7), 963-971.

[8] Fehniger, T. A., Uy, G. L., Trinkaus, K., Nelson, A. D., Domland, J., Abboud, C. N., Cashen, A. F., Stockerl-Goldstein, K. E., Westervelt, P., Di Persio, J. F., & Vij, R. (2011). A phase 2 study of high-dose lenalidomide as initial therapy for older patients with acute myeloid leukemia. *Blood*, 117(6), 1828-1833.

[9] Sekeres, M. A., Gundacker, H., Lancet, J., Advani, A., Petersdorf, S., Liesveld, J., Mulford, D., Norwood, T., Willman, C. L., Appelbaum, F. R., & List, A. F. (2011). A phase 2 study of lenalidomide monotherapy in patients with deletion 5q acute myeloid leukemia: Southwest Oncology Group Study S0605. *Blood*, 118(3), 523-528.

[10] Prebet, T., & Vey, N. (2011). Vorinostat in acute myeloid leukemia and myelodysplastic syndromes. *Expert Opinion on Investigational Drugs*, 20(2), 287-295.

[11] Quintás-Cardama, A., Santos, F. P., & Garcia-Manero, G. (2011). Histone deacetylase inhibitors for the treatment of myelodysplastic syndrome and acute myeloid leukemia. *Leukemia*, 25(2), 226-235.

[12] Ornstein, M. C., & Sekeres, M. A. (2012). Combination strategies in myelodysplastic syndromes. *International Journal of Hematology*, 95(1), 26-33.

[13] Ozbalak, M., Cetiner, M., Bekoz, H., Atezoglu, E. B., Ar, C., Salihoglu, A., Tuzuner, N., & Ferhanoglu, B. (2012). Azacitidine has limited aktivity in 'real life' patiens with MDS and AML: a single centre experience. *Hematological Oncology*, 30(2), 76-81.

[14] Pollyea, D. A., Kohrt, H. E., Gallegos, L., Figueroa, M. E., Abdel-Wahab, O., Zhang, B., Battacharya, S., Zehnder, J., Liedtke, M., Gotlib, J. R., Coutre, S., Berube, C., Melnick, A., Levine, R., Mitchell, B. S., & Medeiros, B. C. (2012). Safety, efficacy and biological predictors of response to sequential azacitidine and lenalidomide for elderly patients with acute myeloid leukemia. *Leukemia,*, 26(5), 893-901.

[15] Schecter, J., Galili, N., & Raza, A. (2012). MDS: Refining existing therapy through improved biologic insights. *Blood Reviews*, 26(2), 73-80.

[16] Fazi, F., Racanicchi, S., Zardo, G., Starnes, L. M., Mancini, M., Travaglini, L., Diverio, D., Ammatuna, E., Cimino, G., Lo-Coco, F., Grignani, F., & Nervi, C. (2007). Epigenetic silencing of the myelopoiesis regulator microRNA-223 by the AML1/ETO oncoprotein. *Cancer Cell*, 12(5), 457-466.

[17] Nervi, C., Fazi, F., & Grignani, F. (2008). Oncoproteins, heterochromatin silencing and microRNAs: a new link for leukemogenesis. *Epigenetics*, 3(1), 1-4.

[18] Garzon, R., Lin, S., Fabbri, M., Liu, Z., Heaphy, C. E., Callegari, E., Schwind, S., Pang, J., Yu, J., Muthusamy, N., Havelange, V., Volinia, S., Blum, W., Rush, L. J., Perrotti, D., Andreeff, M., Bloomfield, C. D., Byrd, J. C., Chan, K., Wu, L. C., Croce, C. M., & Marcucci, G. (2009). MicroRNA-29b induces global DNA hypomethylation and tumor suppressor gene reexpression in acute myeloid leukemia by targeting directly DNMT3A and 3B and indirectly DNMT1. *Blood*, 113(25), 6411-6418.

[19] Sato, F., Tsuchiya, S., Meltzer, S. J., & Shimizu, K. (2011). MicroRNAs and epigenetics. *FEBS Journal*, 278(10), 1598-1609.

[20] Chim, C. S., Wong, K. Y., Leung, C. Y., Chung, L. P., Hui, P. K., Chan, S. Y., & Yu, L. (2011). Epigenetic inactivation of the has-miR-203 in haematological malignancies. *Journal of Cellular and Molecular Medicine*, 15(12), 2760-2767.

[21] Wong, K. Y., So, C. C., Loong, F., Chung, L. P., Lam, W. W., Liang, R., Li, G. K., Jin, D. Y., & Chim, C. S. (2011). Epigenetic inactivation of the miR-1241in haematological malignancies. *PLOS One* 6 (4): e 19027.

[22] Rager, J. E., & Fry, R. C. (2012). The aryl hydrocarbon receptor pathway: a key component of the microRNA-mediated AML signalisome. *International Journal of Environmental Research and Public Health*, 9(5), 1939-1953.

[23] Kantarjian, H., Issa, J. P., Rosenfeld, C. S., Bennett, J. M., Albitar, M., Di Persio, J., Klimek, V., Slack, J., de Castro, C., Ravandi, F., & Helmer, R. (2006). 3rd, Shen L, Nimer SD, Leavitt R, Raza A, Saba H. Decitabine improves patient outcomes in myelodysplastic syndromes: results of a phase III randomized study. *Cancer*, 106(8), 1794-1803.

[24] Issa, J. P., & Kantarjian, H. M. (2009). Targeting DNA methylation. *Clinical Cancer Research*, 15(12), 3938-3946.

[25] Lübbert, M., Suciu, S., Baila, L., Rüter, B. H., Platzbecker, U., Giagounidis, A., Selleslag, D., Labar, B., Germing, U., Salih, H. R., Beeldens, F., Muns, P., Pflüger, K. H., Coens, C., Hagemeijer, A., Eckart, Schaefer. H., Ganser, A., Aul, C., de Witte, T., & Wijermans, P. W. (2011). Low-dose decitabine versus best supportive care in elderly patiens with intermediate- or high-risk myelodysplastic syndrome (MDS) ineligible for intensit chemotherapy: final results of the randomized phase III study of the European Organisation for Research and Treatment of Cancer Leukemia Group and the German MDS Study Group. *Journal of Clinical Oncology*, 29(15), 1987-1996.

[26] Estey E.H. (2012). Acute myeloid leukemia: update on diagnosis, risk stratification, and management. *American Journal of Hematology 2012*, 87(1), 89-99.

[27] Garcia-Manero, G. (2012). Myelodysplastic syndromes: 2012 update on diagnosis, risk stratification, and management. *American Journal of Hematology*, 87(7), 692-701.

[28] Keating, G.M. (2012). Azacitidine: a review of its use in the management of myelodysplastic syndromes/ acute myeloid leukaemia. *Drugs*, 72(8), 1111-1136.

[29] Al-Ali, H. K., Jaekel, N., Junghanss, C., Maschmeyer, G., Krahl, R., Cross, M., Hoppe, G., & Niederwieser, D. (2012). Azacitidine in patients with acute myeloid leukemia medically unfit for or resistant to chemotherapy: a multicenter phase I/II study. *Leukemia and Lymphoma*, 53(1), 110-117.

[30] Marks, P.W. (2012). Decitabine for acute myeloid leukemia. *Expert Review of Anticancer Therapy*, 12(3), 299-305.

[31] Itzykson, R., & Fenaux, P. (2012). Optimizing hypomethylating agents in myelodysplastic syndromes. *Current Opinion of Hematology*, 19(2), 65-70.

[32] Blum, W., Garzon, R., Klisovic, R. B., Schwind, S., Walker, A., Geyer, S., Liu, S., Havelange, V., Becker, H., Schaaf, L., Mickle, J., Devine, H., Kefauver, C., Devine, S. M., Chan, K. K., Heerema, N. A., Bloomfield, C. D., Grever, M. R., Byrd, J. C., Villalona-Calero, M., Croce, C. M., & Marcucci, G. (2010). Clinical response and miR-29b predictive significance in older AML patients treated with a 10-day schedule of decitabine. *Proceedings of the National Academy of Sciences of the United States of America*, 107(16), 7473-7478.

[33] Lübbert, M., Rüter, B. H., Claus, R., Schmoor, C., Schmid, M., Germing, U., Kuendgen, A., Rethwisch, V., Ganser, A., Platzbecker, U., Galm, O., Brugger, W., Hell, G., Hackanson, B., Deschler, B., Döhner, K., Hagemeijer, A., Wijermans, P. W., & Döhner, H. (2012). A multicenter phase II trial of decitabine as first-line treatment for old-

er patiens with acute myeloid leukemia judged unfit for induction chemotherapy. *Haematologica*, 97(3), 393-401.

[34] Kantarjian, H. M., Thomas, X. G., Dmoszynska, A., Wierzbowska, A., Mazur, G., Mayer, J., Gan, J. P., Chou, W. C., Buckstein, R., Cermak, J., Kuo, C. Y., Oriol, A., Ravandi, F., Faderl, S., Delaunay, J., Lysák, D., Minden, M., & Arthur, C. (2012). Multicenter, randomized, open-label phase III trial of decitabine versus patient choice, with physician advice, of either supportive care of low-dose cytarabine for the treatment of older patients with newly diagnosed acute myeloid leukemia. *Journal of Clinical Oncology* published online before print on June 11 doi:JCO.2011.38.9429.

[35] Negrotto, S., Ng, K. P., Jankowska, A. M., Bodo, J., Gopalan, B., Guinta, K., Mulloy, J. C., Hsi, E., Maciejewski, J., & Saunthararajah, Y. (2012). CpG methylation patterns and decitabine treatment response in acute myeloid ledukemia cells and normal hematopoietic precursors. *Leukemia*, 26(2), 244-254.

[36] Fabiani, E., Leone, G., Giachelia, M., D′, Alo′. F., Greco, M., Criscuolo, M., Guidi, F., Rutella, S., Hohaus, S., & Voso, M. T. (2010). Analysis of genome-wide methylation and gene expression induced by 5-aza-2′-deoxycytidine identifies BCL2L10 as a frequent methylation target in acute myeloid leukemia. *Leukemia and Lymphoma*, 51(12), 2275-2284.

[37] Stresemann, C., Brueckner, B., Musch, T., Stopper, H., & Lyko, F. (2006). Functional diversity of DNA methyltransferase inhibitors in human cancer cell lines. *Cancer Research*, 66(5), 2794-2800.

[38] Foulks, J. M., Parnell, K. M., Nix, R. N., Chan, S., Swierczek, K., Saunders, M., Wright, K., Hendrickson, T. F., Ho, K. K., Mc Cullar, M. V., & Kanner, S. B. (2012). Epigenetic drug discovery: targeting DNA methyltransferases. *Journal of Biomolecular Screening*, 17(1), 2-17.

[39] Gore, S.D., & Hermes-De Santis, E.R. (2008). Future directions in myelodysplastic syndrome: newer agents and the role of combination approaches. *Cancer Control* 15 (Suppl), 40-49.

[40] Goodyear, O., Agathanggelon, A., Novitzky-Basso, I., Siddique, S., Mc Skeane, T., Ryan, G., Vyas, P., Cavenagh, J., Stankovic, T., Moss, P., & Craddock, C. (2010). Induction of a CD8+T-cell response to the MAGE cancer testis antigen by combined treatment with azacitidine and sodium valproate in patients with acute myeloid leukemia and myelodysplasia. *Blood*, 116(11), 1908-1918.

[41] Komrokji, R. S., & List, A. F. (2010). Lenalidomide for treatment of myelodysplastic syndromes: current status and future directions. *Hematology/Oncology Clinics of North America*, 24(2), 377-388.

[42] Heise, C., Carter, T., Schafer, P., & Chopra, R. (2010). Pleiotropic mechanisms of action of lenalidomide efficacy in del (5q) myelodysplastic syndromes. *Expert Review of Anticancer Therapy*, 10(10), 1663-1672.

[43] Wei, S., Chen, X., Mc Graw, K., Zhang, L., Komrokji, R., Clark, J., Caceres, G., Billingsley, D., Sokol, L., Lancet, J., Fortenbery, N., Zhou, J., Eksioglu, E. A., Sallman, D., Wang, H., Epling-Burnette, P. K., Djeu, J., Sekeres, M., Maciejewski, J. P., & List, A. (2012). Lenalidomide promotes 53degradation by inhibiting MDM2 auto-ubiquitination in myelodysplastic syndrome with chromosome 5q deletion. *Oncogene 2012* published online before print on April 23 onc.2012.139.

[44] Rice, K. L., Hormaeche, I., & Licht, J. D. (2007). Epigenetic regulation of normal and malignant hematopoiesis. *Oncogene*, 26(47), 6697-6714.

[45] Xu, F., Mao, C., Ding, Y., Rui, C., Wu, L., Shi, A., Zhang, H., Zhang, L., & Xu, Z. (2010). Molecular and enzymatic profiles of mammalian DNA methyltransferases: structures and targets for drugs. *Current Medicinal Chemistry*, 17(33), 4052-4071.

[46] Jin, B., Li, Y., & Robertson, K. D. (2011). DNA methylation: superior or subordinate in the epigenetic hierarchy. *Genes and Cancer*, 2(6), 607-617.

[47] Jurkowska, R. Z., Jurkowski, T. P., & Jeltsch, A. (2011). Structure and function of mammalian DNA methyltransferases. *ChemBioChem.*, 12(2), 206-222.

[48] Figueroa, M. E., Skrabanek, L., Li, Y., Jiemjit, A., Fandy, T. E., Paietta, E., Fernandez, H., Tallman, M. S., Greally, J. M., Carraway, H., Licht, J. D., Gore, S. D., & Melnick, A. (2009). MDS and secondary AML display unique patterns and abundance of aberrant DNA methylation. *Blood*, 114(16), 3448-3458.

[49] Uchida, T., Kinoshita, T., Nagai, H., Nakahara, Y., Saito, H., Holta, T., & Murate, T. (1997). Hypermethylation of the 15INK4Bgene in myelodysplastic syndromes. *Blood* 90 (4) 1403-1409.

[50] Quesnel, B., Guillerm, G., Verecque, R., Wattel, E., Preudhomme, C., Bauters, F., Vanrumbeke, M., & Fenaux, P. (1998). Methylation of the 15INK4b) gene in myelodysplastic syndromes is frequent and acquired during disease progression. *Blood* 91 (8) 2985-2990.

[51] Tien, H. F., Tang, J. H., Tsay, W., Liu, M. C., Lee, F. Y., Wang, C. H., Chen, Y. C., & Shen, M. C. (2001). Methylation of the 15INK4b) gene in myelodysplastic syndrome: it can be detected early at diagnosis or during disease progression and is highly associated with leukaemic transformation. *British Journal of Haematology* 112 (1) 148-154.

[52] Christiansen, D. H., Andersen, M. K., & Pedersen-Bjergaard, J. (2003). Methylation of 15INK4B) is common, is associated with deletion of genes on chromosome arm 7q and predicts a poor prognosis in therapy- related myelodysplasia and acute myeloid leukemia. *Leukemia* 17 (9) 1813-1819.

[53] Cechova, H., Lassuthova, P., Novakova, L., Belickova, M., Stemberkova, R., Jencik, J., Stankova, M., Hrabakova, P., Pegova, K., Zizkova, H., & Cermak, J. (2012). Monitoring of methylation changes in 921region in patients with myelodysplastic syndromes and acute myeloid leukemia. *Neoplasma* 59 (2) 168-174.

[54] Issa, J.P. (2010). Epigenetic changes in the myelodysplastic syndrome. *Hematology/ Oncology Clinics of North America*, 24(2), 317-330.

[55] Valencia, A., Cervera, J., Such, E., Ibanez, M., Gómez, I., Luna, I., Senent, L., Oltra, S., Sanz, M. A., & Sanz, G. F. (2011). Aberrant methylation of tumor suppressor genes in patients with refractory anemia with ring sideroblasts. *Leukemia Research*, 35(4), 479-483.

[56] Yang, Y., Zhang, Q., Xu, F., Wu, L., He, Q., & Li, X. (2012). Tumor suppressor gene BLU is frequently downregulated by promoter hypermethylation in myelodysplastic syndrome. *Journal of Cancer Research and Clinical Oncology*, 138(5), 729-737.

[57] Tran, H. T. T., Kim, H. N., Lee, I. K., Kim, Y. K., Ahn, J. S., Yang, D. H., Lee, J. J., & Kim, H. J. (2011). DNA methylation changes following 5-azacitidine treatment in patients with myelodysplastic syndrome. *Journal of Korean Medical Science*, 26(2), 207-213.

[58] Graubert, T., & Walter, M. J. (2011). Genetics of myelodysplastic syndromes: new insights. *Hematology*, 2011(543), 549.

[59] Fathi, A. T., & Abdel-Wahab, O. (2012). Mutations in epigenetic modifiers in myeloid malignancies and the prospect of novel epigenetic-targeted therapy. *Advances in Hematology* 2012, 469592.

[60] Nikolski, G., van der Reijden, B.A., & Jansen, J.H. (2012). Mutations in epigenetic regulators in myelodysplastic syndromes. *International Journal of Hematology*, 95(1), 8-16.

[61] McDevitt, M.A. (2012). Clinical applications of epigenetic markers and epigenetic profiling in myeloid malignancies. *Seminars in Oncology*, 39(1), 109-122.

[62] Varier, R. A., & Timmers, H. T. (2011). Histone lysine methylation and demethylation pathways in cancer. *Biochimica et Biophysica Acta*, 1815(1), 75-89.

[63] Morishita, M., & di Luccio, E. (2011). Cancers and the NSD family of histone lysine methyltransferases. *Biochimica et Biophysica Acta*, 1816(2), 158-163.

[64] Di Lorenzo, A., & Bedford, M.T. (2011). Histone arginine methylation. *FEBS Letters*, 585(13), 2024-2031.

[65] Wei, Y., Gaňán, Gómez. I., Salazar-Dimicoli, S., Mc Cay, S. L., & Garcia-Manero, G. (2011). *Epigenomics*, 3(2), 193-205.

[66] Shen, X., & Orkin, S. H. (2009). Glimpses of the epigenetic landscape. *Cell Stem Cell* 4 (1), 1-2.

[67] Mochizuki-Kashio, M., Mishima, Y., Miyagi, S., Negishi, M., Saraya, A., Konuma, T., Shinga, J., Koseki, H., & Iwama, A. (2011). Dependency on the polycomb gene Ezh2 distinguishes fetal from adult hematopoietic stem cells. *Blood*, 118(25), 6553-6561.

[68] Agger, K., Cloos, P. A., Christensen, J., Pasini, D., Rose, S., Rappsilber, J., Issaeva, I., Canaani, E., Salcini, A. E., & Helin, K. (2007). UTX and JMJD3 demethylases involved in HOX gene regulation and development. *Nature*, 449(7163), 731-734.

[69] Nikolski, G., Langemeijer, S. M., Kniper, R. P., Knops, R., Massop, M., Tönnissen, E. R., van der Heijden, A., Scheele, T. N., Vandenberghe, P., de Witte, T., van der Reijden, B. A., & Jansen, J. H. (2010). Somatic mutations of the histone methyltransferase gene EZH2 in myelodysplastic syndromes. *Nature Genetics*, 42(8), 665-667.

[70] Xu, F., Li, X., Wu, L., Zhang, Q., Yang, R., Yang, Y., Zhang, Z., He, Q., & Chang, C. (2011). Overexpression of the EZH2, RING1 and BMI1 genes is common in myelodysplastic syndromes: relation to adverse epigenetic alteration and poor prognostic scoring. *Annals of Hematology*, 90(6), 643-653.

[71] Szpurka, H., Jankowska, A. M., Przychodzen, B., Hu, Z., Sauntharajah, Y., Mc Devitt, M. A., & Maciejewski, J. P. (2010). UTX mutations and epigenetic changes in MDS/MPN and related myeloid malignancies. *Blood* (ASH Annual Meeting Abstracts) 116 (21) 121.

[72] Jankowska, A. M., Makishima, H., Tiu, R. V., Szpurka, H., Huang, Y., Traina, F., Visconte, V., Sugimoto, Y., Prince, C., O′, Keefe. C., His, E. D., List, A., Sekeres, M. A., Rao, A., Mc Devitt, M. A., & Maciejewski, J. P. (2011). Mutational spectrum analysis of chronic myelomonocytic leukemia includes genes associated with epigenetic regulation: UTX, EZH2, and DNMT3A. *Blood*, 118(14), 3932-3941.

[73] Jankowska, A. M., & Szpurka, H. (2012). Mutational determinants of epigenetic instability in myeloid malignancies. *Seminars in Oncology*, 39(1), 80-96.

[74] Glozak, M. A., & Seto, E. (2007). Histone deacetylases and cancer. *Oncogene*, 26(37), 5420-5432.

[75] Yang, X. J., & Seto, E. (2007). HATs and HDACs: from structure, function and regulation to novel strategies for therapy and prevention. *Oncogene*, 26(37), 5310-5318.

[76] Rasheed, W. K., Johnstone, R. W., & Prince, H. M. (2007). Histone deacetylase inhibitors in cancer therapy. *Expert Opinion on Investigational Drugs*, 16(5), 659-678.

[77] Dokmanovic, M., Clarke, C., & Marks, P. A. (2007). Histone deacetylase inhibitors: overview and perspectives. *Molecular Cancer Research*, 5(10), 981-989.

[78] Marks, P. A., & Breslow, R. (2007). Dimethyl sulfoxide to vorinostat: development of this histone deacetylase inhibitor as an anticancer drug. *Nature Biotechnology*, 25(1), 84-90.

[79] Glaser, K.B. (2007). HDAC inhibitors: clinical update and mechanism-based potential. *Biochemical Pharmacology*, 74(5), 659-671.

[80] Sato, F., Tsuchiya, S., Meltzer, S. J., & Shimizu, K. (2011). MicroRNAs and epigenetics. *FEBS Journal* , 278(10), 1598-1609.

[81] Starczynowski, D. T., Morin, R., Mc Pherson, A., Lam, J., Chan, R., Wegrzyn, J., Kuchenbauer, F., Hirst, M., Tohyama, M., Humphries, R. K., Lam, W. L., Marra, M., & Karsan, A. (2011). Genome-wide identification of human microRNAs located in leukemia-associated genomic alterations. *Blood*, 117(2), 595-607.

[82] Garzon, R., Heaphy, C. E., Havelange, V., Fabbri, M., Volinia, S., Tsao, T., Zanesi, N., Kornblau, S. M., Marcucci, G., Calin, G. A., Andreef, M., & Croce, C. M. (2009). MicroRNA 29b functions in acute myeloid leukemia. *Blood*, 114(26), 5331-5341.

[83] Marcucci, G., Mrózek, K., Radmacher, M. D., Garzon, R., & Bloomfield, C. D. (2011). The prognostic and functional role of microRNAs in acute myeloid leukemia. *Blood*, 117(4), 1121-1129.

[84] Duursma, A. M., Kedde, M., Schrier, M., le Sage, C., & Agami, R. (2008). miR-148 targets human DNMT3b protein coding region. *RNA*, 14(5), 872-877.

[85] Sander, S., Bullinger, L., Klapproth, K., Fiedler, K., Kestler, H. A., Barth, T. F., Moller, P., Stilgenbauer, S., Pollack, J. R., & Wirth, T. (2008). MYC stimulates EZH2 expression by repression of its negative regulator miR-26a. *Blood*, 112(10), 4202-4212.

[86] Swierczek, S., Yoon, D., Hickman, K., & Prchal, J. T. (2010). MicroRNA-101 is down-regulated in PV and ET granulocytes and its decrease is associated with over-expression of histone methyltransferase in EZH2 in MPN patients. *Blood* (ASH Annual Meeting Abstracts) 116 (21) 1989.

[87] Varambally, S., Cao, Q., Mani, R. S., Shankar, S., Wang, X., Ateeq, B., Laxman, B., Cao, X., Jing, X., Ramnarayanan, K., Brenner, J. C., Yu, J., Kim, J. H., Han, B., Tan, P., Kumar-Sinha, C., Lonigro, R. J., Palanisamy, N., Maher, C. A., & Chinnaiyan, A. M. (2008). Genomic loss of microRNA-101 leads to overexpression of histone methyltransferase EZH2 in cancer. *Science*, 322(5908), 1695-1699.

[88] Friedman, J. M., Liang, G., Liu, C. C., Wolff, E. M., Tsai, Y. C., Ye, W., Zhou, X., & Jones, P. A. (2009). The putative tumor suppressor microRNA-101 modulates the cancer epigenome by repressing the polycomb group protein EZH2. *Cancer Research*, 69(6), 2623-2629.

[89] Gandellini, P., Folini, M., Longoni, N., Pennati, M., Binda, M., Colecchia, M., Salvioni, R., Supino, R., Moretti, R., Limonta, P., Valdagni, R., Daidone, M. G., & Zaffaroni, N. (2009). miR-205 exerts tumor-suppressive functions in human prostate through down-regulation of protein kinase Cepsilon. *Cancer Research*, 69(6), 2287-2295.

[90] Juan, A. H., Kumar, R. M., Marx, J. G., Young, R. A., & Sartorelli, V. (2009). Mir-214-dependent regulation of the polycomb protein Ezh2 in skeletal muscle and embryonic stem cells. *Molecular Cell*, 36(1), 61-74.

[91] Dostalova, Merkerova. M., Krejcik, Z., Votavova, H., Belickova, M., Vasikova, A., & Cermak, J. (2011). Distinctive microRNA expression profiles in CD34+ bone marrow cells from patients with myelodysplastic syndrome. *European Journal of Human Genetics*, 19(3), 313-319.

[92] Jólkowska, J., & Witt, M. (2000). The EVI-1 gene-its role in pathogenesis of human leukemias. *Leuk Res*, 24, 553-558.

[93] Buonamici, S., Chakraborty, S., Senyuk, V., & Nucifora, G. (2003). The role of EVI1 in normal and leukemic cells. *Blood Cells, Molecules & Diseases*, 31(2), 206-212.

[94] Wieser, R. (2007). The oncogene and developmental regulator EVI1 expression, biochemical properties, and biological functions. *Gene*, 396(2), 346-357.

[95] Fuchs, O. (2009). Zinc finger protein EVI1 and its role in normal development and in oncogenesis. Chapter 18 in Focus on Zinc Finger Protein Research, ed. K Yoshida,, 303-319.

[96] Senyuk, V., Premanand, K., Xu, P., Qian, Z., & Nucifora, G. (2011). The oncoprotein EVI1 and the DNA methyltransferase Dnmt3 co-operate in binding and de novo methylation of target DNA. *PLOS One* 6 (6), e20793.

[97] Yoshimi, A., & Kurokawa, M. (2011). Evi1 forms a bridge between the epigenetic machinery and signalling pathway. *Oncotarget*, 2(7), 575-586.

[98] Yoshimi, A., Goyama, S., Watanabe-Okochi, N., Yoshiki, Y., Nannya, Y., Nitta, E., Arai, S., Sato, S., Shimabe, M., Nakayama, M., Imai, Y., Kitamura, T., & Kurokawa, M. (2011). Evi1 represses PTEN expression and activates PI3K/AKT/mTOR via interactions with polycomb proteins. *Blood*, 117(13), 3617-3628.

[99] van Waalwijk, Barjesteh, van Doorn-Khosrovani, S., Erpelinck, C., van Putten, W.L.J., & Valk, P.J.M. (2003). High EVI1 expression predicts poor survival in acute myeloid leukemia: a study of 319 de novo AML patients. *Blood*, 101(3), 837-845.

[100] Breccia, M., Cannella, L., Santopietro, M., Loglisci, G., Federico, V., Salaroli, A., Nanni, M., Mancini, M., & Alimena, G. (2011). Azacitidine in myelodysplastic syndromes with inversion of chromosome 3. *Leukemia*, 25(4), 736-737.

[101] Garcia-Manero, G., & Fenaux, P. (2011). Hypomethylating agents and other novel strategies in myelodysplastic syndromes. *Journal of Clinical Oncology*, 29(5), 516-523.

[102] Curik, N., Burda, P., Vargova, K., Pospisil, V., Belickova, M., Vlckova, P., Savvulidi, F., Necas, E., Hajkova, H., Haskovec, C., Cermak, J., Krivjanska, M., Trneny, M., Laslo, P., Jonasova, A., & Stopka, T. (2012). 5azacitidine in aggressive myelodysplastic syndromes regulates chromatin structure at PU.1 gene and cell differentiation capacity. *Leukemia* DOI:leu.2012.47.

[103] Kagey, J. D., Kapoor-Vazirani, P., Mc Cabe, M. T., Powell, D. R., & Vertino, P. M. (2010). Long-term stability of demethylation after exposure to 5-aza-2′-deoxycytidine correlates with sustained RNA polymerase II occupancy. *Molecular Cancer Research*, 8(7), 1048-1059.

[104] Sorm, F., Pískala, A., Cihák, A., & Veselý, J. (1964). azacytidine, a new, highly effective cancerostatic. *Experientia*, 20(4), 202-203.

[105] Veselý, J., Cihák, A., & Sorm, F. (1968). Characteristics of mouse leukemic cells resistant to 5-azacytidine and 5-aza-2′-deoxycytidine. *Cancer Research*, 28(10), 1995-2000.

[106] Hollenbach, P. W., Nguyen, A. N., Brady, H., Williams, M., Ning, Y., Richard, N., Krushel, L., Aukerman, S. L., Heise, C., & Mac Beth, K. J. (2010). A comparison of azacytidine and decitabine activities in acute myeloid leukemia cell lines. *PLOS One*, 5 (2) e9001.

[107] Silverman, L. R., Demakos, E. P., Peterson, B. L., Kornblith, A. B., Holland, J. C., Odchimar-Reissig, R., Stone, R. M., Nelson, D., Powell, B. L., De Castro, C. M., Ellerton, J., Larson, L. A., Schiffer, C. A., & Holland, J. F. (2002). Randomized controlled trial of azacitidine in patients with the myelodysplastic syndrome: a study of the cancer and leukemia group B. *Journal of Clinical Oncology*, 20(10), 2429-2440.

[108] Fenaux, P., Mufti, G. J., Hellström-Lindberg, E., Santini, V., Finelli, C., Giagounidis, A., Schoch, R., Gattermann, N., Sanz, G., List, A., Gore, S. D., Seymour, J. F., Bennett, J. M., Byrd, J., Backstrom, J., Zimmerman, L., Mc Kenzie, D., Beach, C., & Silverman, L. R. (2009). Efficacy of azacitidine compared with that of conventional care regimens in the treatment of higher-risk myelodysplastic syndromes, a randomised, open-label, phase III study. *Lancet Oncology*, 10(3), 223-232.

[109] Silverman, L. R., Fenaux, P., Mufti, G. J., Santini, V., Hellström-Lindberg, E., Gattermann, N., Sanz, G., List, A., Gore, S. D., & Seymour, J. F. (2011). Continued azacitidine therapy beyond time of first response improves quality of response in patients with higher-risk myelodysplastic syndromes. *Cancer*, 117(12), 2697-2702.

[110] Itzykson, R., Thépot, S., Beyne-Rauzy, O., Ame, S., Isnard, F., Dreyfus, F., Salanoubat, C., Taksin, A. L., Chelgoum, Y., Berthon, C., Malfuson, J. V., Legros, L., Vey, N., Turlure, P., Gardin, C., Bohrer, S., Ades, L., & Fenaux, P. (2012). Does addition of erythropoiesis stimulating agents improve the outcome of higher-risk myelodysplastic syndromes treated with azacytidine. *Leukemia Research* 36 (4), 397-400.

[111] Van der Helm, L. H., Alhan, C., Wijermans, P. W., van Marwijk, Kooy. M., Schaafsma, R., Biemond, B. J., Beeker, A., Hoogendoorn, M., van Rees, B. P., de Weerd, O., Wegman, J., Libourel, W. J., Luykx-de, Bakker. S., Minnema, M. C., Brouwer, R. E., Croon-de, Boer. F., Eefting, M., Jie, K. S., van de Loosdrecht, A. A., Koedam, J., Veeger, N.J., Veeger, E., & Huls, G. (2011). Platelet doubling after the first azacitidine cycle is a promising predictor for response in myelodysplastic syndromes (MDS), chronic myelomonocytic leukaemias (CMML) and acute myeloid leukaemia (AML) patients in the Dutch azacitidine compassionate named patient programme. *British Journal of Haematology*, 155(5), 596-606.

[112] Pollyea, D. A., Raval, A., Kusler, B., Gotlib, J. R., Alizadeh, A. A., & Mitchell, B. S. (2011). Impact of TET2 mutations on mRNA expression and clinical outcomes in MDS patients treated with DNA methyltransferase inhibitors. *Hematological Oncology*, 29(3), 157-160.

[113] Hájková, H., Marková, J., Haškovec, C., Šárová, I., Fuchs, O., Kostečka, A., Cetkovský, P., Michalová, K., & Schwarz, J. (2012). Decreased methylation in acute myeloid leukemia patients with DNMT3A mutations and prognostic implications of DNA methylation. *Leukemia Research 2012* doi:j.leukres.05.012.

[114] Sekeres, M. A., List, A. F., Cuthbertson, D., Paquette, R., Ganetzky, R., Latham, D., Paulic, K., Afable, M., Saba, H. I., Loughran, T. P., & Maciejewski, J. P. (2010). Phase I combination trial of lenalidomide and azacitidine in patients with higher-risk myelodysplastic syndromes. *Journal of Clinical Oncology*, 28(13), 2253-2258.

[115] Van den, Berghe. H., Cassiman, J. J., David, G., Fryns, J. P., Michaux, J. L., & Sokal, G. (1974). Distinct haematological disorder with deletion of long arm of no. 5 chromosome. *Nature*, 251(5474), 437-438.

[116] Van den Berghe, H., & Michaux, L. (1997). 5q-, twenty-five years later: a synopsis. *Cancer Genetics and Cytogenetics*, 94(1), 1-7.

[117] Boultwood, J., Pellagatti, A., Mc Kenzie, A. N., & Wainscoat, J. S. (2010). Advances in the 5q- syndrome. *Blood*, 116(26), 5803-5811.

[118] Corral, L. G., Haslett, P. A., Muller, G. V., Chen, R., Wong, L. M., Ocampo, C. J., Patterson, R. T., Stirling, D. I., & Kaplan, G. (1999). Differential cytokine modulation and T cell activation by two distinct classes of thalidomide analogues that are potent inhibitors of TNF-alpha. *Journal of Immunology*, 163(1), 380-386.

[119] Vallet, S., Palumbo, A., Raje, N., Boccadoro, M., & Anderson, K. C. (2008). Thalidomide and lenalidomide: mechanism-based potential drug combinations. *Leukemia & Lymphoma*, 49(7), 1238-1245.

[120] Kotla, V., Goel, S., Nischal, S., Heuck, C., Vivek, K., Das, B., & Verma, A. (2009). Mechanism of action of lenalidomide in haematological malignancies. *Journal of Hematology and Oncology* 2, 36.

[121] List, A., Kurtin, S., Roe, D. J., Buresh, A., Mahadevan, D., Fuchs, D., Rimsza, L., Heaton, R., Knight, R., & Zeldis, J. B. (2005). Efficacy of lenalidomide in myelodysplastic syndromes. *The New England Journal of Medicine*, 352(6), 549-557.

[122] List, A., Dewald, G., Bennett, J., Giagounidis, A., Raza, A., Feldman, E., Powell, B., Greenberg, P., Thomas, D., Stone, R., Reeder, C., Wride, K., Patin, J., Schmidt, M., Zeldis, J., & Knight, R. (2006). Myelodysplastic Syndrome-003 Study Investigators. Lenalidomide in the myelodysplastic syndrome with chromosome 5q deletion. *The New England Journal of Medicine*, 355(14), 1456-1465.

[123] Giagounidis, A., Fenaux, P., Mufti, G. J., Muus, P., Platzbecker, U., Sanz, G., Cripe, L., Von-Toal, Lilienfeld., , M., & Wells, R. A. (2008). Practical recommendations on the use of lenalidomide in the management of myelodysplastic syndromes. *Annals of Hematollogy*, 87(5), 345-352.

[124] Giagounidis, A. A., Kulasekararaj, A., Germing, U., Radkowski, R., Haase, S., Petersen, P., Göhring, G., Büsche, G., Aul, C., Mufti, G. J., & Platzbecker, U. (2012). Long-

term transfusion independence in del(5q) MDS patients who discontinue lenalidomide. *Leukemia*, 26(4), 855-858.

[125] Göhring, G., Lange, K., Hofmann, W., Nielsen, K. V., Hellström-Lindberg, E., Roy, L., Morgan, M., Kreipe, H., Büsche, G., Giagounidis, A., & Schlegelberger, B. (2012). Telomere shortening, clonal evolution and disease progression in myelodysplastic syndrome patients with 5q deletion treated with lenalidomide. *Leukemia*, 26(2), 356-358.

[126] Jädersten, M., Saft, L., & Pellagatti, A. (2009). Clonal heterogeneity in the 5q- syndrome: 53expressing progenitors prevail during lenalidomide treatment and expand at disease progression. *Haematologica* 94 (12) 1762-1766.

[127] Jädersten, M., Saft, L., Smith, A., Kulasekararaj, A., Pomplun, S., Göhring, G., Hedlund, A., Hast, R., Schlegelberger, B., Porwit, A., Hellström-Lindberg, E., & Mufti, G. J. (2011). TP53 mutations in low-risk myelodysplastic syndromes with del(5q) predict disease progression. *Journal of Clinical Oncology*, 29(15), 1971-1979.

[128] Tehranchi, R., Woll, P. S., & Anderson, K. (2010). Persistent malignant stem cells in del(5q) myelodysplasia in remission. *The New England Journal of Medicine*, 363(11), 1025-1037.

[129] Ebert, B. L., Prety, J., Bosco, J., Chang, C. Y., Tamazo, P., Galili, N., Raza, A., Root, D. E., Attar, E., Ellis, S. R., & Golub, T. R. (2008). Identification of RPS14 as a 5q- syndrome gene by RNA interference screen. *Nature*, 451(7176), 335-339.

[130] Ebert B.L. (2009). Deletion 5q in myelodysplastic syndrome: a paradigm for the study of hemizygous deletions in cancer. *Leukemia*, 23(7), 1252-1256.

[131] Narla, A., & Ebert, B. L. (2010). Ribosomopathies: human disorders of ribosome dysfunction. *Blood*, 115-3196.

[132] Czibere, A. G., Bruns, I., Junge, B., Singh, R., Kobbe, G., Haas, R., & Germing, U. (2009). Low RPS14 expression is common in myelodysplastic syndromes without 5q- aberration and defines a subgroup of patients with prolonged survival. *Haematologica*, 94(10), 1453-1455.

[133] Ebert, B. L., Galili, N., Tamayo, P., Bosco, J., Mak, R., Pretz, J., Tanguturi, S., Ladd-Acosta, C., Stone, R., Golub, T. R., & Raza, A. (2008). An erythroid differentiation signature predicts response to lenalidomide in myelodysplastic syndrome. *PLoS Medicine* 5 (2) e35.

[134] Fenaux, P., Giagounidis, A., Selleslag, D., Beyne-Rauzy, O., Mufti, G., Mittelman, M., Muus, P., Te, Boekhorst. P., Sanz, G., Del Canizo, C., Guerci-Bresler, A., Nilsson, L., Platzbecker, U., Lübbert, M., Quesnel, B., Cazzola, M., Ganser, A., Bowen, D., Schlegelberger, B., Aul, C., Knight, R., Francis, J., Fu, T., & Hellström-Lindberg, E. (2011). MDS-004 Lenalidomide del 5q Study Group. A randomized phase 3 study of lenalidomide versus placebo in RBC transfusion-dependent patients with low-/intermediate-1-risk myelodysplastic syndromes with del5q. *Blood*, 118(14), 3765-3776.

[135] Le Bras, F., Sebert, M., Kelaidi, C., Lamy, T., Dreyfus, F., Delaunay, J., Banos, A., Blanc, M., Vey, N., Schmidt, A., Visanica, S., Eclache, V., Turlure, P., Beyne-Rauzy, O., Guerci, A., Delauer, A., de Botton, S., Rea, D., Fenaux, P., & Adés, L. (2011). Treatment by lenalidomide in lower risk myelodysplastic syndrome with 5q deletion-the GFM experience. *Leukemia Research*, 35(11), 1444-1448.

[136] Park, S., Vassilieff, D., Bardet, V., Viguié, F., & Dreyfus, F. (2010). Efficacy of the association of lenalidomide to erythropoiesis-stimulating agents in del (5q) MDS patients refractory to single-agent lenalidomide. *Leukemia*, 24(11), 1960-1977.

[137] Narla, A., Dutt, S., Mc Auley, J. R., Al-Shahrour, F., Hurst, S., Mc Conkey, M., Neuberg, D., & Ebert, B. L. (2011). Dexamethasone and lenalidomide have distinct functional effects on erythropoiesis. *Blood*, 118(8), 2296-2304.

[138] Cmejlova, J., Dolezalova, L., Pospisilova, D., Petrtylova, K., Petrak, J., & Cmejla, R. (2006). Translational efficiency in patients with Diamond-Blackfan anemia. *Haematologica*, 91(11), 1456-1464.

[139] Pospisilova, D., Cmejlova, J., Hak, J., Adam, T., & Cmejla, R. (2007). Successful treatment of a Diamond-Blackfan anemia patient with amino acid leucine. *Haematologica* 92 (5) e, 66-67.

[140] Payne, E., Virgilio, M., Narla, A., Sun, H., Levine, M., Paw, B. H., Berliner, N., Look, A. T., Ebert, B., & Khanna-Gupta, A. (2011). L-leucine improves the anemia and developmental defects associated with Diamond-Blackfan anemia and del(5q) MDS by activating the mTOR pathway. *Blood 2012* 10.1182/ blood-10-382986

[141] Yip, B. H., Pellagatti, A., Vuppusetty, C., Giagounidis, A., Germing, U., Lamikanra, A. A., Roberts, D. J., Fernandez-Mercado, M., Mc Donald, E. J., Killick, S., Wainscoat, J. S., & Boultwood, J. (2012). Effects of L-leucine in RPS14deficient erythroid cells. *Leukemia* leu.2012.82.

[142] Voutsadakis, I. A., & Cairoli, A. (2012). A critical review of the molecular pathophysiology of lenalidomide sensitivity in 5q- myelodysplastic syndromes. *Leukemia & Lymphoma*, 53(5), 779-788.

[143] Wei, S., Chen, X., Rocha, K., Epling-Burnette, P. K., Djeu, J. Y., Liu, Q., Byrd, J., Sokol, L., Lawrence, N., Pireddu, R., Dewald, G., Williams, A., Maciejewski, J., & List, A. (2009). A critical role for phosphatase haplodeficiency in the selective suppression of deletion 5q MDS by lenalidomide. *Proceedings of the National Academy of Sciences of the United States of America*, 106(31), 12974-12979.

[144] Moutouh-de, Parseval. L. A., Verhelle, D., Glezer, E., Jensen-Pergakes, K., Ferguson, G. D., Corral, L. G., Morris, C. L., Muller, G., Brady, H., & Chan, K. (2008). Pomalidomide and lenalidomide regulate erythropoiesis and fetal hemoglobin production in human CD34+ cells. *Journal of Clinical Investigation*, 118(1), 248-258.

[145] Starczynowski, D. T., & Karsan, A. (2010). Innate immune signaling in the myelodysplastic syndromes. *Hematology/Oncology Clinics of North America*, 24(2), 343-359.

[146] Siva, K., Jaako, P., Miharada, K., Miharada, K., Rörby, E., Ehinger, M., Karlsson, G., & Karlsson, S. (2012). SPARC is dispensable for murine hematopoiesis, despite its suspected pathophysiological role in 5q- myelodysplastic syndrome. *Leukemia* leu. 2012.97.

[147] Steensma, D. P., & Stone, R. M. (2011). Lenalidomide in AML: del(5q) or who? *Blood,* 118(3), 481-482.

[148] Sugimoto, Y., Sekeres, M. A., & Makishima, H. (2012). Cytogenetic and molecular predictors of response in patients with myeloid malignancies without del(5q) treated with lenalidomide. *Journal of Hematology and Oncology* 5, 4.

Chapter 6

Minimal Residual Disease and Leukemic Stem Cells in Acute Myeloid Leukemia

W. Zeijlemaker and G.J. Schuurhuis

Additional information is available at the end of the chapter

http://dx.doi.org/10.5772/52080

1. Introduction

Acute myeloid leukemia (AML) is the most common type of acute leukemia in adults. With current treatment strategies, almost 80% of AML patients (18-60 years) will achieve complete remission (CR). However, approximately 50% of these patients will experience a relapse, resulting in a five-year survival rate of only 35%-40% [1]. This implies that despite CR, in these patients a number of cancer cells survive treatment and can grow out to cause a relapse. Efforts towards development of more sensitive methods to accurately determine CR and detect residual cancer cells are necessary to improve risk-adapted management to eventually prolong overall survival rates.

2. Minimal residual disease and acute myeloid leukemia

In AML patients, morphologic assessment is performed to evaluate chemotherapy response and to define remission status. By definition, patients are in CR when less than 5% blast cells are present in the bone marrow (BM) concurrent with evidence of normal erythropoiesis, granulopoiesis and megakaryopoiesis. In addition, neutrophils and platelets in peripheral blood should be at least 1.0 x 10^9/l and 100 x 10^9/l, respectively [2]. Since about 50% of patients in CR will eventually experience a relapse, for prognostic purposes more precise assessment of the quality of CR is necessary. To this end residual disease detection could be of high importance. This so-called minimal residual disease (MRD) is thus defined as the persistence of leukemic cells after chemotherapy treatment and thought to be responsible for the emergence of relapse (Figure 1). Quantitative MRD frequency assessment could give important prognostic information after chemotherapy treatment. Two highly sensitive methods for MRD detection in leukemia are multiparameter flow cytometry (MFC) and real-time quantitative polymerase chain reaction (RQ-PCR). Both methods and their clinical applications will be reviewed in this chapter.

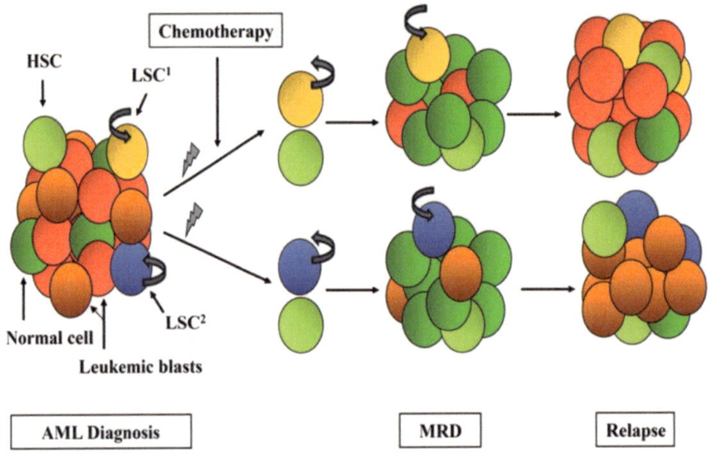

Figure 1. The role of minimal residual disease and leukemic stem cells in the emergence of relapse. HSC, normal hematopoietic stem cell, LSC, leukemic stem cell. At AML diagnosis a heterogeneous population of cells often coexist, including different subpopulations of LSCs. MRD frequency assessment focuses on the detection of leukemic cells present after treatment. Different subpopulations of chemotherapy resistant LSCs can grow out and cause relapse (discussed in section 3).

2.1. Immunophenotypic MRD detection

2.1.1. Principles of immunophenotypic MRD detection

One of the most frequently used techniques to assess MRD in leukemia is based on assessment of immunophenotypic aberrant antigen expression using flow cytometry. For practical purposes, in most cases, this approach is restricted to cell surface antigen expression. At diagnosis, so-called leukemia associated (immuno)phenotypes (LA[I]Ps, further referred to as LAPs) are determined. Such a LAP consists of (an) aberrantly expressed cell surface marker(s), usually combined with a myeloid marker (CD13/CD33) and with a normal progenitor antigen, i.e. CD34, CD117 or CD133. LAPs are grouped into (1) cross-lineage antigen expression (e.g. expression of lymphoid markers in myeloid blasts), (2) asynchronous antigen expression (co-expression of antigens that are not concomitantly present during normal differentiation), (3) lack of antigen expression and (4) antigen overexpression [3]. Such aberrancies can subsequently be used to detect MRD (Figure 2).

Due to large heterogeneity of immunophenotypes in AML, determination of LAPs has to be performed for each individual patient. These LAPs are not, or only in very low frequencies, present on normal BM cells in remission BM. Sensitivities have been reported to be in a range of 10^{-3} down to 10^{-5} (1 leukemic cell in 1,000 to 100,000 normal cells) [4-9]. Besides these relatively high sensitivities, it is also a very rapid technique. Main advantage of flow cytometric MRD assessment is its broad applicability: in 80%-95% of all AML patients one or more LAPs can be defined. [4,5,9-11]. There are, however, potential pitfalls/disadvantages that should be taken into account. *Firstly,* blast cells at diagnosis are often characterized by subpopulations with different immunophenotypes. For this reason a LAP defined at diagnosis, is often not a characteristic of the total population of leukemic blast cells. Since only the LAP positive (LAP$^+$) cells can be identified at follow-up, this may thus result in under-estimation of cell frequency of *all* leukemic blast cells, referred to as MRD. To approach the real MRD cell frequency, there is the possibility to correct LAP$^+$ frequency at follow-up for the LAP$^+$ frequency, as percentage of blasts, at diagnosis. *Secondly,* the presence of low percentages of normal cells that express a particular LAP may result in over-estimation of MRD cell frequency. This background staining may even lead to false-positive results. A relatively low background staining can be achieved by including a primitive marker in the definition of a LAP, since these cells are only present at low frequencies in normal BM. *Thirdly,* immunophenotypic shifts may occur in the course of treatment and result in false-negativity [6,12,13]. To avoid this, it is recommended to use multiple LAPs. *Finally,* due to the large number of different LAPs, MRD analysis is quite complex and needs vast experience in discriminating leukemic cells from cells with normal differentiation patterns.

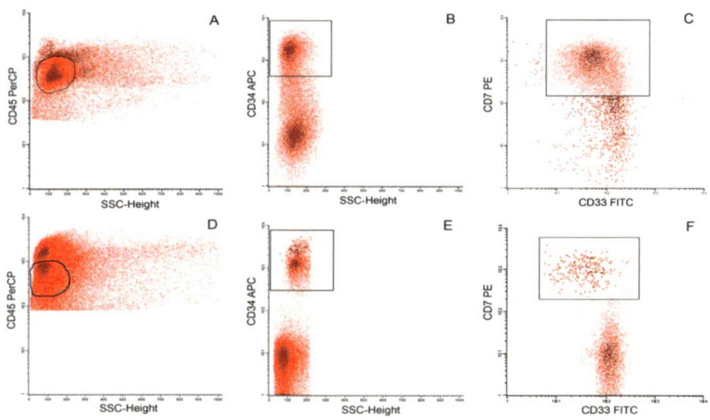

Figure 2. Example of MRD detection in BM using the aberrant phenotype of CD34$^+$CD7$^+$ cells at AML diagnosis (A-C) and during follow-up (D-F). Gating of the blast cells with CD45dim expression and low sideward scatter (SSC) (A, D), gating of the CD34 positive progenitors cells (B, E) and gating of the leukemic blast population with aberrant expression of CD7 on the myeloid progenitor cells (C, F). After chemotherapy treatment a residual population of leukemic blasts can be detected (F).

2.1.2. Prognostic value of immunophenotypic MRD in bone marrow

The likelihood of achieving CR after therapy and the duration of CR depend on different factors. Important prognostic risk factors available at diagnosis are: history of previous leukemia or myelodysplastic syndrome, age, white blood cell (WBC) count, percentage of BM blast cells and the presence of particular cytogenetic and/or molecular aberrancies [14]. Besides these pre-treatment prognostic factors, it is suggested that MRD detection in BM shortly after treatment offers an important post-treatment prognostic factor. To evaluate the impact of MRD frequencies on relapse rate and overall survival (OS), MRD was related to outcome parameters using survival analyses such as Kaplan Meier curves. For these analyses, most studies set a threshold to define MRD negative (or low) and MRD positive (or high) patients. Different laboratories use different optimal cut-off values after both induction and consolidation therapy (Table 1). However, it should be emphasized that usually, it is not a single cut-off point, but a range of cut-off values that significantly predict clinical outcome.

Author	Patients (n)	Cut-off post-induction	Cut-off post-consolidation	Reference
San Miguel *et al.*	126	<0.01%, 0.01-0.1%, 0.1-1%, >/1%	not available	[15]
Feller *et al.*	52	0.14%	0.11%	[6]
Kern *et al.*	62	Log difference 1.70	Log difference 2.94	[5]
Maurillo *et al.*	142	0.035%	0.035%	[16]
Al-Mawali *et al.*	54	0.15%	0.15%	[10]

Table 1. Overview of studies in adult AML with cut-off values used for analyzing relapse free and overall survival.

San Miguel *et al.* were the first to show the prognostic impact of MRD in a group of 53 AML patients [4]. Later they extended the study to 126 patients. An overview of three-year relapse rates for three distinct patient risk groups with considerable patient numbers is given in Table 2. Univariate analysis of prognostic factors revealed five disease characteristics that had significant impact on relapse-free survival (RFS); these included cytogenetic abnormalities, number of chemotherapy cycles needed to achieve CR, WBC count, absolute peripheral blood (PB) blast cell count and MRD levels. In a multivariate analysis only cytogenetics (p =.03) and MRD levels (p =.002) were independent prognostic factors for RFS [15]. These results are in line with other studies. Results from Feller *et al.*, showed a relative risk of relapse of 3.4 after induction therapy (p =.003) and 7.2 after consolidation therapy (p =.004) in the patient group with high MRD levels [6].

MRD level	Patients (n)	Relapse rate ± standard error
< 0.1 %	16	9% ± 7%
0.1% - 1%	45	56% ± 9%
"/1%	21	83% ± 10%

Table 2. Overview of three-year relapse rates for three distinct risk groups based on MRD levels determined after induction therapy (p =.006) [15].

Al-Mawali *et al.* demonstrated in a multivariate analysis that post-induction positive MRD status was an independent prognostic factor for both RFS and OS (p =.037 and p =.026, respectively) MRD positivity after induction therapy was also associated with increased risk of relapse (Hazard ratio [HR] 4.7, 95% confidence interval [CI] 1.1-20.5) [10]. Maurillo *et al.*, in a study following their original report [7], have reported similar results in a study of 142 AML patients. In a multivariate analysis of RFS, cytogenetics (p =.0001), multidrug resistance-1 phenotype (p =.03) and MRD positivity after consolidation therapy (p =.001) were independent prognostic factors. In multivariate analysis of OS, post-consolidation MRD positivity (p =.004) was the only independent prognostic factor [16]. Kern and colleagues, in an approach that established log reduction of blast cells as a measure for MRD, showed that after induction therapy < 1.7 log reduction (p =.006) and unfavorable karyotype (p =.0001) were independent prognostic factors for relapse [5]. After consolidation therapy < 2.94 log reduction (p =.006) and unfavorable karyotype (p =.015) were found to be independent factors for relapse. Although above-mentioned study results are promising and consistent, the clinical importance of MRD in adult AML still has to be validated in a prospective study. Terwijn *et al.* studied the value of MRD monitoring in a large cohort of 462 AML patients. Multivariate analysis, performed with conventional prognostic factors, demonstrated that MRD frequency was an independent prognostic factor for RFS after every cycle (first cycle p =.010, second cycle p<.00001 and consolidation p<.00001) and for OS after the first cycle (p =. 023) and second cycle (p =.01). To our knowledge, this is the first study that demonstrates the importance of MRD monitoring in a prospective study [17]. Because of these prospective data, the next step would be to implement MRD status in clinical decision-making.

2.2. Molecular MRD detection

Although flow cytometry is an attractive technique for MRD detection, the limitations, including background staining, immunophenotypic switches, complexity of analysis and LAP expression on only part of the leukemic cells, give rise to alternative approaches for MRD detection, including molecular MRD monitoring using the Polymerase Chain Reaction (PCR) technique. This approach allows for the detection of mutations, translocations, inversions, deletions and polymorphisms. Real-time-(qRT-) PCR is the most sensitive technique for MRD detection: it allows detecting MRD with sensitivities that have been reported in a range of 10^{-4} to 10^{-6} [18-21]. QRT-PCR is now extensively being studied as approach for MRD detection. Common targets for molecular MRD monitoring, including fusion genes, overexpressed genes and gene mutations, will be reviewed in this section.

2.2.1. Fusion genes

Fusion genes are among the best potential targets for molecular MRD detection. In AML the most common chromosomal rearrangements, producing fusion genes, are t(8;21), t(15;17) and inv(16)/t(16;16). The corresponding fusion genes are *AML1-ETO*, *PML-RARα* and *CBFβ-MYH11*, respectively. Depending on geographics, these occur in about 15%-45% of all AML cases and are associated with favorable prognosis [22]. Molecular MRD studies performed for *AML1-ETO* and *CBFβ-MYH11* are relatively scarce and have included relatively few patients.

In t(8;21) rearrangement, the AML1 gene on chromosome 21 fuses with the MTG8(ETO) gene on chromosome 8 to produce the fusion gene *AML1-MTG8*, also called *AML1-ETO* [23]. Tobal *et al.* studied 25 t(8;21) patients and demonstrated a 2 to 3 log reduction in the level of *AML1-MTG8* after induction chemotherapy and a further 2 to 3 log reduction after consolidation therapy. In all patients with durable CR (n = 20), *AML1-MTG8* transcripts levels in BM were ≤ 1 x 10^3 molecules/μg (median 227 molecules/μg). On the other hand, levels of ≥ 0.71 x 10^5 molecules/μg were predictive of relapse within 3 to 6 months (n = 5, median 1.49 x 10^5 molecules/μg) [24]. Krauter *et al.* retrospectively studied 37 AML patients with t(8;21) (n = 22) or inv(16) (n = 15) using RT-PCR. Levels of *AML1/MTG8* and *CBFβ/MYH11* were quantified relative to expression of a housekeeping gene. This resulted in significantly lower MRD levels in non-relapsing patients (median 0%, range 0%-1.5%) compared to patients who did experience relapse (median 0.14%, range 0%-15.6%, p<.01). Furthermore, RFS was significantly shorter in patients with high MRD levels (≥ 1% of the pre-treatment value) compared to patients without relapse (p<.001), with a similar trend for OS (p = 0.12) [25]. Guerrasio *et al.* retrospectively studied a cohort of 16 AML patients with *CBFβ/MYH11* rearrangements. Analysis in first CR revealed a significantly higher mean copy number of *CBFβ/MYH11* transcripts in patients who relapsed (mean 151) than in patients with stable remission (mean 9, p<.0001) [20]. Buonamici and colleagues also retrospectively studied 21 patients with inv(16) rearrangements and found that patients who relapsed always had *CBFβ/MYH1*:control ratios > 0.12% during CR (median 0.54%, range 0.12%-7.1%). Patients without subsequent relapse, on the other hand, always had ratios < 0.25% (median 0%, range 0%-0.25%), suggesting a cut-off point of 0.25% above which relapse is probable. Despite these promising results, two patients with MRD levels below the cut-off of 0.25% still experienced a relapse [26]. It thus seems that quantitation of both *AML1/MTG8* and *CBFβ/MYH11* can detect important changes in the level of fusion transcripts and that it can give prognostic information. However, it is important that these results still have to be confirmed in larger studies. Despite the advantages, MRD monitoring using *AML1/MTG8* and *CBFβ/MYH11* is possible in only a minority of AML patients.

More research has been done on the *PML-RARA* transcript in acute promyelocytic leukemia (APL). Although the outcome for APL patients has significantly improved with the development of targeted therapies, including all-trans-retinoic acid (ATRA) and arsenic trioxide (ATO), still 10%-15% of APL patients will suffer from relapse. Therefore MRD monitoring to predict clinical outcome could also be of importance in this subgroup of AML patients. In a large prospective study, including 406 APL patients, MRD, monitored by *PML-RARA* transcript analysis, was used to direct pre-emptive therapy with ATO and to guide use of transplantation. In this study, MRD was identified as most powerful prognostic factor for RFS (HR 17.87, 95% CI 6.88-46.41, p<.0001) in a multivariate analysis. Furthermore, increases in *PML-RARA* transcript levels were used to guide pre-emptive therapy and this resulted in a cumulative relapse incidence of only 5% at 3 years [27]. This showed that detection of APL fusion transcripts after chemotherapy treatment is a valid strategy for MRD guided pre-emptive therapy, a strategy that allows reduction of relapse rates. This approach, however, is only applicable in approximately 5%-30% of AML patients.

Mixed-lineage leukemia (*MLL*) fusion genes, which are the result of 11q23 rearrangements, occur in around 10% of both acute lymphocytic leukemia (ALL) and AML and are associated with adverse clinical outcome [28,29]. MRD detection using *MLL* transcripts is challenging, since up to 50 different translocations, resulting in different *MLL* fusion genes, have been described. Most common 11q23 abnormalities are t(9;11)(p22;q23), t(11;19)(q23;p13.3) and t(6;11)(q27;q23) [30]. Mittelbauer *et al.* studied 209 patients at AML diagnosis and detected *MLL* gene rearrangements in 27 patients (12.9%). The *MLL-AF6* fusion transcript, caused by t(6;11)(q27;q23), was detected by RT-PCR in 6 of those 27 patients. All 6 patients achieved hematological CR, however, only one patient achieved molecular CR and that patient was still in stable CR 33 months after diagnosis. The other 5 patients did not reach molecular CR and they all relapsed 2.6-8.3 months after achieving hematological CR. The authors suggest that a reduction of positive blasts below the RT-PCR detection limit of 10^{-5} to 10^{-6} seems to be a prerequisite for long term CR. Unfortunately the incidence of *MLL-AF6* was only 3% in the whole group of 209 patients, resulting in low applicability of this assay [21]. To summarize, levels of *MLL* fusion transcripts may be useful to evaluate treatment response and predict clinical outcome. However, large prospective studies have to be performed to confirm the clinical importance. A major drawback is the limited applicability due to the relatively low incidence of 11q23 rearrangements, also characterized by high numbers of different translocations.

2.2.2. Overexpressed genes

Since in only a small fraction of patients, fusion transcripts are present, overexpressed genes might offer a potential alternative target for molecular MRD monitoring. Such overexpressed genes are either silenced or expressed at very low levels in normal hematopoietic cells. Commonly overexpressed genes are *WT1, EVI1* and *PRAME.* In particular for *WT1*, which has originally been described in the development of Wilms tumor [31], multiple studies have been performed. This gene was shown to be also highly expressed in leucocytes of several hematopoietic malignancies, including AML [32,33]. Although the mechanisms of this overexpression are poorly understood, *WT1* overexpression could be a suitable candidate as molecular marker for MRD monitoring. However, the potential use of this marker may be hampered by the overexpression of *WT1* in normal regenerating BM [34-36]. In a large study by Cilloni *et al.*, 504 patients were studied at diagnosis and *WT1* was found to be overexpressed in 86% of the cases. Of these, 129 patients were analysed during follow-up and it was demonstrated that after the first chemotherapy cycle a larger than 2-log reduction in *WT1* levels was an independent prognostic factor for decreased risk of relapse (HR 0.54, range 0.36-0.83, p =.004). After consolidation therapy low *WT1* levels also predicted decreased risk of relapse (p =.004) [37]. Hämäläinen and co-workers analysed *WT1* expression at diagnosis in BM of 100 AML patients and found no prognostic significance as such (cut-off 9.7%, compared with K562 cell *WT1* gene expression). Although *WT1* expression levels were constantly detectable during the remission period, they nevertheless found that an increase in *WT1* expression levels may be a predictor for relapse [38]. Although these results show that *WT1* overexpression for MRD monitoring is a potentially useful marker that can be used in the majority of AML patients, despite multiple studies having been performed, the clinical utility of *WT1* monitoring remains somewhat controversial [37,38].

Another potential marker is *PRAME*, a gene originally recognized in melanoma patients, which is expressed in 35%-64% of AML patients [39-41]. In a study by Qin *et al.*, using BM material from 204 newly diagnosed patients, *PRAME* overexpression was found in 55.4% of the cases. In follow-up patients who achieved continuous haematological CR (n = 20), *PRAME* levels had decreased but never reached the normal range in 6/20 patients. All of these patients ultimately relapsed. In seven patients *PRAME* levels decreased down to normal levels, but thereafter rose again above normal values; all of these patients eventually relapsed within 4 months. In the remaining patients (7/20) *PRAME* levels decreased down to the normal range and these patients remained in continuous CR. This suggests that the *PRAME* gene may be a useful marker for MRD monitoring [42]. Although these results are promising, a few potential pitfalls should be taken into account. Both *WT1* and *PRAME* are expressed in relatively high levels in normal hematopoietic cells, which result in high levels of background expression before and after treatment. *WT1* and *PRAME* are thus not highly specific markers, with risk on false-positive results [37,38]. To avoid this, PB may be used as an alternative source of cells, since both *WT1* and *PRAME* levels are much lower in circulating normal PB cells, than in normal BM cells [37,42]. Furthermore, a more general disadvantage for gene overexpression is the risk of RNA degradation during isolation procedures that might result in false-negativity. Since overexpression of *WT1* is more frequent in AML cells than *PRAME, WT1* is probably the most useful target for MRD monitoring.

The ecotropic virus integrations-1 (*EVI1*) proto-oncogene is associated with chromosome 3q26 rearrangements and high expression at diagnosis predicts poor clinical outcome [43]. *EVI1* overexpression has been demonstrated in approximately 8% of the AML patients [44]. To our knowledge, no MRD studies using *EVI1* overexpression have been performed thus far. At least 4 different splice forms have been identified (*EVI1-1A, -1B, -1C and -3L*) [45]. Seen the low frequency of cases with overexpression, *EVI1* based MRD detection would add significantly to MRD detection if all splice variants could be detected. Since *EVI1* positive patients have an extremely poor prognosis it may be suggested that MRD based pre-emptive therapy in *EVI1* positive patients would allow therapeutic intervention at an earlier time point and thereby possibly improve clinical outcome. Future studies will have to confirm if *EVI1* is indeed a useful and stable MRD marker.

2.2.3. Gene mutations

Since fusion genes are only present in 15%-45% of AML patients and overexpressed genes seem to be less specific MRD markers, gene mutations may offer another attractive group of targets for MRD monitoring.

A decade ago, fms-like tyrosine kinase 3 (*FLT3*) mutations were found to be present in approximately 30% of AML patients. Different *FLT3* mutations exist; however, the most common is the *FLT3*-internal tandem duplication (*ITD*) in the juxtamembrane region. This *ITD* results in an extra sequence that varies between 3 and 400 base pairs and is thought to cause a constant activation of the tyrosine kinase receptor, resulting in advantages for cell survival. The *FLT3-ITD* occurs in approximately 23% of adult AML patients and is associated with poor prognosis [46-48]. Since *FLT3-ITD* is suggested as potential MRD marker, several studies have been performed to confirm this. Chou *et al.* demonstrated that both OS and disease free survival (DFS) were significantly longer in CR patients who obtained a > 3-log reduction compared to the CR patients with less reduction (OS not reached v. 14.7 months, p =. 016, DFS 7.5 v. 3.0 months, p<.001). Moreover, a > 3-log reduction of *FLT3-ITD* was an independent prognostic factor for DFS (HR 0.264, p =.002) with a trend for OS (HR 0.308, p =.057) [49]. Thus, MRD monitoring by *FLT3-ITD* can provide prognostic information [49-52]. However, a serious limitation of the use of a *FLT3-ITD*, is its instability during disease. In part of the AML samples that harbor a *FLT3-ITD* at diagnosis, it has changed or disappeared at relapse [49,53-55], which would result in false-negative MRD results. Furthermore, because of the heterogeneity in *FLT3-ITD* lengths and molecular sequence, no common qRT-PCR can be developed, which offers a serious problem in regular diagnostics [46,51,56].

Mutations in the nucleophosmin (*NPM1*) gene have also been identified as frequent genetic alterations, occurring in approximately 35% of all AML patients. This mutation occurs most frequently in exon 12 of the gene, resulting in loss of one or both C-terminal tryptophan residues leading to an aberrant localization of the protein in the cytoplasm [57,58]. The presence is strongly associated with a normal karyotype, where *NPM1* mutations occur in approximately 60% of patients [59]. When not accompanied by a *FLT3* mutation, it has been described as a favorable factor in patients with normal cytogenetics [60,61]. Quantitative monitoring of *NPM1* mutations after treatment has shown to give important prognostic information [50,62-66]. Although stability of this marker has been reported in several studies [50,62,63,65], loss of the *NPM1* mutation at relapse has also been found [67,68]. It has to be taken into account that more than 30 different types of *NPM1* mutations have been described, but fortunately two types (type A and type B) are by far the most common [57,58]. It can be concluded that MRD assessment by *NPM1* mutations is a suitable, stable and sensitive marker. However, more prospective studies are warranted to validate these results and to confirm stability of *NPM1* during disease.

CCAAT/enhancer binding protein alpha (*CEBPα*) is a transcription factor involved in the regulation of myeloid differentiation and cellular growth arrest [69]. *CEBPA* mutations have been reported in 8% to 19% of cytogenetically normal AML patients and are associated with favorable prognosis [70-72]. There are two major types of *CEBPA* mutations, including C-terminal mutations that occur in the bZIP domain and N-terminal mutations. Furthermore, some patients carry biallelic mutations, whereas others are heterozygous for different kind of mutations [72]. Although *CEBPA* is a potential suitable target for MRD monitoring, to our knowledge, no studies have been reported thus far. Seen the low frequency of cases with a *CEBPA* mutation, *CEBPA* based MRD detection would have limited applicability in AML patients. Future clinical trials have to demonstrate if *CEBPA* is indeed a suitable and stable marker for MRD detection.

2.3. Clinical applications of MRD

As discussed above, MRD frequency assessment using immunophenotypic and molecular parameters in patients with AML in clinical remission has important prognostic value and can predict forthcoming relapses. Therefore, it would be of potential importance to monitor MRD cell frequency for risk stratification. Current AML risk stratification is based on a number of parameters determined at diagnosis, including origin of leukemia (secondary AML, AML after myelodysplastic syndrome), age, WBC count, and presence of certain cytogenetic and/or molecular aberrancies [14]. Novel AML risk stratification should not only be based on risk assessment at diagnosis, but also on MRD cell frequency as a "response to treatment" parameter. Including MRD in AML risk stratification could help identify CR patients after induction therapy with increased MRD levels and therefore high risk of relapse. For instance, good risk patients with high MRD levels after induction therapy may benefit from allogeneic stem cell transplantation, while on the other hand intermediate risk group patients with low MRD levels could be spared from an allogeneic transplantation and the accompanying toxicity. Especially in this intermediate risk group, MRD monitoring would be of great help, since the prognosis of these patients is difficult to estimate. Therefore, MRD based clinical decision making after induction therapy may contribute to better RFS and OS rates.

Also after consolidation therapy, MRD based clinical intervention is promising. Even after an allogeneic transplantation, still a proportion of 20%-40% of the patients will relapse [73-75]. Therapeutic options in the case of post-transplant relapse consist of withdrawal or decrease of dose of immune-suppressive drugs, or immunotherapeutic intervention with a donor lymphocyte infusion. As these approaches intend to boost the graft versus leukemia effect, they are most effective when the leukemic cell load is small. Therefore early detection of impending post-transplant relapses is essential and would allow immunotherapeutic intervention at a low leukemic burden. The current standard to guide post-transplant treatment is the level of donor chimerism. This refers to the percentage of donor cells in PB or BM and it can be determined using short tandem repeat (STR)-PCR. Although mixed chimerism (< 95% of donor cells) has been associated with a higher incidence of relapse [76,77], patients with full chimerism (> 95% donor cells) can still suffer from relapse [77]. Additional monitoring of MRD levels in these transplanted patients could improve successful prediction of relapse, since MRD analysis directly detects the neoplastic part of the patient cell population, while STR analysis reflects total donor and total patient populations. Multiple studies have shown that MRD monitoring after an allogeneic transplantation indeed correlates with clinical outcome and identifies patients who are likely to relapse [78-81]. Therefore, it can be suggested that MRD based pre-emptive immunotherapy after transplantation could reduce relapse and improve survival. Standardization of treatment, based on MRD and chimerism analysis in the post-transplant period, seems therefore warranted. In conclusion, since MRD frequency assessment gives important prognostic information after both induction and consolidation therapy, it seems likely that using MRD for therapeutic intervention in the post-remission phase might reduce relapse rates en prolong OS. To confirm this hypothesis, large prospective studies with MRD based clinical intervention in the post-remission phase are essential.

2.4. Improvement of and alternatives for bone marrow MRD detection

2.4.1. Improvements for immunophenotypic and molecular MRD detection

Although flow cytometric MRD monitoring has many advantages, one of the difficulties is the complexity of MRD analysis. Nowadays, more advanced data analysis programs, that aid to distinguish between normal and malignant cells, are available [82]. This might simplify the analysis and result in more objective results. Notwithstanding the high prognostic value of MRD monitoring, in almost all studies 20%-40% of the patients with immunophenotypic defined low MRD levels still suffer from a relapse [5-7,10,16]. There are several potential reasons for missing these MRD cells. Normal BM cells express LAPs at low frequencies. Counting these cells as leukemic might result in false-positivity. This background expression thus seriously hinders specific identification of leukemic cells. On the other hand, subtracting background levels might under-estimate MRD frequencies and this could result in false-negatives. High specificity and thereby high sensitivity can be achieved when only the most specific immunophenotypic aberrancies are used, i.e. with no expression in normal cells. Inclusion of markers/marker combinations that allow excluding non-specific events in a multi-color approach may increase specificity. This is already shown for the transition of a four to five-color flow cytometric approach [83]. Another explanation for MRD misclassification is low sensitivity of the aberrant immunophenotype. Marker expression may be highly heterogeneous in an AML sample: LAPs may thereby often not be expressed on the total population of blast cells, thereby, at follow up, preventing the identification of all leukemic cells. Improvements can only be expected with the discovery of new aberrancies that cover larger parts of diagnosis blast cells. At present, with the large differences in specificity and sensitivity of LAPs the level of detection of MRD varies between patients: 1:10,000 or even better may be reached in one patient, while in another patient 1:1,000 may be the best attainable. Besides misclassification, immunophenotype shifts can also contribute to false-negative observations. To reduce this, it is recommended to use multiple LAPs for MRD monitoring [6,12,13]. Recently, it has become clear that such shifts may occur through clonal selection: while major molecular clones may disappear upon therapy, minor diagnosis clones may survive chemotherapy treatment, and grow out to relapse [84]. This may be accompanied by immunophenotype changes [84]. More efforts towards recognition of minor clones at diagnosis, that potentially can expand to cause relapse, may identify emerging molecular clones and immunophenotypes instead of disappearing molecular clones and immunophenotypes only. For molecular MRD, in fact most of the pitfalls for immunophenotypic MRD hold here as well. Similar to MFC, multiple molecular MRD studies have reported patients with low molecular MRD levels that still suffer from relapse [25,26,37,38,42]. Underlying causes may include 1) as argued earlier for different LAPs, Q-PCRs for different mutations and fusion genes reach different sensitivities as well; 2) part of the blasts may only be characterized by the molecular aberrancy of interest; and 3) molecular clone shifts occur between diagnosis and relapse. To avoid these false-negative results different molecular markers, if present in the patient, could be quantified for MRD monitoring. There are no real solutions for these problems unless more generally applicable, specific and stable markers are discovered. Until then, combining as many molecular and immunophenotypic targets may contribute to accurate MRD based prediction of relapse. Another possible explanation for finding false-negative MRD results is the fact that it may not only be the number of leukemic blasts that determines the chance for relapse, but more specifically the number of leukemic stem cells (LSCs). These LSCs can cause tumor outgrowth, thereby leading to MRD and finally resulting into overt disease relapse [85]. Although these stem cells are much less frequent than whole blast MRD, LSC frequency assessment may offer an additional specific and biologically relevant determinant of risk on relapse. In section 3 the role of leukemic stem cells in acute myeloid leukemia will be further discussed.

2.4.2. Alternative parameters for risk stratification

Perhaps the conceptually simplest method to evaluate treatment response is calculating the decrease rate of peripheral blasts shortly after treatment. As shown previously for childhood acute lymphocytic leukemia [86], this may directly reflect the chemosensitivity of individual patients. The big advantage would be that it is applicable independent of the initial immunophenotype of the blasts. To accurately calculate such a blast cell decrease rate, blast frequencies have to be measured every day of chemotherapy treatment. Lacombe *et al.* reported two different modalities to evaluate blast cell decrease: 1) calculation of the blast cell decrease slope by linear regression between day 0 and the first day when at least 90% of the initial blast load has disappeared, 2) assessment of the total time period needed to reach 90% blast decrease. All patients (n = 74) who reached a 90% blast reduction within 6 days achieved CR. The authors also showed a strong correlation for both modalities with patients' clinical outcome [87]. Since leukemic blasts at diagnosis in most cases are present in the PB too, it has been proposed that PB may represent an alternative specific source for immunophenotypic MRD detection. Since aspiration of BM is an invasive procedure, MRD detection in the PB would offer significant advantages over BM-MRD both for patients and physicians. Furthermore, the BM contains immature normal populations that resemble LAPs, while these are thought to be largely absent in PB. The latter would clearly have advantages for the easiness of interpreting MRD. Although MRD frequencies in PB are lower than in BM, PB-MRD frequencies correlated with BM-MRD frequencies and turned out to have prognostic value [88]. Once the value of PB-MRD is validated in other studies and once it has been confirmed that BM-MRD is positive in all PB-MRD positive cases, PB-MRD may replace BM-MRD, provided that PB is MRD positive. In case of PB-MRD negativity, it will probably remain necessary to perform BM acquisition, since BM-MRD is more sensitive. Another alternative parameter for risk stratification is the presence of B-lymphocyte precursors in AML BM. A high level of B-lymphocyte precursors after first CR thereby predicts for DFS [89]. Furthermore, an abnormal high $CD34^+$ myeloid / $CD34^+$ lymphoid ratio (≥ 10) is associated with worse outcome [90]. The development of an algorithm including not only BM-MRD, but also other parameters, including PB-MRD, blast reduction rate, $CD34^+$ myeloid/ lymphoid ratio and the percentage of B-lymphocyte precursors, may contribute to improved accurate prediction of relapses.

3. Leukemic stem cells and acute myeloid leukemia

3.1. Definition of leukemic stem cells

It was hypothesized that a small population of cells, distinct from the bulk of tumor cells, is responsible for tumor initiation and growth in various cancers, including AML [91,92]. These cells are referred to as leukemic stem cells (LSCs) or leukemia-initiating cells (LICs). It is assumed that similar to normal hematopoiesis, leukemia is hierarchically structured. In many respects LSCs resemble normal hematopoietic stem cells (HSCs). Similar to HSCs, LSCs are defined by their ability to undergo self-renewal and the capacity to differentiate to a limited, although highly variable, extent [93,94]. Furthermore, the immunophenotype of LSCs resembles the immunophenotype of normal HSCs. The majority of HSCs are present in the $CD34^+CD38^-$ immunophenotypic compartment [95,96] and initial AML studies demonstrated leukemia initiating capacity also to be in the $CD34^+CD38^-$ compartment [97]. This small subpopulation of $CD34^+CD38^-$ cells was able to engraft and cause leukemia in non-obese diabetic/sever combined immune-deficient (NOD/SCID) mice. These cells were present at a frequency of only 0.2 to 100 cells per 10^6 mononuclear cells [97]. Nowadays it is known that AML LSCs can also reside within the $CD34^+CD38^+$ or the $CD34^-$ immunophenotypic compartment [98-102]. There is growing evidence that the transformation of a normal human cell into a LSC not only can occur in a normal HSC, but also in a normal progenitor cell [103]. Mutations in a normal progenitor cell may confer self-renewal properties to progenitors. A recent study demonstrated that $CD34^+CD38^-$ LSCs, despite the immunophenotypic similarities with normal HSCs, are most related to normal progenitors instead of normal stem cells [102]. In addition, it has been demonstrated that within a patient, the pool of LSCs at diagnosis is often largely heterogeneous. This implies that different subpopulations of LSCs often coexist at diagnosis [84,101] (Figure 1). In CD34 positive patients often both $CD34^+CD38^-$ cells, $CD34^+CD38^+$ and $CD34^-$ cells are present and all are able to show leukemic engraftment when infused separately in NOD/SCID mice. However, no information exists on possible competition between these compartments in leukemogenesis. Moreover, the $CD34^+CD38^-$ compartment has been shown to be less immunogenic compared to the other compartments [104], which may explain why it was almost exclusively the $CD34^+CD38^-$ compartment that engrafted in NOD/SCID mice with residual immunity [97], while in the severely immunocompromised later mouse models, the other compartments engrafted as well. In CD34 negative AML by definition, the $CD34^-$ compartment and in particular the $CD34^-CD38^+$ compartment contain LSCs [100]. For clinical treatment and patient survival it is important to know which putative LSC will survive therapy. In that respect it is important to realize that the $CD34^+CD38^-$ compartment has been shown to be most therapy resistant *in vitro* [104]. In line with this, it has been reported that in CD34 positive relapsed patients a $CD34^+CD38^-$ subpopulation is most likely to survive chemotherapy treatment and expand towards development of relapse [84].

In the course of time other compartments enriched for LSCs have been identified. These are based on functional properties and include aldehyde dehydrogenase (ALDH) activity and drug efflux (Hoechst) capacity. ALDH is a group of cytosolic enzymes that catalyze the oxidation of aldehydes. It plays an important role in the retinoid metabolism, since it is required for the conversion of retinol (Vitamin A) to retinoic acids. For maturation, loss of quiescence and differentiation of HSCs, these retinoic acids are important [105,106]. Furthermore, ALDH activity is supposed to protect cells from the toxic effects of cyclophosphamide and therefore high ALDH expression in leukemic cells may play a role in chemotherapy resistance [107,108]. Recently it has been shown that leukemic cells and normal hematopoietic cells differ in ALDH activity. Normal stem- and progenitor cells have high ALDH expression [109-112]. It has to be emphasized that it has recently been demonstrated that the population of cells with intermediate ALDH activity appeared to be enriched for leukemic $CD34^+CD38^-$ cells [113-115]. Several authors have confirmed the leukemia initiating capacity of these cells in NOD/SCID mice [116-118].

Another functional stem cell compartment is the so-called side population (SP). These SP cells are primarily defined by their capability of efficient Hoechst 33342 dye efflux and especially by the way in which fluorescence emission of Hoechst is recorded. In normal BM a population of $CD34^+CD38^-$ cells was found in the SP [119,120]. In AML, it has been demonstrated that the SP compartment contains a heterogeneous population of cells, containing HSCs, LSCs, LSC progenitors and early lymphocytes [121]. AML SP cells have shown to be able to initiate acute leukemia in NOD/SCID mice [122,123]. All these immunophenotypic and functional findings are important for gaining insight in the process of leukemogenesis and especially for the development of new therapies aiming at eradication of LSCs.

Besides the ability of LSCs to initiate and sustain the initial AML, there is increasing evidence pointing towards the importance of LSCs in the occurrence of MRD and the emergence of a relapse. LSCs are thought to be more resistant to standard chemotherapy compared to the total population of malignant blast cells and therefore these LSCs are able to escape apoptosis. Other essential LSC features are their acquired capacity for self-renewal and proliferation. Such properties allow LSCs to survive chemotherapy treatment, to divide and to grow out and cause a relapse (Figure 1). Consequently, identification and characterization of LSCs is fundamental to gain insight in the mechanisms that underlie relapse and how to evade relapse.

3.2. Identification of leukemic stem cells

Since the assumed role of LSC in the emergence of an AML relapse, identification of these probably most malignant cells becomes imperative. The hypothesis would thus be that quantitation of LSCs in AML patients would give important information about treatment response and risk of relapse. Similar to MRD identified by flow cytometry, LSCs in BM can be identified using cell surface antigen expression. As mentioned before, LSCs can reside in different immunophenotypic compartments, but, as argued before, the $CD34^+CD38^-$ defined LSCs may be most malignant/resistant [84,104]. Since both HSCs and LSCs reside within this compartment, discrimination between $CD34^+CD38^-$ HSCs and LSCs is challenging. Immunophenotypic LSC detection is often possible making use of the fact that the lineage marker combinations used for MRD detection, are frequently aberrantly expressed on $CD34^+CD38^-$ cells too [124]. These lineage markers include CD2, CD7, CD11b, CD13, CD15, CD19, CD22

http://dx.doi.org/10.5772/52080

CD33, CD56 and HLA-DR. Combinations of lineage markers could also be used, like CD33⁺CD13⁻ and CD15⁺HLA-DR⁻. Besides these lineage markers, a growing number of other markers is now available to discriminate between LSCs and HSCs. These include CLL-1 CD25, CD32, CD33, CD44, CD47, CD96, CD123 and TIM-3 (Figure 3). An overview of LSC markers is given in Table 3.

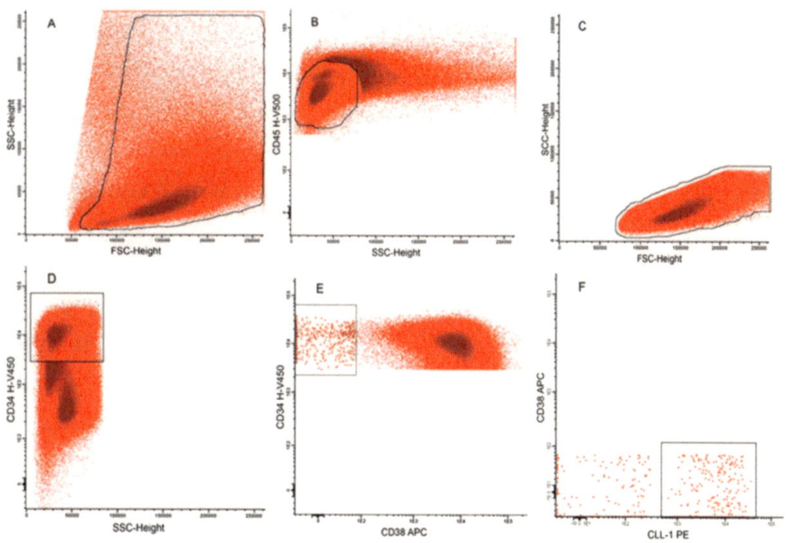

Figure 3. Gating strategy for $CD34^+CD38^-$ LSC detection at diagnosis in AML bone marrow. Gating of viable white blood cells (A). Gating of blast cells with CD45dim expression and low sideward scatter (SSC) (B, C). CD34 positive progenitors cells (D). Gating of the CD34 positive and CD38 negative blasts (E). The $CD34^+CD38^-$ cells gated against CLL-1. Two populations of stem cells are shown: a CLL-1 negative stem cell population, containing the HSCs and the $CD34^+CD38^-$ cells with positive expression of CLL-1. These stem cells with aberrant expression of CLL-1 are defined as LSCs (F).

It is important to realize that there is a large heterogeneity in marker expression. This implies that marker expression differs between AML patients and even within an individual patient different stem cell markers are often differentially expressed (Figure 4). Thus, none of the individual markers are expressed in all AML cases. For accurate LSC detection, high specificity of stem cell markers is essential. Both CLL-1 and lineage markers have proven to be highly specific, since these are present on leukemic $CD34^+CD38^-$ cells in a substantial part of the AML patient population, but absent on normal $CD34^+CD38^-$ cells, also after chemotherapy [124,125]. For the other stem cell markers high specificity and stability during treatment/disease still have to be confirmed. The established differences in ALDH activity between $CD34^+CD38^-$ LSCs and $CD34^+CD38^-$ HSCs were confirmed using this aberrant marker approach [114,115], thereby strengthening that the functional ALDH assay offers an alternative tool for $CD34^+CD38^-$ LSC identification, which importantly, could be applied in absence of aberrant antigen expression. In contrast, the SP phenotype does not discriminate between HSCs and LSCs since both may be present in the SP compartment. Here the immunophenotypic marker approach is necessary to discriminate between LSCs and HSCs [121].

Both ALDH and SP assays not only identify leukemia initiating cells with the $CD34^+CD38^-$ immunophenotype, but also other cell types, like $CD34^+CD38^+$ progenitors or $CD34^-$ cells [114,115,117].

Although functional assays, like ALDH and SP, are complex and time-consuming compared to standard immunophenotypic LSC detection, they may offer promising alternatives for $CD34^+$ AML patients without detectable $CD34^+CD38^-$ cells, as well as for AML patients who are defined as CD34 negative. The latter patients usually have less than 1% expression of CD34 on the leukemic blast cells which all are of non-neoplastic origin [133]. However, also for cases with $CD34^+CD38^-$ LSCs present, these functionally defined compartments may be important: since the frequency of SP cells is far lower compared to the frequency of $CD34^+CD38^-$ stem cells [121], an interesting possibility would be that combination of both assays may narrow the real stem cell compartment [121]. In contrast to the immunophenotypic definition, ALDH activity and dye efflux ability are likely directly related to drug response and in that sense may predict which stem cells will survive therapy. Together with the observations that immunophenotypically defined $CD34^+CD38^-$ cells are *in vitro* therapy resistant too [104] and that most likely a $CD34^+CD38^-$ subpopulation grows out to relapse [84], the possibility that relapses are caused by functionally defined subpopulations of the $CD34^+CD38^-$ compartment can be suggested.

Antigen	Function	Reference
CLL-1	C-type lectin-like molecule-1	[125]
Lineage markers	Lymphoid lineage and myeloid lineage markers	[124]
CD25	Interleukin-2 receptor α-chain	[126]
CD32	Fc fragement of IgG, low affinity IIa receptor	[126]
CD33	Myeloid marker	[127]
CD44	Receptor for hyaluronan	[128]
CD47	Integrin associated protein	[129]
CD96	T cell-activated increased late expression protein	[130]
CD123	Interleukin 3 receptor alpha chain	[131]
TIM-3	T-cell Ig mucin-3	[132]

Table 3. Overview of stem cell markers.

Seen the large clonal heterogeneity at diagnosis [84,101], and the possibility that not just the major clone at diagnosis, but often low-frequency $CD34^+CD38^-$ clones may grow out [84], this suggests that identification of functionally defined minor subpopulations present at diagnosis may offer clues how to predict relapse in a very early stage and thereby ultimately how to circumvent such relapses.

$CD34^+CD38^-$ population was analyzed for the expression of six aberrant markers: CD2 (A), CLL-1 (B), CD22 (C), CD96 (D), CD123 (E), CD11b (F). Expressions percentages for marker positive and marker negative $CD34^+CD38^-$ cells are shown for each marker.

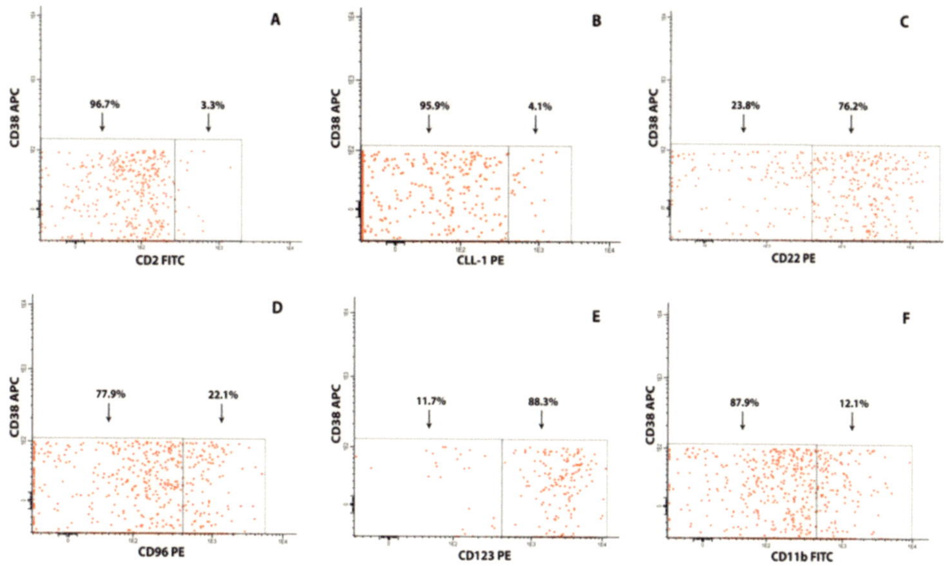

Figure 4. Heterogeneity in expression of different stem cell markers in one AML case at diagnosis.

3.3. Prognostic value of LSC frequency

Since it has been hypothesized that the subpopulation of chemotherapy resistant LSCs is responsible for relapse, LSC frequency, similar to MRD frequency, should have direct prognostic impact.

Van Rhenen *et al.* were the first to study the correlation between the frequency of $CD34^+CD38^-$ cells at diagnosis and clinical outcome in 92 AML patients. In a multivariate analysis, including known risk factors, the frequency of the $CD34^+CD38^-$ compartment (% of blast cells) turned out to be an independent prognostic factor for RFS ($p = 0.004$) and DFS ($p = 0.05$) [134]. In a small group of pediatric AML patients, Witte *et al.* found that the $CD34^+CD38^-$ subpopulation was significantly lower in patients with 5-year DFS ($n = 8$) compared to patients with relapse and/or death ($n = 9$) (0.45% ± 0.61% v. 1.52% ± 1.52%, $p = 0.04$) [135]. Moreover, Hwang and colleagues have demonstrated, in a group of 54 AML patients, that the proportion of $CD34^+CD38^-$ cells at diagnosis was significantly lower in patients achieving CR compared to patients who did not achieve CR (median 0.7% v. 6.9%, $p = 0.006$) [136]. Lastly, using the ALDH activity assay, Ran *et al.* have shown a significant difference in OS and RFS between patients with high and low LSC frequencies (OS, $p = 0.04$, RFS, $p = 0.01$). Multivariate Cox regression for OS showed LSC frequency and WBC count at diagnosis to be the only significant prognostic factors (HR 10.5 for LSCs, $p = 0.05$), with borderline significance for RFS (HR 3.8, $p = 0.05$) [118]. In our recent study we refined the definition used in aforementioned papers by including markers that enabled to discriminate LSC from HSC [137]. In total, 101 patients were monitored for LSC frequency. Again, differences in prognosis were found between patients groups defined by different cut offs (Table 4.)

	Cut-off	Number of patients above cut-off	Relative risk of relapse	95% C.I.
First cycle	5×10^{-6}	14	5.0	1.8-14.0
Second cycle	5×10^{-6}	18	4.7	2.2-10.1
Consolidation	2×10^{-6}	14	8.5	1.8-41.4

Table 4. Relative risk of relapse defined by LSC frequency [137].

All together, several studies showed $CD34^{+}CD38^{-}$ LSC frequency to be an independent prognostic risk factor. Important to emphasize, however, is that these studies focus on LSC detection and quantification at AML diagnosis. Because LSCs are hypothesized to be chemotherapy resistant and to grow out after treatment and then cause a relapse, it would be of utmost importance to study the frequency of these LSCs during follow-up. For the first time we also demonstrated that the frequencies of LSCs after different courses of therapy significantly correlated with clinical outcome [137]. More effort is needed to identify LSCs and their prognostic value in immunophenotypic compartments other than $CD34^{+}CD38^{-}$, like the $CD34^{+}CD38^{+}$ and $CD34^{-}$ compartment using the ALDH and SP assay. Ultimately, when the clinical importance of different stem cell compartments have been prospectively confirmed, this, together with MRD based strategies, should offer new diagnostic tools to guide clinical intervention and to monitor effectiveness of therapy and, moreover, to design new therapies that specifically target LSCs while leaving the normal HSCs intact.

3.4. Leukemic stem cell targeted therapy

Apart from the clinical application of LSCs, characterization of these malignant cells offers the design of new therapies that specifically target LSCs while leaving the normal HSCs intact. The most direct example of such therapy is the application of antibodies that are used to specifically discriminate between LSC and HSC. CD123 and CD33 are examples. It has been reported, using NOD/SCID mice, that treatment with the anti-CD123 antibody 7G3 improved mouse survival [138]. A humanized version of the anti-CD123 antibody (CLS360) has been studied in a phase 1 study in relapsed, refractory and high-risk AML patients. Interim analysis showed no treatment related toxicity, besides two mild infusion reactions and one infection possibly related to the treatment. Of eight patients treated with CLS360, one CR had been observed [139]. Further clinical studies are needed to determine the efficacy of this antibody in AML patients.

CD33 is expressed on leukemic blasts in 85%-90% of AML patients and therefore, already years ago, it had been suggested as a potential target for anti-AML therapy. The CD33 immunoconjugate gemtuzumab ozogamicin (Mylotarg) has been studied in several trials and, after initial disappointment relating to toxicity, new studies with altered treatment schedules suggest that Mylotarg is beneficial in certain subgroups of AML patients, including patients with favorable cytogenetics [140]. However, it is important to emphasize that no studies so far determined the correlation between the efficacy of Mylotarg and the presence of CD33 positive LSCs. It may be speculated that subgroups of patients with CD33 positive LSCs may benefit from this additional therapy. Further clinical trials will also have to determine if other stem cell markers are potential targets as well.

4. Conclusions and future perspectives

MRD frequency assessments by RQ-PCR and MFC in AML patients are more sensitive methods to define remission status compared to current morphologic assessment. Although RQ-PCR is in general the most sensitive technique, MFC is applicable in almost all AML patients. Since the importance of flow cytometric MRD detection has now been validated in a first prospective study, it is of utmost importance that, when these data are confirmed in other prospective studies, MRD status will be implemented in clinical decision-making. We have described that alternatives for BM MRD may include MRD assessment in peripheral blood and blast reduction, frequency of B-lymphocytes precursors and $CD34^{+}$ myeloid/lymphoid ratios. It thus seems that development of algorithms including all such parameters may ultimately contribute to improved detection of residual therapy resistant cells and early and accurate prediction of relapses. Also, based on the observation of immunophenotypic and molecular shifts, occurring between diagnosis and relapse, a new issue in MRD research may be that not only disappearing phenotypes, but also emerging "new" phenotypes have to be monitored. An alternative, probably more specific method to predict clinical outcome is LSC frequency assessment. Results so far on the clinical importance of LSCs are limited, but very promising, especially since for the first time the correlation between the presence of LSCs after treatment and clinical outcome has been reported. When the value of LSC assessment is confirmed in other retrospective and eventually prospective studies, it may be hypothesized that in the future, not only MRD, but also LSC frequency assessment may be implemented in clinical decision-making.

Hopefully, using the suggested approaches in this chapter, it will become possible to significantly improve clinical outcome of acute myeloid leukemia patients.

Acknowledgements

We thank J. Cloos for reviewing the manuscript and A. Kelder for assistance in figure preparation.

Author details

W. Zeijlemaker* and G.J. Schuurhuis*

*Address all correspondence to:

*Address all correspondence to: GJ.Schuurhuis@vumc.nl

Department of Hematology, VU University Medical Center, Amsterdam, The Netherlands

References

[1] Cornelissen, J. J., van Putten, W. L. J., Verdonck, L. F., Theobald, M., Jacky, E., Daenen, S. M., et al. (2007). Results of a HOVON/SAKK donor versus no-donor analysis of myeloablative HLA-identical sibling stem cell transplantation in first remission acute myeloid leukemia in young and middle-aged adults: benefits for whom? *Blood*, 109(9), 3658-66.

[2] Cheson, B. D., Bennett, J. M., Kopecky, K. J., Büchner, T., Willman, C. L., Estey, E. H., et al. (2003). Revised recommendations of the International Working Group for Diagnosis, Standardization of Response Criteria, Treatment Outcomes, and Reporting Standards for Therapeutic Trials in Acute Myeloid Leukemia. *J Clin Oncol*, 21(24), 4642-9.

[3] Kern, W., Haferlach, C., Haferlach, T., & Schnittger, S. (2008). Monitoring of minimal residual disease in acute myeloid leukemia. *Cancer*, 112(1), 4-16.

[4] San, Miguel. J. F., Martinez, A., Macedo, A., Vidriales, M. B., López-Berges, C., González, M., et al. (1997). Immunophenotyping investigation of minimal residual disease is a useful approach for predicting relapse in acute myeloid leukemia patients. *Blood*, 90(6), 2465-70.

[5] Kern, W., Voskova, D., Schoch, C., Hiddemann, W., Schnittger, S., & Haferlach, T. (2004). Determination of relapse risk based on assessment of minimal residual disease during complete remission by multiparameter flow cytometry in unselected patients with acute myeloid leukemia. *Blood*, 104(10), 3078-85.

[6] Feller, N., van der Pol, M. A., van Stijn, A., Weijers, G. W. D., Westra, A. H., & Evertse, B. W. et al. (2004). MRD parameters using immunophenotypic detection methods are highly reliable in predicting survival in acute myeloid leukaemia. *Leukemia* , 18(8), 1380-90.

[7] Venditti, A., Buccisano, F., Del Poeta, G., Maurillo, L., Tamburini, A., Cox, C., et al. (2000). Level of minimal residual disease after consolidation therapy predicts outcome in acute myeloid leukemia. *Blood*, 96(12), 3948-52.

[8] Diez-Campelo, M., Pérez, J., Alcoceba, M., Richtmon, J., Vidriales, B., & San, Miguel. J. (2009). Minimal residual disease monitoring after allogeneic transplantation may help to individualize post-transplant therapeutic strategies in acute myeloid malignancies. *Am J Hematol*, 84(3), 149-52.

[9] Buccisano, F., Maurillo, L., Spagnoli, A., Del Principe, M. I., Ceresoli, . E., Lo, Coco. F., et al. (2009). Monitoring of minimal residual disease in acute myeloid leukemia. *Curr Opin Oncol*, 21(6), 582-8.

[10] Al-Mawali, A., Gillis, D., Lewis, I., & 20, . (2009). The use of receiver operating characteristic analysis for detection of minimal residual disease using five-color multiparameter flow cytometry in acute myeloid leukemia identifies patients with high risk of relapse. *Cytometry B Clin Cytom*, 76(2), 91-101.

[11] Vidriales, M. B., San-Miguel, J. F., Orfao, A., Coustan-Smith, E., & Campana, D. (2003). Minimal residual disease monitoring by flow cytometry. *Best Pract Res Clin Haematol*, 16(4), 599-612.

[12] Baer, M. R., Stewart, C. C., Dodge, R. K., Leget, G., Sulé, N., Mrózek, K., et al. (2001). High frequency of immunophenotype changes in acute myeloid leukemia at relapse: implications for residual disease detection (Cancer and Leukemia Group B Study 8361). *Blood*, 97(11), 3574-80.

[13] Macedo, A., San, Miguel. J. F., Vidriales, M. B., López-Berges, M. C., García-Marcos, M. A., Gonzales, M., et al. (1996). Phenotypic changes in acute myeloid leukaemia: implications in the detection of minimal residual disease. *J Clin Pathol*, 49(1), 15-8.

[14] Grimwade, D., & Hills, R. K. (2009). Independent prognostic factors for AML outcome. *Hematology Am Soc Hematol Educ Program:*, 385-95.

[15] San, Miguel. J. F., Vidriales, M. B., López-Berges, C., Diaz-Mediavilla, J., Guttiérrez, N., Cañizo, C., et al. (2001). Early immunophenotypical evaluation of minimal residual disease in acute myeloid leukemia identifies different patient risk groups and may contribute to postinduction treatment stratification. *Blood*, 98(6), 1746-51.

[16] Maurillo, L., Buccisano, F., Del Principe, M. I., Del Poeta, G., Spagnoli, A., Panetta, P., et al. (2008). Toward optimization of postremission therapy for residual disease-positive patients with acute myeloid leukemia. *J Clin Oncol*, 26(30), 4944-51.

[17] Terwijn, M., Kelder, A., van Putten, W. L. J., Snel, A. N., van der Velden, V. H. J., & Brooimans, R. A. et al. (2010). High prognostic impact of flowcytometric minimal residual disease detection in acute myeloid leukemia: prospective data from the HOVON/SAKK 42a study. *Blood* (ASH Annual Meeting Abstracts)116:760.

[18] Sugimoto, T., Das, H., Imoto, S., Murayama, T., Gomyo, H., Chakraborty, S., et al. (2000). Quantitation of minimal residual disease in t(821)-positive acute myelogenous leukemia patients using real-time quantitative RT-PCR. *Am J Hematol*, 64(2), 101-6.

[19] Tobal, K., & Liu, Yin J.A. (1996). Monitoring of minimal residual disease by quantitative reverse transcriptase-polymerase chain reaction for AML1-MTG8 transcripts in AML-M2 with t(821). *Blood*, 88(10), 3704-9.

[20] Guerrasio, A., Pilatrino, C., De Micheli, D., Cilloni, D., Serra, A., Gottardi, E., et al. (2002). Assessment of minimal residual disease (MRD) in CBFbeta/MYH11-positive acute myeloid leukemias by qualitative and quantitative RT-PCR amplification of fusion transcripts. *Leukemia*, 16(6), 1176-81.

[21] Mitterbauer, G., Zimmer, C., Pirc-Danoewinata, H., Haas, O. A., Hojas, S., Schwarzinger, I., et al. (2000). Monitoring of minimal residual disease in patients with MLL-AF6-positive acute myeloid leukaemia by reverse transcriptase polymerase chain reaction. *Br J Haematol*, 109(3), 622-8.

[22] Grimwade, D., Hills, R. K., Moorman, A. V., Walker, H., Chatters, S., Goldstone, A. H., et al. (2010). Refinement of cytogenetic classification in acute myeloid leukemia: determination of prognostic significance of rare recurring chromosomal abnormalities among 5876 younger adult patients treated in the United Kingdom Medical Research Council trials. *Blood*, 116(3), 354-65.

[23] Erickson, P., Gao, J., Chang, K. S., Look, T., Whisenant, E., Raimondi, S., et al. (1992). Identification of breakpoints in t(821) acute myelogenous leukemia and isolation of a fusion transcript, AML1/ETO, with similarity to a drosophila segmentation gene, runt. *Blood*, 80(7), 1825-31.

[24] Tobal, K., Newton, J., Macheta, M., Chang, J., Morgenstern, G., Evans, P. A. S., et al. (2000). Molecular quantitation of minimal residual disease in acute myeloid leukemia with t(821) can identify patients in durable remission and predict clinical relapse. *Blood*, 95(3), 815-9.

[25] Krauter, J., Görlich, K., Ottmann, O., Lübbert, M., Döhner, H., Heit, W., et al. (2003). Prognostic value of minimal residual disease quantification by real-time reverse transcriptase polymerase chain reaction in patients with core binding factor leukemias. *J Clin Oncol*, 21(23), 4413-22.

[26] Buonamici, S., Ottaviani, E., Testoni, N., Montefusco, V., Visani, G., Bonifazi, F., et al. (2002). Real-time quantitation of minimal residual disease in inv(16)-positive acute myeloid leukemia may indicate risk for clinical relapse and may identify patients in a curable state. *Blood*, 99(2), 443-9.

[27] Grimwade, D., Jovanovic, J. V., Hills, R. K., Nugent, E. A., Patel, Y., Flora, R., et al. (2009). Prospective minimal residual disease monitoring to predict relapse of acute promyelocytic leukemia and to direct pre-emptive arsenic trioxide therapy. *J Clin Oncol*, 27(22), 3650-8.

[28] Pui, C. H., Relling, M. V., & Downing, J. R. (2004). Acute lymphoblastic leukemia. *N Engl J Med*, 350(15), 1535-48.

[29] Wetzler, M., Dodge, R. K., Mrozek, K., Carroll, A. J., Tantravahi, R., Block, A. W., et al. (1999). Prospective karyotype analysis in adult acute lymphoblastic leukemia: the cancer and leukemia Group B experience. *Blood*, 93(11), 3983-93.

[30] Scholl, C., Breitinger, H., Schlenk, R. F., Dohner, H., Frohling, S., & Dohner, K. (2003). Development of a real-time RT-PCR assay for the quantification of the most frequent MLL/AF9 fusion types resulting from translocation t(911)(22q23) in acute myeloid leukemia. *Genes Chromosomes Cancer* 38(3):274-80.

[31] Yang, L., Han, Y., Suarez, F., & Minden, M. D. (2007). A tumor suppressor and oncogene: The WT1 story. *Leukemia*, 21(5), 868-76.

[32] Sugiyama, H. (2001). Wilms' tumor gene WT1: its oncogenic function and clinical application. *Int J Hematol*, 73(2), 177-87.

[33] Inoue, K., Ogawa, H., Sonoda, Y., Kimura, T., Sakabe, H., Oka, Y., et al. (1997). Aberrant overexpression of the Wilms tumor gene (WT1) in human leukemia. *Blood*, 89(4), 1405-12.

[34] Béné, M. C., & Kaeda, J. S. (2009). How and why minimal residual disease studies are necessary in leukemia: a review from WP10 and WP12 of the European Leukaemia Net. *Haematologica*, 94(8), 1135-50.

[35] Jacobsohn, D. A., Tse, W. T., Chaleff, S., Rademaker, A., Duerst, R., Olszewski, M., et al. (2009). High WT1 gene expression before haematopoeitic stem cell transplant in children with acute myeloid leukaemia predicts poor event-free survival. *B J Haematol*, 146(6), 669-74.

[36] Candoni, A., Tiribelli, M., Toffoletti, E., Cilloni, D., Chiarvesio, A., Michelutti, A., et al. (2008). Quantitative assessment of WT1 gene expression after allogeneic stem cell transplantation is a useful tool for monitoring minimal residual disease in acute myeloid leukemia. *Eur J Haematol*, 82(1), 61-8.

[37] Cilloni, D., Renneville, A., Hermitte, F., Hills, R. K., Daly, S., Jovanovic, J. V., et al. (2009). Real-time quantitative polymerase chain reaction detection of minimal residual disease by standardized WT1 assay to enhance risk stratification in acute myeloid leukemia: A European LeukemiaNet Study. *J Clin Oncol*, 27(31), 5195-201.

[38] Hämäläinen, M. M., Kairisto, V., Juvonen, V., Johansson, J., Aurén, J., Kohonen, K., et al. (2008). Wilms tumour gene 1 overexpression in bone marrow as a marker for minimal residual disease in acute myeloid leukaemia. *Eur J Haematol*, 80(3), 201-7.

[39] Matsushita, M., Ikeda, H., Kizaki, M., Okamoto, S., Ogasawara, M., Ikeda, Y., et al. (2001). Quantitative monitoring of the PRAME gene for the detection of minimal residual disease in leukaemia. *Br J Haematol*, 112(4), 916-26.

[40] Steinbach, D., Hermann, J., Viehmann, S., Zintl, F., & Gruhn, B. (2002). Clinical implications of PRAME gene expression in childhood acute myeloid leukemia. *Cancer Genet Cytogenet*, 133(2), 118-23.

[41] Greiner, J., Ringhoffer, M., Taniguchi, M., Li, L., Schmitt, A., Shiku, H., et al. (2004). mRNA expression of leukemia-associated antigens in patients with acute myeloid leukemia for the development of specific immunotherapies. *Int J Cancer*, 108(5), 704-11.

[42] Qin, Y., Zhu, H., Jiang, B., Li, J., Lu, X., Li, L., et al. (2009). Expression patterns of WT1 and PRAME in acute myeloid leukemia patients and their usefulness for monitoring minimal residual disease. *Leuk Res*, 33(3), 384-90.

[43] Barjesteh van, Waalwijk., van Doorn-Khosrovani, S., Erpelinck, C., van Putten, W. L. J., Valk, P. J. M., van der Poel-van de, Luytgaarde. S., & Hack, R. et al. (2003). High EVI1 expression predicts poor survival in acute myeloid leukemia: a study of 319 de novo AML patients. *Blood* , 101(3), 837-45.

[44] Lugthart, S., van Drunen, E., van Norden, Y., van Hoven, A., Erpelinck, C. A. J., Valk, P. J. M., et al. (2008). High EVI1 levels predict adverse outcome in acute myeloid leukemia: prevalence of EVI1 overexpression and chromosome 3q26 abnormalities underestimated. *Blood*, 111(8), 4329-37.

[45] Aytekin, M., Vinatzer, U., Musteanu, M., Raynaud, S., & Wieser, R. (2005). Regulation of the expression of the oncogene EVI1 through the use of alternative mRNA 5'-ends. *Gene*, 356, 160-8.

[46] Schnittger, S., Schoch, C., Dugas, M., Kern, W., Staib, P., Wuchter, C., et al. (2002). Analysis of FLT3 length mutations in 1003 patients with acute myeloid leukemia: correlation to cytogenetics, FAB subtype, and prognosis in the AMLCG study and usefulness as a marker for the detection of minimal residual disease. *Blood*, 100(1), 59-66.

[47] Small, D. (2006). FLT3 mutations: biology and treatment. *Hematology Am Soc Hematol Educ Program*, 178-84.

[48] Wagner, K., Damm, F., Thol, F., Göhring, G., Görlich, K., Heuser, M., et al. (2011). FLT3-internal tandem duplication and age are the major prognostic factors in patients with relapsed acute myeloid leukemia with normal karyotype. *Haematologica*, 96(5), 681-6.

[49] Chou, W. C., Hou, H. A., Liu, C. Y., Chen, C. Y., Lin, L. I., Huang, Y. N., et al. (2011). Sensitive measurement of quantity dynamics of FLT3 internal tandem duplication at early time points provides prognostic information. *Ann Oncol*, 22(3), 696-704.

[50] Schnittger, S., Kern, W., Tschulik, C., Weiss, T., Dicker, F., Falini, B., et al. (2009). Minimal residual disease levels assessed by NPM1 mutation-specific RQ-PCR provide important prognostic information in AML. *Blood*, 114(11), 2220-31.

[51] Schiller, J., Praulich, I., Krings, Rocha. C., & Kreuzer, K. A. (2012). Patient-specific analysis of FLT3 internal tandem duplications for the prognostication and monitoring of acute myeloid leukemia. *Eur J Haematol*, 89(1), 53-62.

[52] Abdelhamid, E., Preudhomme, C., Helevaut, N., Nibourel, O., Gardin, C., Rousselot, P., et al. (2012). Minimal residual disease monitoring based on FLT3 internal tandem duplication in adult acute myeloid leukemia. *Leuk Res*, 36(3), 316-23.

[53] Cloos, J., Goemans, B. F., Hess, C. J., van Oostveen, J. W., Waisfisz, Q., Corthals, Q., et al. (2006). Stability and prognostic influence of FLT3 mutations in paired initial and relapsed AML samples. *Leukemia*, 20(7), 1217-20.

[54] Kottaridis, P. D., Gale, R. E., Langabeer, S. E., Frew, M. E., Bowen, D. T., & Linch, D. C. (2002). Studies of FLT3 mutations in paired presentation and relapse samples from patients with acute myeloid leukemia: implications for the role of FLT3 mutations in leukemogenesis, minimal residual disease detection, and possible therapy with FLT3 inhibitors. *Blood*, 100(7), 2393-98.

[55] Bachas, C., Schuurhuis, G. J., Hollink, I. H., Kwidama, Z. J., Goemans, B. F., Zwaan, C. M., et al. (2010). High-frequency type I/II mutational shifts between diagnosis and relapse are associated with outcome in pediatric AML: implications for personalized medicine. *Blood*, 116(15), 2752-8.

[56] Beretta, C., Gaipa, G., Rossi, V., Bernasconi, S., Spinelli, O., Dell'Oro, M. G., et al. (2004). Development of a quantitative-PCR method for specific FLT3/ITD monitoring in acute myeloid leukemia. *Leukemia*, 18(8), 1441-44.

[57] Fallini, B., Bolli, N., Shan, J., Martelli, M. P., Liso, A., Pucciarini, A., et al. (2006). Both carboxy-terminus NES motif and mutated tryptophan(s) are crucial for aberrant nuclear export of nucleophosmin leukemic mutants in NPMc+ AML. *Blood*, 107(11), 4514-23.

[58] Falini, B., Nicoletti, I., Martelli, M. F., & Mecucci, C. (2007). Acute myeloid leukemia carrying cytoplasmic/mutated nucleophosmin (NPMc(+)AML): biologic and clinical features. *Blood*, 109(3), 874-85.

[59] Falini, B., Mecucci, C., Tiacci, E., Alcalay, M., Rosati, R., Pasqualucci, L., et al. (2005). Cytoplasmic nucleophosmin in acute myelogenous leukemia with a normal karyotype. *N Engl J Med*, 352(3), 254-66.

[60] Dohner, K., Schlenk, R. F., Habdank, M., Scholl, C., Rücker, F. G., Corbacioglu, A., et al. (2005). Mutant nucleophosmin (NPM1) predicts favorable prognosis in younger adults with acute myeloid leukemia and normal cytogenetics: interaction with other gene mutations. *Blood*, 106(12), 3740-6.

[61] Schneider, F., Hoster, E., Schneider, S., Dufour, A., Benthaus, T., Kakadia, P. M., et al. (2012). Age-dependent frequencies of NPM1 mutations and FLT3-ITD in patients with normal karyotype AML (NK-AML). *Ann Hematol*, 91(1), 9-18.

[62] Dvorakova, D., Racil, Z., Jeziskova, I., Palasek, I., Protivankova, M., Lengerova, M., et al. (2010). Monitoring of minimal residual disease in acute myeloid leukemia with frequent and rare patient-specific NPM1 mutations. *Am J Hematol*, 85(12), 926-9.

[63] Chou, W. C., Tang, J. L., Wu, S. J., Tsay, W., Yao, M., Huang, S. Y., et al. (2007). Clinical implications of minimal residual disease monitoring by quantitative polymerase chain reaction in acute myeloid leukemia patients bearing nucleophosmin (NPM1) mutations. *Leukemia*, 21(5), 998-1004.

[64] Barragan, E., Pajuelo, J. C., Ballester, S., Fuster, O., Cervera, J., Moscardo, F., et al. (2008). Minimal residual disease detection in acute myeloid leukemia by mutant nucleophosmin (NPM1): comparison with WT1 gene expression. *Clinica Chimica Acta*395(1-2):120-3.

[65] Kristensen, T., Møller, M. B., Friis, L., Bergmann, O. J., & Preiss, B. (2011). NPM1 mutation is a stable marker for minimal residual disease monitoring in acute myeloid leukaemia patients with increased sensitivity compared to WT1 expression. *Eur J Haematol*, 87(5), 400-8.

[66] Gorello, P., Cazzaniga, G., Alberti, F., Dell'Oro, M. G., Gottardi, E., Specchia, G., et al. (2006). Quantitative assessment of minimal residual disease in acute myeloid leukemia carrying nucleophosmin (NPM1) gene mutations. *Leukemia*, 20(6), 1103-8.

[67] Papadaki, C., Dufour, A., Seibl, M., Schneider, S., Bohlander, S. K., Zellmeier, E., et al. (2009). Monitoring minimal residual disease in acute myeloid leukaemia with NPM1 mutations by quantitative PCR: clonal evolution is a limiting factor. *Br J Haematol*, 144(4), 517-23.

[68] Suzuki, T., Kiyoi, H., Ozeki, K., Tomita, A., Yamaji, S., Suzuki, R., et al. (2005). Clinical characteristics and prognostic implications of NPM1 mutations in acute myeloid leukemia. *Blood*, 106(8), 2854-61.

[69] Nerlov. (2004). C/EBPalpha mutations in acute myeloid leukemias. *Nature Rev Cancer*, 4(5), 394-400.

[70] Schlenk, R. F., Dohner, K., Krauter, J., Fröhling, S., Corbacioglu, A., Bullinger, L., et al. (2008). Mutations and treatment outcome in cytogenetically normal acute myeloid leukemia. *N Engl J Med*, 358(18), 1909-18.

[71] Benthaus, T., Schneider, F., Mellert, G., Zellmeier, E., Schneider, S., Kakadia, P. M., et al. (2008). Rapid and sensitive screening for CEBPA mutations in acute myeloid leukaemia. *Br J Haematol*, 143(2), 230-9.

[72] Fröhling, S., Schlenk, R. F., Stolze, I., Bihlmayr, J., Benner, A., Kreitmeier, S., et al. (2004). CEBPA mutations in younger adults with acute myeloid leukemia and normal cytogenetics: prognostic relevance and analysis of cooperating mutations. *J Clin Oncol*, 22(4), 624-33.

[73] Mohty, M., Labopin, M., Volin, L., Gratwohl, A., Socié, G., Esteve, J., et al. (2010). Reduced-intensity versus conventional myeloablative conditioning allogeneic stem cell transplantation for patients with acute lymphoblastic leukemia: a retrospective study from the European Group for Blood and Marrow Transplantation. *Blood*, 116(22), 4439-43.

[74] Kröger, N., Brand, R., van Biezen, A., Zander, A., Dierlamm, J., Niederwieser, D., et al. (2009). Risk factors for therapy-related myelodysplastic syndrome and acute myeloid leukemia treated with allogeneic stem cell transplantation. *Haematologica*, 94(4), 542-9.

[75] Klingebiel, T., Cornish, J., Labopin, M., Locatelli, F., Darbyshire, P., Handgretinger, R., et al. (2010). Results and factors influencing outcome after fully haploidentical hematopoietic stem cell transplantation in children with very high-risk acute lymphoblastic leukemia: impact of center size: an analysis on behalf of the Acute Leukemia and Pediatric Disease Working Parties of the European Blood and Marrow Transplant group. *Blood*, 115(17), 3437-46.

[76] Bader, P., Kreyenberg, H., Hoelle, W., Dueckers, G., Handgretinger, R., Lang, P., et al. (2004). Increasing mixed chimerism is an important prognostic factor for unfavorable outcome in children with acute lymphoblastic leukemia after allogeneic stem-cell transplantation: possible role for pre-emptive immunotherapy? *J Clin Oncol*, 22(9), 1696-705.

[77] Rettinger, E., Willasch, A. M., Kreyenberg, H., Borkhardt, A., Holter, W., Kremens, B., et al. (2011). Preemptive immunotherapy in childhood acute myeloid leukemia for patients showing evidence of mixed chimerism after allogeneic stem cell transplantation. *Blood*, 118(20), 5681-8.

[78] Díez-Campelo, M., Pérez-Simón, J. A., Pérez, J., Alcoceba, M., Richtmon, J., Vidriales, B., et al. (2009). Minimal residual disease monitoring after allogeneic transplantation may help to individualize post-transplant therapeutic strategies in acute myeloid malignancies. *Am J Hematol*, 84(3), 149-52.

[79] Rubnitz, J. E., Inaba, H., Dahl, G., Ribeiro, R. C., Bowman, P., Taub, J., et al. (2010). Minimal residual disease-directed therapy for childhood acute myeloid leukemia: results of the AML02 multicenter trial. *Lancet Oncol*, 11(6), 543-52.

[80] Miyazaki, T., Fujita, H., Fujimaki, K., Hosoyama, T., Watanabe, R., Tachibana, T., et al. (2012). Clinical significance of minimal residual disease detected by multidimensional flow cytometry: Serial monitoring after allogeneic stem cell transplantation for acute leukemia. *Leuk Res*, 36(8), 998-1003.

[81] Yan, C. H., Liu, D. H., Liu, K. Y., Xu, L. P., Liu, Y. R., Chen, H., et al. (2012). Risk stratification-directed donor lymphocyte infusion could reduce relapse of standard-risk acute leukemia patients after allogeneic hematopoietic stem cell transplantation. *Blood*, 119(14), 3256-62.

[82] Pyne, S., Hu, X., Wang, K., Rossin, E., Lin, T. I., Maier, L. M., et al. (2009). Automated high-dimensional flow cytometric data analysis. *Proc Natl Acad Sci U S A*, 106(21), 8519-24.

[83] Voskova, D., Schnittger, S., Schoch, C., Haferlach, T., & Kern, W. (2007). Use of five-color staining improves the sensitivity of multiparameter flow cytometric assessment

of minimal residual disease in patients with acute myeloid leukemia. *Leuk Lymphoma*, 48(1), 80-8.

[84] Bachas, C., Schuurhuis, G. J., Assaraf, Y. G., Kwidama, Z. J., Kelder, A., Wouters, F., et al. (2012). The role of minor subpopulations within the leukemic blast compartment of AML patients at initial diagnosis in the development of relapse. *Leukemia*, 26(6), 1313-20.

[85] Becker, M. W., & Jordan, C. T. (2011). Leukemia stem cells in 2010: Current understanding and future directions. *Blood rev*, 25(2), 75-81.

[86] Panzer-Grümayer, E. R., Schneider, M., Panzer, S., Fasching, K., & Gadner, H. (2000). Rapid molecular response during early induction chemotherapy predicts a good outcome in childhood acute lymphoblastic leukemia. *Blood*, 95(3), 790-4.

[87] Lacombe, F., Arnoulet, C., Maynadie, M., Lippert, E., Luquet, I., Pigneux, A., et al. (2009). Early clearance of peripheral blasts measured by flow cytometry during the first week of AML induction therapy as new independent prognostic factor: a GOELAMS study. *Leukemia*, 23(2), 350-7.

[88] Maurillo, L., Buccisano, F., Spagnoli, A., Del Poeta, G., Panetta, P., Neri, B., et al. (2007). Monitoring of minimal residual disease in adult acute myeloid leukemia using peripheral blood as an alternative source to bone marrow. *Haematologica*, 92(5), 605-11.

[89] Chantepie, S. P., Salaün, V., Parienti, J. J., Truquet, F., Macro, M., Cheze, S., et al. (2011). Hematogenes: a new prognostic factor for acute myeloblastic leukemia. *Blood*, 117(4), 1315-8.

[90] Martinez, A., San, Miguel. J. F., Vidriales, M. B., Ciudad, J., Caballero, M. D., López-Berges, M. C., et al. (1999). An abnormal CD34+ myeloid/CD34+ lymphoid ratio at the end of chemotherapy predicts relapse in patients with acute myeloid leukemia. *Cytometry*, 38(2), 70-5.

[91] McCulloch E.A. (1983). Stem cells in normal and leukemic hemopoiesis (Henry Stratton Lecture, 1982). *Blood*, 62(1), 1-13.

[92] Griffin, J. D., & Löwenberg, B. (1986). Clonogenic cells in acute myeloblastic leukemia. *Blood*, 68(6), 1185-95.

[93] Luo, L., & Han, Z. C. (2006). Leukemia stem cells. *Int J Hematol*, 84(2), 123-7.

[94] Testa, U. (2011). Leukemia stem cells. *Ann Hematol*, 90(3), 245-71.

[95] Bhatia, M., Wang, J. C., Kapp, U., Bonnet, D., & Dick, J. E. (1997). Purification of primitive human hematopoietic cells capable of repopulating immune-deficient mice. *Proc Natl Acad Sci U S A*, 94(10), 5320-5.

[96] Civin, C. I., Almeida-Porada, G., Lee, M. J., Olweus, J., Terstappen, L. W., & Zanjani, E. D. (1996). Sustained, retransplantable, multilineage engraftment of highly purified adult human bone marrow stem cells in vivo. *Blood*, 88(11), 4102-9.

[97] Bonnet, D., & Dick, J. E. (1997). Human acute myeloid leukemia is organized as a hierachy that originates from a primitive hematopoeitic cell. *Nat Med*, 3(7), 730-7.

[98] Hogan, C. J., Shpall, E. J., & Keller, G. (2002). Differential long-term and multilineage engraftment potential from subfractions of human CD34+ cord blood cells transplanted into NOD/SCID mice. *Proc Natl Acad Sci U S A*, 99(1), 413-8.

[99] Taussig, D. C., Miraki-Moud, F., Anjos-Alsonso, F., Pearce, D. J., Allen, K., Ridler, C., et al. (2008). Anti-CD38 antibody-mediated clearance of human repopulating cells masks the heterogeneity of leukemia-initiating cells. *Blood*, 112(3), 568-75.

[100] Taussig, D. C., Vargaftig, J., Miraki-Moud, F., Griessinger, E., Sharrock, K., Luke, T., et al. (2010). Leukemia-initiating cells from some acute myeloid leukemia patients with mutated nucleophosmin reside in the $CD34^-$ fraction. *Blood*, 115(10), 1976-84.

[101] Sarry, J. E., Murphy, K., Perry, R., Sanchez, P. V., Secreto, A., Keefer, C., et al. (2011). Human acute myelogenous leukemia stem cells are rare and heterogeneous when assayed in NOD/SCID/IL2Rγc-deficient mice. *J Clin Invest*, 121(1), 384-95.

[102] Goardon, N., Marchi, E., Atzberger, A., Quek, L., Schuh, A., Soneji, S., et al. (2011). Coexistence of LMPP-like and GMP-like leukemia stem cells in acute myeloid leukemia. *Cancer cell*, 19(1), 138-52.

[103] Krivtsov, A. V., Twomey, D., Feng, Z., Stubbs, M. C., Wang, Y., Faber, J., et al. (2006). Transformation from committed progenitor to leukaemia stem cell initiated by MLL-AF9. *Nature*, 442(7104), 818-22.

[104] Costello, R. T., Mallet, F., Gaugler, B., Sainty, D., Arnoulet, C., Gastaut, J. A., et al. (2000). Human acute myeloid leukemia CD34+/CD38- progenitor cells have decreased sensitivity to chemotherapy and Fas-induced apoptosis, reduced immunogenicity, and impaired dendritic cell transformation capacities. *Cancer Res*, 60(16), 4403-11.

[105] Chute, J. P., Muramoto, G. G., Whitesides, J., Colvin, M., Safi, R., Chao, N. J., et al. (2006). Inhibition of aldehyde dehydrogenase and retinoid signaling induces the expansion of human hematopoietic stem cells. *Proc Natl Acad Sci U S A*, 103(31), 11707-12.

[106] Duester, G. (2000). Families of retinoid dehydrogenases regulating vitamin A function: production of visual pigment and retinoic acid. *Eur J Biochem*, 267(14), 4315-24.

[107] Magni, M., Shammah, S., Schiró, R., Mellado, W., Dalla-Favera, R., & Gianni, A. M. (1996). Induction of cyclophosphamide-resistance by aldehyde-dehydrogenase gene transfer. *Blood*, 87(3), 1097-1103.

[108] Takebe, N., Zhao, S. C., Adhikari, D., Mineishi, S., Sadelain, M., Hilton, J., et al. (2001). Generation of dual resistance to 4-hydroperoxycyclophosphamide and methotrexate by retroviral transfer of the human aldehyde dehydrogenase class 1 gene and a mutated dihydrofolate reductase gene. *Mol Ther*, 3(1), 88-96.

[109] Storms, R. W., Trujillo, A. P., Springer, J. B., Shah, L., Colvin, O. M., Ludeman, S. M., et al. (1999). Isolation of primitive human hematopoietic progenitors on the basis of aldehyde dehydrogenase activity. *Proc Natl Acad Sci U S A*, 96(16), 9118-23.

[110] Armstrong, L., Stojkovic, M., Dimmick, I., Ahmad, S., Stojkovic, P., Hole, N., et al. (2004). Phenotypic characterization of murine primitive hematopoietic progenitor cells isolated on basis of aldehyde dehydrogenase activity. *Stem Cells*, 22(7), 1142-51.

[111] Christ, O., Lucke, K., Imren, S., Leung, K., Hamilton, M., Eaves, A., et al. (2007). Improved purification of hematopoietic stem cells based on their elevated aldehyde dehydrogenase activity. *Haematologica*, 92(9), 1165-72.

[112] Gentry, T., Deibert, E., Foster, S. J., Haley, R., Kurtzberg, J., & Balber, A. E. (2007). Isolation of early hematopoietic cells, including megakaryocyte progenitors, in the ALDH-bright cell population of cryopreserved, banked UC blood. *Cytotherapy*, 9(6), 569-76.

[113] Gerber, J. M., Smith, B. D., Ngwang, B., Zhang, H., Vala, M. S., Morsberg, L., et al. (2012). A clinically relevant population of leukemic $CD34^{+}CD38^{-}$ cells in acute myeloid leukemia. *Blood*, 119(15), 3571-7.

[114] Smit, L., Min, L. A., Terwijn, M., Kelder, A., Snel, A. N., Ossenkoppele, G. J., et al. (2009). High Aldehyde Dehydrogenase Activity (ALDH) is a general marker for normal hematopoietic stem cells but not leukemic stem cells in acute myeloid leukemia (AML). *Blood* (ASH Annual Meeting Abstracts)114:4035.

[115] Schuurhuis, G. J., Meel, M. H., Min, L. A., Wouters, F., Terwijn, M., Kelder, A., et al. Consistently high aldehyde dehydrogenase (ALDH) activity is a feature of normal hematopoietic stem cells but not leukemic stem cells in Acute Myeloid Leukemia. *Submitted.*

[116] Cheung, A. M., Wan, T. S., Leung, J. C., Chan, L. Y., Huang, H., Kwong, Y. L., et al. (2007). Aldehyde dehydrogenase activity in leukemic blasts defines a subgroup of acute myeloid leukemia with adverse prognosis and superior NOD/SCID engrafting potential. *Leukemia*, 21(7), 1423-30.

[117] Pearce, D. J., Taussig, D., Simpson, C., Allen, K., Rohatiner, A. Z., Lister, T. A., et al. (2005). Characterization of cells with a high aldehyde dehydrogenase activity from cord blood and acute myeloid leukemia samples. *Stem Cells*, 23(6), 752-60.

[118] Ran, D., Schubert, M., Taubert, I., Eckstein, V., Bellos, F., Jauch, A., et al. (2012). Heterogeneity of leukemia stem cell candidates at diagnosis of acute myeloid leukemia and their clinical significance. *Exp Hematol*, 40(2), 155-65.

[119] Goodell, M. A., Brose, K., Paradis, G., Conner, A. S., & Mulligan, R. C. (1996). Isolation and functional properties of murine hematopoietic stem cells that are replicating in vivo. *J Exp Med*, 183(4), 1797-806.

[120] Goodell, M. A., Rosenzweig, M., Kim, H., Marks, D. F., De Maria, M., Paradis, G., et al. (1997). Dye efflux studies suggest that hematopoietic stem cells expressing low or undetectable levels of CD34 antigen exist in multiple species. *Nat Med*, 3(12), 1337-45.

[121] Moshaver, B., van Rhenen, A., Kelder, A., van der Pol, M., Terwijn, M., & Bachas, C. et al. (2008). Identification of a small subpopulation of candidate leukemia-initiating cells in the side population of patients with acute myeloid leukemia. *Stem Cells* , 26(12), 3059-67.

[122] Wulf, G. G., Wang, R. Y., Kuehnle, I., Weidner, D., Marini, F., Brenner, M. K., et al. (2001). A leukemic stem cell with intrinsic drug efflux capacity in acute myeloid leukemia. *Blood*, 98(4), 1166-73.

[123] Feuring-Buske, M., & Hogge, D. E. (2001). Hoechst 33342 efflux identifies a subpopulation of cytogenetically normal CD34(+)CD38(-) progenitor cells from patients with acute myeloid leukemia. *Blood*, 97(12), 3882-9.

[124] van Rhenen, A., Moshaver, B., Kelder, A., Feller, N., Nieuwint, A. W. M., Zweegman, S., et al. (2007). Aberrant marker expression patterns on the CD34+CD38- stem cell compartment in acute myeloid leukemia allows to distinguish the malignant from the normal stem cell compartment both at diagnosis and in remission. *Leukemia*, 21(8), 1700-7.

[125] Van Rhenen, A., van Dongen, G. A. M. S., Kelder, A., Rombouts, E. J., Feller, N., Moshaver, B., et al. (2007). The novel AML stem cell associated antigen CLL-1 aids in discrimination between normal and leukemic stem cells. *Blood*, 110(7), 2659-66.

[126] Saito, Y., Kitamura, H., Hijikata, A., Tomizawa-Murasawa, M., Tanaka, S., Takagi, S., et al. (2010). Identification of therapeutic targets for quiescent, chemotherapy-resistant human leukemia stem cells, *Sci Transl Med* 2(17):17ra9.

[127] Taussig, D. C., Pearce, D. J., Simpson, C., Rohatiner, A. Z., Lister, T. A., Kelly, G., et al. (2005). Hematopoietic stem cells express multiple myeloid markers: implications for the origin and targeted therapy of acute myeloid leukemia. *Blood*, 106(13), 4086-92.

[128] Jin, L., Hope, K. J., Zhai, Q., Smadja-Joffe, F., & Dick, J. E. (2006). Targeting of CD44 eradicates human acute myeloid leukemic stem cells. *Nat Med*, 12(10), 1167-74.

[129] Majeti, R., Park, C. Y., & Weissman, I. L. (2007). Identification of a hierarchy of multipotent hematopoietic progenitors in human cord blood. *Cell Stem Cell*, 1(6), 635-45.

[130] Hosen, N., Park, C. Y., Tatsumi, N., Oji, Y., Sugiyama, H., Gramatzki, M., et al. (2007). CD96 is a leukemic stem cell-specific marker in human acute myeloid leukemia. *Proc Natl Acad Sci U S A*, 104(26), 11008-13.

[131] Jordan, C. T., Upchurch, D., Szilvassy, S. J., Guzman, M. L., Howard, D. S., Pettigrew, A. L., et al. (2000). The interleukin-3 receptor alpha chain is a unique marker for human acute myelogenous leukemia stem cells. *Leukemia*, 14(10), 1777-84.

[132] Jan, M., Chao, M. P., Cha, A. C., Alizadeh, A. A., Gentles, A. J., Weissman, I. L., et al. (2011). Prospective separation of normal and leukemic stem cells based on differential expression of TIM3, a human acute myeloid leukemia stem cell marker. *Proc Natl Acad Sci U S A*, 108(12), 5009-14.

[133] van der Pol, M. A., Feller, N., Roseboom, M., Moshaver, B., Westra, G., Broxterman, H. J., et al. (2003). Assessment of the normal or leukemic nature of CD34+ cells in acute myeloid leukemia with low percentages of CD34 cells. *Haematologica*, 88(9), 983-93.

[134] Van Rhenen, A., Feller, N., Kelder, A., Westra, A. H., Rombouts, E., Zweegman, S., et al. (2005). High stem cell frequency in acute myeloid leukemia at diagnosis predicts high minimal residual disease and poor survival. *Clin Cancer Res*, 11(18), 6520-7.

[135] Witte, K. E., Ahlers, J., Schäfer, I., André, M., Kerst, G., & , H. H.G.(2011). Scheel-Walter et al. High proportion of leukemic stem cells at diagnosis is correlated with unfavorable prognosis in childhood acute myeloid leukemia. *Pediatr Hematol Oncol* , 28(2), 91-9.

[136] Hwang, K., Park, C. J., Jang, S., Chi, H. S., Kim, D. Y., Lee, J. H., et al. (2012). Flow cytometric quantification and immunophenotyping of leukemic stem cells in acute myeloid leukemia. *Ann Hematol* jun 6.

[137] Terwijn, M., Rutten, A. P., Kelder, A., Snel, A. N., Scholten, W. J., Zweegman, S., et al. (2010). Accurate detection of residual leukemic stem cells in remission bone marrow predicts relapse in acute myeloid leukemia patients. *Blood* (ASH Annual Meeting Abstracts)116:759.

[138] Jin, L., Lee, E. M., Ramshaw, H. S., Busfield, S. J., Peoppl, A. G., Wilkinson, L., et al. (2009). Monoclonal antibody-mediated targeting of CD123, IL-3 receptor α chain, eliminates human acute myeloid leukemic stem cells. *Cell Stem Cell*, 5(1), 31-42.

[139] Roberts, A. W., He, S., Bradstock, K. F., Hertzberg, M. S., Durrant, S. T. S., Ritchie, D., et al. (2008). A Phase 1 and correlative biological study of CSL360 (anti-CD123 mAb) in AML. *Blood* (ASH Annual Meeting Abstracts)112:2956.

[140] Walter, R. B., Appelbaum, F. R., Estey, E. H., & Bernstein, I. D. (2012). Acute myeloid leukemia stem cells and CD33-targeted immunotherapy. *Blood*, 119(26), 6198-208.

Chapter 7

Modern Therapy of Chronic Myeloid Leukemia

M.M. Zaharieva, G. Amudov, S.M. Konstantinov and
M. L. Guenova

Additional information is available at the end of the chapter

http://dx.doi.org/10.5772/55505

1. Introduction

Chronic myeloid leukemia is one of the most thoroughly studied and, undoubtedly, best understood neoplasms. There are about 4000 and 5000 new cases of CML every year in the USA. CML is a hematologic stem cell malignancy that typically evolves in 3 distinct clinical stages: chronic and accelerated phases and blast crisis. The chronic phase lasts several years and is characterized by accumulation of myeloid precursors and mature cells in bone marrow, peripheral blood, and extramedullary sites. The accelerated phase lasts 4 to 6 months and is characterized by an increase in disease burden and in the frequency of progenitor/precursor cells. The blast crisis lasts a few months and is the terminal phase of chronic myelogenous leukemia, characterized by the rapid expansion of a population of myeloid or lymphoid differentiation-arrested blast cells (Calabretta and Perrotti 2004; Radich 2007).

The cytogenetic hallmark of CML is the Philadelphia chromosome (Ph). It is a product of a reciprocal translocation between chromosomes 9 and 22 (t[9;22][q34;q11]). The *Bcr-abl* oncogene, responsible for the deregulated tyrosine kinase, arises out of the conjugation between the breakpoint cluster region gene (*Bcr*) on chromosome 22 and the Abelson kinase (*Abl*) gene on chromosome 9. This oncogene activates multiple signal transduction pathways such as Ras/Raf/mitogen-activated protein kinase [MAPK], phosphatidylinositol 3 kinase, STAT5/Janus kinase, and Myc (Fig. 1). The Bcr-Abl tyrosine kinase activity leads to uncontrolled cell proliferation and significantly reduced apoptosis and so starts the malignant expansion of pluripotent stem cells in the bone marrow. The Wnt/ß-catenin pathway was also found to be critical for the evolution to blast crisis as far as its activation was observed in primary cell samples from patients with CML. Most of the pathways activated by Bcr-Abl are known, but the pathways downstream Bcr-Abl that are critical for oncogenesis and transformation are yet not well understood. For example, several transcription factors like Jun B, MZF1 and δEF1 appear to be involved in CML progression. Jun B has been shown to be down-regulated in CML progression. The transcription factors MZF1 and δEF1 that play key role in hematopoietic stem cell differentiation, including modulation of CD34 and *cMyb* expression, are also deregulated during CML progression (Calabretta and Perrotti 2004; Steelman, Pohnert et al. 2004; Jabbour, Cortes et al. 2007; Radich 2007; Druker 2008; Roychowdhury and Talpaz 2011). All these findings reflect the recent knowledge about the molecular disease pathogenesis and are platform for translating bench research into clinical application of target-driven therapeutic strategies.

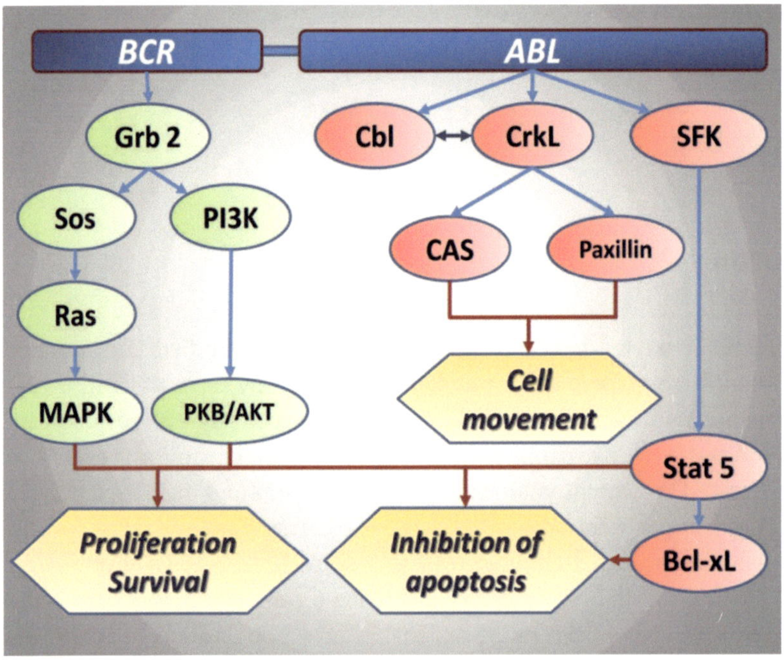

Figure 1. Pathways activated by the fusion oncoprotein Bcr-Abl. The RAS pathway becomes constitutively activated by mechanisms involving the interaction of Bcr-Abl with the growth factor receptor-binding protein (Grb-2)/Gab2 complex. This leads to enhanced activity of the guanosine diphosphate/guanosine triphosphate (GDP/GTP) exchange factor Sos, which promotes the accumulation of the active GTP-bound form of Ras. Bcr-Abl interacts also indirectly with the p85 regulatory subunit of PI3K via various docking proteins including GRB-2/Gab2 and c-cbl. Activation of the PI3K pathway triggers an Akt-dependent cascade that has a critical role in BCR/ABL transformation by regulating the subcellular localization or activity of several targets such as BAD, MDM2, IκB-kinase α, and members of the Forkhead family of transcription factors. Another signaling pathway activated by BCR/ABL is that dependent on signal transducer and activator of transcription 5 (STAT5). The consequence of this activation is inhibition of apoptosis and enhanced survival.

Treatment of this disease improved dramatically with the development of tyrosine kinase inhibitors (TKIs). Recently, the modern therapy of CML includes the use of TKIs (first and second generation), stem cell transplantation and clinical trials with novel agents such as novel multiple kinase inhibitors, Aurora kinase inhibitors, arsenic trioxide, hystone deacetilase inhibitors, proteasome inhibitors, other semi-synthetic drugs (Fig. 2). Imatinib is the golden standard in CML therapy and serves as first-line drug of choice in the chronic phase of CML

http://dx.doi.org/10.5772/55505

(CP-CML) whereas second generation TKIs are taken in consideration after appearance of resistance to imatinib due to Bcr-Abl mutations. Accoridning to de Lavallade et al. only 62,7% of the patients treated with imatinibe achieved complete cytogenetic response (CCyR) and up to 5% of the patients present with advanced disease are poorly responsive to TKIs in general (de Lavallade, Apperley et al. 2008; Roychowdhury and Talpaz 2011). In other words, about one third of CML patients devepole intolerance or resistance to TKIs and therefore they need alternative therapies.

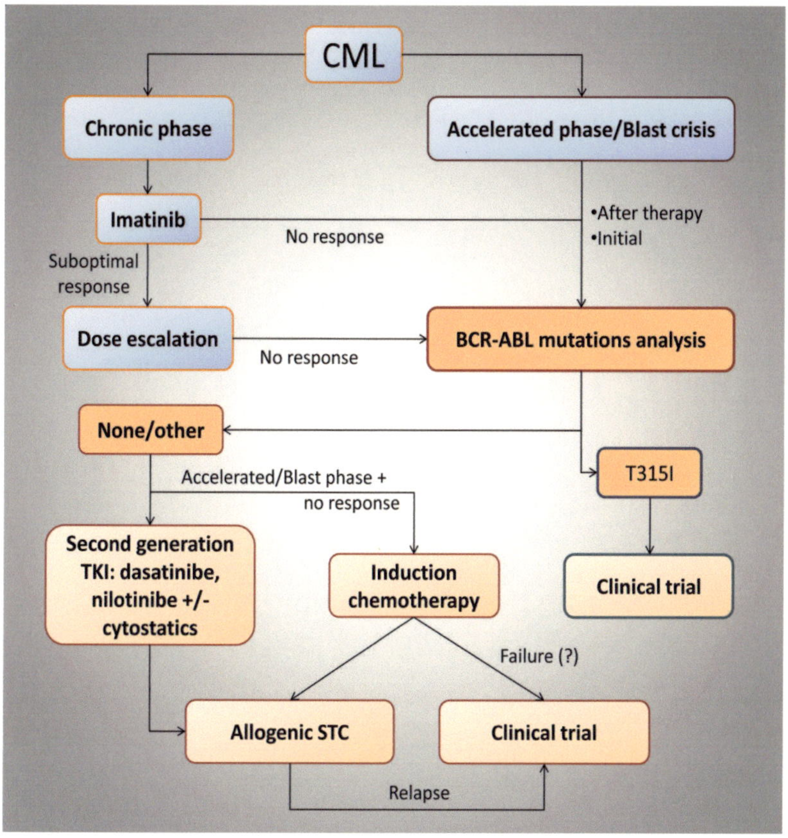

Figure 2. Clinical algorithm for CML therapy: chronic, accelerated and blast phase (adapted from Roychowdhury et al., 2011, 25(6): 279-90).

2. Tyrosine-kinase inhibitors

Imatinib, dasatinib and nilotinib are today the three clinically applied tyrosine kinase inhibitors of the fusion oncoprotein Bcr-BL for the treatment of CML and Ph (+) ALL (Fig. 3, Table 1). The constitutively active Bcr-Abl tyrosine kinase functions by transferring a phosphate group from ATP to tyrosine residues on various substrates (signaking molecules) to cause excess proliferation of myeloid cells typical for CML. Imatinib and the other two tyrosine kinase-inhibitors block the binding of ATP to Bcr-Abl, thus inhibiting its kinase activity (Fig. 4). They also act on other components of the cellular metabolism and signalling, e.g. Abl and ARG (Abl-related gene), C-kit receptor (KIT), receptors for platelet growth factor alpha (PDGFR-α) and beta (PDGFR-β), receptor for colony stimulating factor 1 (c-FMS) etc. (Kantarjian, Cortes et al. 2010). All tyrosine kinase inhibitors have good gastrointestinal absorption, which makes them suitable for oral application.

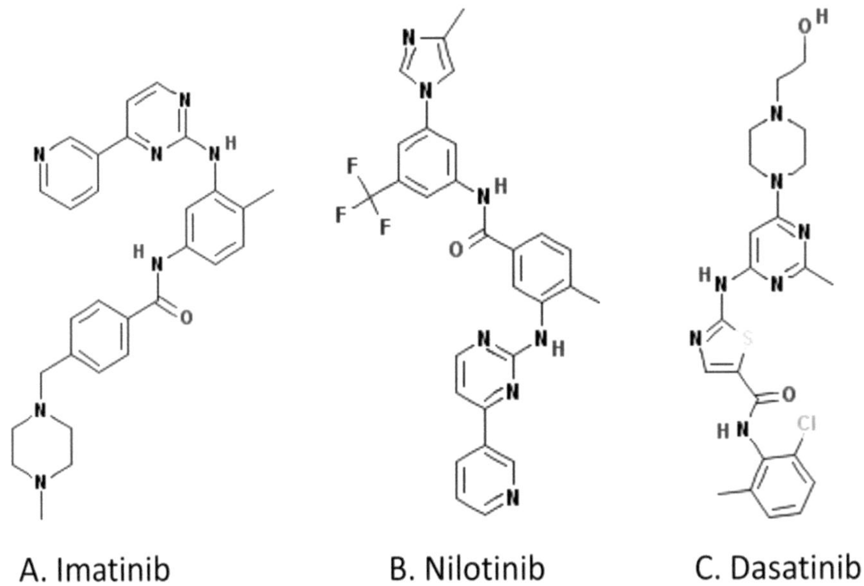

Figure 3. Chemical structures of first and second line tyrosine kinase-inhibitors.

2.1. First generation tyrosine-kinase inhibitors — Imatinib

Imatinib was introduced for clinical use in 1998 for the treatment of CML. It showed high efficacy and revolutionized the disease management. Nowadays, Imatinib is the first-line drug of choice for the treatment of patients with CML in chronic phase and Ph (+) ALL as it induces long lasting remissions and is well tolerated as compared to conventional cytostatics (Fig. 2). Imatinib stops the progression of CML at early stages (Baccarani and Dreyling 2009).

Imatinib reaches C_{max} within 2 to 4 h. Its total bioavailability is 98%. The half-lifes of Imatinib and its main metabolite, N-demethyl derivative (CGP74588), are 18 h and 40 h, respectively. Plasma protein binding (mainly albumin and α1-acid glycoprotein) for imatinib reaches 95%. The drug is primarily metabolized by CYP3A4 and to a lesser extent by CYP1A2, CYP2D6, CYP2C9 and CYP2C19. The main active metabolite of Imatinib is one N-demethylated piperazine derivative, formed by CYP3A4 and has *in vitro* activity similar to that of Imatinib. Imatinib is a potent inhibitor of CYP2C9, CYP2D6 and CYP3A4/5, which is described in *in vitro* studies conducted with human liver microsomes. It is eliminated with the faeces, mainly in the form of respective metabolites. Imatinib clearance in one 50 year-old-patient, weighing 50 kg is 8 L/h, while in patient weighing 100 kg, it increases to 14 L/h (Roychowdhury and Talpaz 2011).

The superiority of Imatinib against IFNα was confirmed in the third phase of the International Randomized Study of Interferon and STI-571 (IRIS). A substantial cytogenetic response was achieved in 87% of the patients receiving Imatinib after 18 months, compared to 35% in those who received IFN. Complete cytogenetic remission was observed in 76.2% of the patients treated with Imatinib, compared to 14.5% of the treated with IFN. Molecular remission with reduction of the Bcr-Abl transcripts was found in 39% of the patients treated with Imatinib, against 2% for IFN. 325 (71%) of 456 patients who had achieved complete cytogenetic remission with Imatinib sustained their remission on the sixth year of treatment. Tracking patients over the 6-year exploration period indicated that Imatinib had a favourable and long-lasting safety profile, as there were no new adverse events during the 5th and 6th year of study. The use of Imatinib as first-line drug for CML did not affect subsequent treatment of patients with allogeneic hematopoietic stem cells transplantation (Kantarjian, O'Brien et al. 2003; Deininger 2008; Baccarani and Dreyling 2009).

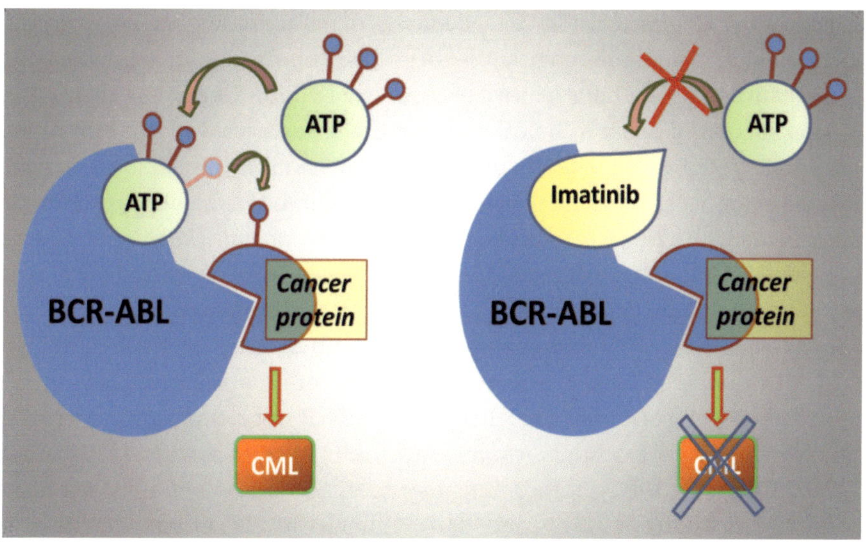

Figure 4. Mode of action of Imatinib. Imatinib blocks the ATP binding center of Bcr-Abl thus inhibiting its phosphorylation activity.

2.2. Second generation tyrosine-kinase inhibitors

2.2.1. Nilotinib

Nilotinib is a highly selective ABL inhibitor and derivative of Imatinib and can overcome some mutations that can cause imatinib resistance with the exception of T315I. During first phase clinical trial, Nilotinib was tested at doses of 50 mg once daily to 600 mg twice daily in 119 Imatinib-resistant CML patients at various stages of the disease. 92% of the patients in chronic phase achieved complete hematologic remission. 72% of the patients in the acute phase of CML presented hematologic remission and 48% of them had a cytogenetic response. 39% of patients with CML in blast crisis demonstrated a hematologic response and 9 of them (27%) had a cytogenetic response. The results of the study defined a recommended dose of 400 mg twice daily (Table 1). Nilotinib adverse reactions include small pleural or pericardial effusions. The most common adverse effects during the study were thrombocytopenia (20% -33%), neutropenia (13% -31%), elevated bilirubin (7%), and increased serum lipase (5% -15%). Grapefruit and other food that inhibits hepatic metabolism (mainly CYP3A4 inhibitors) should be avoided. Nilotinib is not recommended for patients with prolonged QT-segment, and drugs that prolong the QT-segment should not be given during treatment with Nilotinib (Kantarjian, Giles et al. 2007; Olivieri and Manzione 2007; Weisberg, Catley et al. 2007; Melo and Chuah 2008; Giles, Rosti et al. 2010; Kantarjian, Cortes et al. 2010; Kantarjian, Giles et al. 2010; Quintas-Cardama, Kim et al. 2010).

2.2.2. Dasatinib

Dasatinib is another ABL kinase inhibitor that binds to the active conformation of the ABL-kinase domain and to the structurally related kinases of the Src-family. *In-vitro* dasatinib is 300 times more potent than imatinib against Bcr-Abl mutated blasts. Dasatinib inhibited almost all Imatinib-resistant Bcr-Abl mutants with the exception of T315I and was shown to block PDGFRs and KIT. After successful phase II clinical trials dasatinib was approved in North America and Europe and in many other countries. It should be given to patients with imatinib resistance. During the trials some severe hematologic adverse effects were observed in imatinib resistant or imatinib intolerant patients with CML, e.g. thrombocytopenia (48%), anemia (22%), neutropenia (49%), and leukopenia (27%). There were some non-haematological adverse reactions as well, e.g. pleural effusions (6%). In the phase III trials, in order to reduce Dasatinib-related toxicity while maintaining efficacy of treatment, 670 randomly selected imatinib resistant or imatinib intolerant patients with CML in the chronic phase received dasatinib in 1 of 4 dose regimens: 100 mg once daily, 50 mg twice daily, 140 mg once daily, or 70 mg twice daily. It was found that non-hematological and hematological adverse reactions are rarer at a dose of 100 mg once daily (Hochhaus, Kantarjian et al. 2007). Currently, this is the recommended dosage for patients with chronic phase CML, while the 70 mg twice daily or 140 mg once daily regimens are options for patients in the acute phase or blast crisis CML (Table 1).

Nowadays, the choice between treatment with dasatinib and nilotinib in imatinib resistant patients is made on the basis of the history of comorbidities, since no such very important comparative study of both drugs has been made so far. Therefore, patients with a history of lung disease may be more suitable for treatment with nilotinib, while patients with pancreatic disease could benefit from treatment with dasatinib. Patients bearing the T315I mutation are resistant to treatment with both dasatinib and nilotinib. Such patients should be offered the option for inclusion in clinical trials or allogeneic bone marrow transplantation (Kantarjian, Cortes et al. 2010).

1. Chronic phase of CML:			
a Initial therapy:			
Imatinib	400 mg	p.o.	Daily
b Salvage therapy:			
Dasatinib	70 mg 100 mg	b.i.d.p.o. p.o.	Daily
Nilotinib	400 mg	b.i.d.p.o.	Daily
Imatinib (high-dose)	400 mg	b.i.d.p.o.	Daily
2. Accelerated phase and blast crisis of CML:			
Imatinib	400-600 mg	p.o.	Daily
Dasatinib	70 mg	b.i.d.p.o.	Daily
Nilotinib	400 mg	b.i.d.p.o.	Daily
3. Pediatric patients with CML:			
Imatinib	260 mg/m^2/d 340 mg/m^2/d	p.o p.o..	daily daily

Table 1. Treatment schedule with tyrosine kinase-inhibitors.

2.3. Resistance towards TKI — Mechanisms and management

The most important problem in the target therapy of CML today is the development of resistance towards TKIs. Lucas et al. reported after a population-based study in Northern England that about 50% of the patients treated with imatinib developed intolerance or failure up to two years after initiation (Lucas, Wang et al. 2008). Responses obtained in patients with advanced desease were also not durable. CCyR at 6 years after initiating imatinib therapy is determined by 57% patients and 55% remain on the treatment after 8 years (Burke, Swords et al. 2011). Even nilotinib at best achieved CCyR in 80% of the treated patients (Rosti, Palandri et al. 2009). In summary, there is a significant minority of patients developing resistance towards imatinib and second generation TKIs. Investigators distinguish between primary and secondary resistance. Secondary treament failure or desease replase is characterized by the loss of already achieved complete cytogenetic or hematological response and is dependent on different factors such as age, stage of disease, duration of INF therapy and duration of response to initial therapy. In contrast, primary resistance is the failure to achieve CCyR or hematologic response and is not very well investigated and understood. Concernig leukemic cell proliferation and survival two other models of imatinib resintance could be outlined: on one hand leukemic cells became independent from the fusion oncoprotein for their survuval and proliferation and, on the other hand the tyrosine kinase Bcr-Abl circuvented the inhibition by imatinib or other TKIs, e.g. appearance of the mutation T315I (Burke, Swords et al. 2011; Roychowdhury and Talpaz 2011).

The mechanisms of imatinib resistance could be classified as either Bcr-Abl dependent or Bcr-Abl independent. Bcr-Abl dependent mechnisms include Bcr-Abl amplification, kinase domain mutations and Bcr-Abl induced genomic instability. Bcr-Abl independent mechanisms are usually related to drug complience and metabolism, drug transport, clonal evolution, escape of the primitive progenitors from therapy and activation of alternative signal transduction pathways.

Kinase domain mutations belong to the most important mechanisms of resistance towards TKIs. They were identified in clinical studies with patients with imatinib resistance (initial or developed during the therapy) where 30% of the patients had primary resistance and 57% - secondary resistance (Shah, Nicoll et al. 2002; Soverini, Martinelli et al. 2005). Today over a 90 mutations in the Bcr-Abl fusion gene are described and they affect 57% of the amino-acid residues. Some of these mutations cause a direct steric interference to drug-enzyme binding or alter allosterically the kinase domain activity and are reported to be the main reason for treatment failure in many clinical trials. Mutations in the P-loop are assigned as poor prognistic factor. In particular, the T315I mutation accounts for the majority of secondary resistance (Burke, Swords et al. 2011). The T315I mutation is a single amino-acid substitution of isoleucine with threonine at position 315 on c-Abl. It alters the ATP-binding site of the tyrosine kinase, confers cross-resistance to nearly all clinically applied TKIs and correlates with decreased cytogenetic response and progression free survival rates. In summary, in clinical studies about 50% incidence of this mutation had been reported for patients with secondary resistance. Therefore, introduction of new drugs is substantially needed (Bradeen, Eide et al. 2006). However, there are studies reporting that kinase domain mutations were found also in patients with CCyR and in remission, but only few of them eventually developed disease relapse. It is evident that not all kinds of resistance are due to Abl-mutations and not all mutaions could lead to resistance (Branford, Melo et al. 2009; Roychowdhury and Talpaz 2011). Correlations based on *in vitro* sensitivity have not been consistent in all studies. Thus Bcr-Abl induced genimic instability or unknown Bcr-Abl independent mechanisms are suspected to be also responsible for disease resistance development.

In vitro studies showed that Bcr-Abl could promote genomic instability and resistance. There are additional facts that support the hypothesis that Bcr-Abl can affect the mismatch repair activity. The fusion protein caused down-regulation of nucleotide excision repair in leukemic cell lines and promoted double-stranded DNA breaks through single strand annealing (Stoklosa, Poplawski et al. 2008; Fernandes, Reddy et al. 2009).

Pharmacokinetic characteristics of the TKIs were also demonstrated to be important for better clinical outcomes. Imatinib is substrate for the liver enzyme CYP3A4 which converts it into active metabolite. A higher enzyme acitivity correlated with higher rate of complete molecular responses (Green, Skoglund et al. 2010). The α-1-acid glycoprotein directly binds imatinib, thus increasing its clearance. Therefore, patients with high levels of this protein demonstrated lower plasma concentrations of imatinib which worsened the therapeutic response (Delbaldo, Chatelut et al. 2006). Through *in vitro* experiments with radio-labeled imatinib it was demonstrated that cellular mechanisms for drug transport (influx and efflux) are also important determinants of the drug sensitivity. The imatinib influx is an active process which involves the human organic cation transporter 1 (hOCT1). In a study with 56 patients it was reported that high activity of hOCT1 is associated with significantly improved overall survival and response rates (Giles, Kantarjian et al. 1999; Roychowdhury and Talpaz 2011). The P-glycoprotein (MDR1 or ABCB1) which is responsible for the drug efflux out of the leukemic cells also mediated resistance but did not appear to be essential for the development of imatinib resistance even in primitive CD34+ CML progenitors *in vitro*.

Another reason for developing resistance towards targeted CML therapy is provided by the stem cell hypothesis. According to some investigators there is a reservoir of primitive progenitors that are capable of self-renewal or progression *in vitro* or *in vivo* in immunodeficient mice. Another proof for this hypothesis is the fact that patients with deep remissions in the chronic phase of CML can relapse after discontinuation of imatinib therapy. There are different biological mechanisms responsible for the behavior of the stem cell compartment. The Wnt/ß-catenin signal pathway and the Foxo transcription factors were found to be involved in the renewal of malignant and normal haematopoietic stem cells. Additionally, the Hedgehog signaling pathway seems to be important for CML stem renewal. Thus far, it is clear that CML biology involves a stem cell component, but its exact role and biological mechanisms have not yet been determined.

The strategies to overcome resistance include first optimization of the front line therapy with imatinib such as escalation of the daily dose up to 800 mg and second the introduction of second generation TKIs such as dasatinib, nilotinib (Table 1) and other new compounds that are still in clinical trials (Jabbour, Kantarjian et al. 2009; Roychowdhury and Talpaz 2011). Dasatinib and nilotinib were successfully used in patients in accelerated phase or blast crisis after Bcr-Abl mutation analysis that demonstrated other mutations than T315I. Ponatinib, a new multiple kinase inhibitor, showed high activity against T315I mutants *in vitro* and low toxicity in vivo during a Phase I clinical trial and is a very promising new TKI for the treatment of patients bearing the T315I mutation. There have been no randomized studies to evaluate the predictive value of kinase domain mutations for response to specific TKIs until now. However, a summary of the data can be taken from retrospective studies. Dasatinib is recommended for patients with the following mutations: Y253H, E255K/V and F359V/C. Nilotinib is beneficial for pytients with F317L and V299L mutations. The side effect profile and patient's characteristics are also important for the choice of an appropriate TKI (Hughes, Saglio et al. 2009; Jabbour, Jones et al. 2009; Roychowdhury and Talpaz 2011).

After failure of imatinib and a second generation TKI, most patients could be included in ongoing clinical trials. Next, some of the novel agents beeing evaluated in Ph(+) leukemias are listed.

3. Experimental drugs for CML therapy

3.1. Tyrosine kinase inhibitors

3.1.1. Bosutinib

Bosutinib was developed to overcome the resistance to first and second generation TKIs and is still in clinical trials. It was shown to possess a high antiproliferative activity *in vitro* and in xenografts against most of the Bcr-Abl mutants except T315I. It is a dual Abl and Src kinase inhibitor and binds to both active and intermediate conformations of the fusion oncoprotein Bcr-Abl. Bosutinib was found to inhibit the proliferation of CML progenitors about 200 times better than imatinib. However, it was not able to eliminate all mutant populations and was moderately effective in inducing apoptosis. The Phase II studies with bosutinib showed that about 36% of all patients in chronic pahse, 22% in accelerated pahse and 9% in blast crisis achieved complete cytogenetic responses. Preliminary data indicate that bosutinib was well tolerated and the most common adverse events were gastrointestinal discomfort and grade 3-4 myelosuppression which occurred in the advanced disease phases (Melo and Chuah 2008; Roychowdhury and Talpaz 2011).

3.1.2. Other experimental tyrosine kinase inhibitors

There are also new types of compounds inhibiting pathobiochemical pathways, resulting from the *bcr-abl* oncogene. These allosteric inhibitors use a newly described allosteric, non-ATP competitive mechanism, potentially involving binding to the myristate pocket in the C-lobe of the Bcr-Abl kinase domain. The most promising of these compounds is the GNF-2. It has practically no activity against most kinases, including Kit, PDGFR and SFK. GNF-2 inhibited the growth of cells with the Y253F and E255V mutations, but not the other P-loop mutants, the T315I or F317L mutants. Another promising new agent is INNO-406 (Bafetinib) which is Abl/Lyn kinase inhibitor and is about 55 times more potent than imatinib *in vitro*. It has been shown to inhibit numerous Bcr-Abl muitants except T315I. The drug underwent a Phase I study in patients with resistance to imatinib. It was well tolerated and 2 of 7 patients achieved complete cytogenetic response. The novel multiple kinase inhibitor, the purine derivate AP24534 (ponatinib) inhibits FLT3, Src kinases, Bcr-Abl and multipule Bcr-Abl mutants, including the T315I mutation. During the preclinical studies it was evidenced that ponatinib is highly effective mutant Bcr-Abl inhibitor *in vitro* and *in vivo* in mouse models. Interestingly, no dose-limiting toxicity was found in a dose-escalating Phase I clinical trial. Ponatinib was effective in patients who had failed to respond to all other approved theprapies, including patients with the T315I mutation of the fusion oncoprotein Bcr-Abl. Therefore ponatinib is fastly moving to phase II studies in patients with Ph+ leukemias.

Other new TKIs are the SFK/Abl kinase inhibitor, the anilino-quinazoline AZD0530; the purine derivates AP23464 and its analogue AP23848; the pyrido-pyrimidines, PDI66326, PDI73955 and PDI180970; thje pyrazolo-pyrimidines, PP1 and PP2; the acetylanes AC22 and K1P. These compounds have not been developed for clinical use yet (Melo and Chuah 2008; Bixby and Talpaz 2009; Burke, Swords et al. 2011).

3.2. Aurora kinase inhibitors

The Aurora kinase familiy consists of serine-threonine kinases that are crucial for different stages of the mitosis. There are two family members Aurira A and B and are overexpressed in some neoplasias. Following Aurora kinase inhibitors are in pre-clinical and clinical evaluation: PHA-739358 (danusertib), AT9283, MLN8237XL-228, KW-2449 and MK-0457. Danusetib showed safety profile and efficacy in patients bearing the T315I mutation in phase I clinical study. AT9238 is a multi-kinase inhibitor which also inhibited cells with the T315I mutation.

http://dx.doi.org/10.5772/55505

It was well-tolerated during phase I clinical trial and shwed promising anti-leukemic activity (Cortes-Franco, Dombret et al. 2009; Howard, Berdini et al. 2009; Moore, Blagg et al. 2010; Tanaka, Squires et al. 2010; Burke, Swords et al. 2011).

3.3. Heat shock protein 90 inhibitor

As a molecular chaperone that interacts with various proteins (Raf, Akt, FLT-3 and Bcr-Abl) Hsp90 maintains those proteins in a stable and functional conformation. Geldanamycin and its derivative, 17-allylamino-17-demethoxygeldanamycin (17-AAG) bind to the ATP-binding pocket of Hsp90 and inhibit its chaperone activity. This leads to downregulation of Bcr-Abl and also induction of apoptosis in CML cell lines. Gledanamycin and 17-AAG inhibited the cell growth of some mutant lines (E255K and T315I). Hsp90 has its limits and there are some cross-resistant types. Combination therapy with imatinib and 17-AAG led to synergistic inhibition of growth and induction of apoptosis in cross-resistant cell lines but not in the imatinib-sensitive counterparts. 17-AAG may also block the imatinib efflux (Melo and Chuah 2008; Burke, Swords et al. 2011).

3.4. Arsenic trioxide

Another compound that induces apoptosis in Bcr-Abl-positive cell lines and reduces proliferation of CML blasts without affecting the CD34+ progenitors, is the arsenic trioxide (As_2O_3). The combination of As_2O_3 with imatinib exerted additive to synergistic effect. This combination induced cell death in imatinib-resistant cell lines with overexpressed Bcr-Abl or bearing M351T or Y253F mutations, but it does not affect the T315I mutants (Melo and Chuah 2008; Roychowdhury and Talpaz 2011).

3.5. Homoharringtonine

Homoharringtonine (HHT), a by-product of a plant alkaloid, inhibits protein synthesis and induces apoptosis. The combination of HHT with imatinib is synergistic or additive on CML derived cell lines. Omacetaxine and chemgenex are semisynthetic HHT derivatives that combined with imatinib showed promising activities. Omacetaxine is now in phase II trials with TKIs-resistant patients with or without the T315I mutation (Melo and Chuah 2008; Burke, Swords et al. 2011).

3.6. Histone deacetylase inhibitors

Histone deacetylases (HDAC) are the catalysts in deacetylation of lysine residues at the amino termini of core nucleosomal histones. Histone deacetylase inhibitors (HDI) such as suberoylanilide hydroxamic acid (SAHA, vorinostat), generate hyperacetylated histones, causing transcriptional upregulation of the cyclin-dependent kinase inhibitor, p21, cell-cycle arrest and apoptosis in tumor cells. SAHA also induces expression of a key cell-cycle regulator p27, and its application is associated with downregulation of the p210 Bcr-Abl protein. There is a synergetic interaction between SAHA and imatinib on CML cell lines. The mentioned combination induces apoptosis in imatinib-resistant CML cell lines as well. The co-treatment with nilotinib and the HDI LBH589 (panobinostat) was very effective in inducing apoptosis in K-562 and LAMA-84 CML cell lines. LBH589 showed efficacy in imatinib-resistant cell lines bearing the T315I and E255K mutations and this was associated with depletion of Bcr-Abl. A published study showed that when combined with imatinib, the HDI valproate can increase the antileukemic efficacy and sensitize imatinib-resistant CML cells (Kantarjian, O'Brien et al. 2003; Melo and Chuah 2008; Burke, Swords et al. 2011).

3.7. Proteasome inhibitors

Proteasomes are responsible for the degradation of different cellular proteins. The proteasome inhibitor bortezomib was shown to inhibit proliferation, to stop the cell cycle in the G_2/M phase and to promote apoptosis in imatinib-sensitive and imatinib-resistant CML cell lines. Co-treatment with bortezomib and imatinib isn't recommended because there are some antagonistic interactions. However, if a low dose bortezomib exposure of CML cell lines is followed by imatinib, there are some additive effects. Synergistic interactions between bortezomib and the HDI SAHA are reported, and between bortezomib and flavopiridol in *in vitro* as well (Melo and Chuah 2008).

3.8. Semi-synthetic drugs

Semi-synthetic drugs flavone and flavopiridol are going through clinical trials. They target multiple cyclin-dependent kinases. Flavopiridol showed a very promising activity in combination with imatinib for inducing apoptosis in Bcr-Abl-positive CML cell lines (Melo and Chuah 2008).

3.9. Farnesyl Transferase Inhibitors (FTIs)

Current FTIs under investigation and with a potential as antileukemic agents are tipifarnib and lonafarnib. They are inhibitors of the Ras-MAPK signal pathway which was shown to couple to Bcr.Abl through protein-protein interactions and to play a central role in leukemogenic transformation. Tipifarnib is in Phase II trial involving 22 patients with CML. Complete or partial hematological response was achieved in 32% of the patients. The combination imatinib and tipifarnib was well tolerated and active in patients with imatinib-resistnat CML – a partial cytogenetic response was achieved in patients harboring the T315I mutant. Lonafarnib is a selective inhibitor of primary progenitor cells derived from CML patients. It reduced colony formation of progenitor cells and showed activity in imatinib-resitant CML cell lines. However, the reports from a pilot study demonstrated that only 2 of 13 patients achieved a clinical response.

3.10. Raf-1 inhibitors

Sorafenib (BAY 43-9006) is a multi kinase inhibitor of the RAS/Raf pathway which is involved in leukemogenesis downstream from Bcr-Abl. Drug concetrations of 5-10 μM were found to induce apoptosis via the mitochondrial pathway in imatinib-rsistant cell lines. The combination between sorafenib and vorinostat (HDAC inhibitor) triggers cell dysfunction through

Mcl-1 downregulation and p21 inhibition. Sorafenib is approved for the treatment of hepatocellular and renal cancers and Phase I and Phase II trials are carried out in CML patients (Burke, Swords et al. 2011).

3.11. MEK inhibitors

CI-1040 was the first MEK inhibitor which entered a clinical trial in CML patients. It has been studied in combinations with imatinib, dasatinib, HDAC inhibitors, arsenic trioxide and HSP 90 inhibitors. The last two combinations were tested with a positive effect in patients with T315I mutation. Because of the challenging pharamokinetic properties, clinical advancement is unlikely, but a derivate (PD0325901) is under development (Burke, Swords et al. 2011).

3.12. mTOR inhibitors

The protein kinase, mTOR (mammalian target of rapamycin), is a downstream mediator in the PI3K/Akt pathway which controls cell growth and survival. Rapamycin (sirolimus) is the prototype compound of this group, but it has poor aqueous solubility and chemical stability, limiting its clinical usefulness. However, in a small clinical trial four out of six patients with imatinib-resistant disease responded to oral rapamycin. Rapamycin also significantly inhibited the cell growth in Ph+ cell lines with or without the T315I mutation. The combination between imatinib and another mTOR inhibitor, everolimus, was associated with an increased expression of c-Abl and inhibition of Bcr-Abl. In the presence of inhibited Bcr-Abl, c-Abl enetrs the nucleus an modulates apoptosis. A Phase I trial with imatinib and everolimus has been completed while a study with temsirolimus is currently in accrual (Burke, Swords et al. 2011).

4. Interferons

Before the era of TKIs and since the 1980s interferon-α had constituted the first-line therapy for CML patients in the chronic phase of the disease. Interferon induced long-lasting remissions in up to 80% of the patients with complete cytogenetic response. After interferon therapy they had disease-free survival beyond 10 years. There are some clinical trials that showed succesful combinations between TKIs and interferon which provided an adjunct immunologic response during induction or maintenance therapies. Treatment with interferon after imatinib was shown to be followed by a possible remission status (Burchert, Muller et al. 2010; Roychowdhury and Talpaz 2011). Howerver, additional data are required in order to clarify the role of interferon in conjunction to the TKI therapy.

5. Stem cell transplantation

Allogeneic stem cell transplantation (ASCT) was first line therapy for CML patients for many years. In the imatinib era, however, ASCT is becomning second or even third option for these patients if hematological, cytogenetic or molecular remission with imatinib is not achieved after 3,12 and 18 months, respectively (Baccarani and Dreyling 2009). ASCT is still the only treatment that offers a definitive cure. The risks of ASCT are some mortality rate, graft-versus-host disease (GVHD), potentially lethal acute or chronic infections death and risk of second malignancy. There are no data about negative influence on ASCT of pre-treatment with tyrosine-kinase inhibitors. In a single institution in the USA between 1995 and 2000 131 CP CML patients underwent allogeneic SCT with bone marrow or perpheral blood from related donors. In the 3 year long period, the probability of disease-free survival was 78%. The survival and disease recurrence rates were estimated at 86% and 8% respectively. The Chronic Leukemia Working Party of the European Group for Blood and Marrow Transplantation (EBMT) published own data. In the period between 2000 and 2003 3018 patients were treated with ASCT for CML. The 2-year survival rate was 61%, the transplant-related mortality rate was 30%, and the rate of disease recurrence was 22%. Better results were observed in patients who underwent ASCT at the time of first CP using as a donor an HLA-identical sibling. The 2-year survival rate in this case was 74%, transplant-related mortality rate 22% and disease recurrence rate 18%. This confirms the fact that the outcome of ASCT is highly dependent on risk factors. EBMT study showed that favorable factors are sibling donor, treatment at early stage of the disease, under 12 months after diagnosis, and younger age of the patient (age under 20 years is better than 20-40 years, and above 40 the risks are higher). If successful, ASCT can lead to long-lasting results. In a 10-year study of patients transplantated with an allogeneic bone marrow from siblings, the mean time of hematologic or cytogenetic disease recurrence was 7.7 years and 46% of the long-term survivors never developed disease recurrence.

One of the main problems standing in front of ASCT is that most of the patients don't have a suitable HLA-matched sibling. National Marrow Donor Program institutions in the U.S. conducted a study in the period between 1988 and 1999 that compared results from 2464 unrelated donor bone marrow transplantations with 450 HLA-identical sibling donor transplantations. The results from this study confirm that patients transplantated with bone marrow from a non-relative donor have greater risk of complications. However it is important to mention that data from this study didn't show a significant difference in the 5-year survival rate between the two types of donors if the transplantion was made within 1 year after diagnosis (Jabbour, Cortes et al. 2007).

6. Conclusion

Imatinib is now the most common first line drug for the treatment of CML and is a hallmark of target drug therapies for malignant diseases. However resistance to this drug is a major problem that can't be overcome by increasing the dosage (Jabbour, Kantarjian et al. 2007; O'Hare, Eide et al. 2007). Single agent therapy with imatinib may not be the best long-term option in many of the CML patients and other approaches should be considered. There are many novel compounds that are in development and in preclincal and clinical trials, some of them showed very promising results. Dasatinib, nilotinib and bosutinib are representatives of the newer generation TKIs which are effective and safe to use in imatinib-resistant and/or -intolerant CML patients. It is very likely that new Bcr-Abl mutants will become resistant to these small-molecule inhibitors. Therefore, other therapeutic approaches are required. The combination of TKIs with other inhibitors of non-Bcr-Abl targets is needed to overcome the resistance.

Author details

M.M. Zaharieva[1,2], G. Amudov[3], S.M. Konstantinov[2,4] and M. L. Guenova[2,5]

1 Institute of Microbilogy-BAS, Sofia, Bulgaira

2 Center of Excellence – Translational Research in Haematology, National Specialised Hospital for Active Treatment of Haematological Diseases, Sofia, Bulgaria

3 Faculty of Medicine, Sofia University „St. Kl. Ohridski", Sofia, Bulgaria

4 Faculty of Pharmacy, Medical University of Sofia, Sofia, Bulgaria

5 Laboratory of Haematopathology and Immunology, National Specialised Hospital for Active Treatment of Haematological Diseases, Sofia, Bulgaria

References

[1] Baccarani, M, & Dreyling, M. (2009). Chronic myelogenous leukemia: ESMO clinical recommendations for diagnosis, treatment and follow-up." *Ann Oncol* 20 Suppl , 4, 105-7.

[2] Bixby, D, & Talpaz, M. (2009). Mechanisms of resistance to tyrosine kinase inhibitors in chronic myeloid leukemia and recent therapeutic strategies to overcome resistance." *Hematology Am Soc Hematol Educ Program*: , 461-76.

[3] Bradeen, H. A, Eide, C. A, et al. (2006). Comparison of imatinib mesylate, dasatinib (BMS-354825), and nilotinib (AMN107) in an N-ethyl-N-nitrosourea (ENU)-based mutagenesis screen: high efficacy of drug combinations." *Blood* , 108(7), 2332-8.

[4] Branford, S, Melo, J. V, et al. (2009). Selecting optimal second-line tyrosine kinase inhibitor therapy for chronic myeloid leukemia patients after imatinib failure: does the BCR-ABL mutation status really matter?" *Blood* , 114(27), 5426-35.

[5] Burchert, A, Muller, M. C, et al. (2010). Sustained molecular response with interferon alfa maintenance after induction therapy with imatinib plus interferon alfa in patients with chronic myeloid leukemia." *J Clin Oncol* , 28(8), 1429-35.

[6] Burke, A. C, Swords, R. T, et al. (2011). Current status of agents active against the T315I chronic myeloid leukemia phenotype." *Expert Opin Emerg Drugs* , 16(1), 85-103.

[7] Calabretta, B, & Perrotti, D. (2004). The biology of CML blast crisis." *Blood* , 103(11), 4010-22.

[8] Cortes-franco, J, Dombret, H, et al. (2009). Danusertib hydrochloride (PHA-739358), a multi-kinase aurora inhibitor, elicts clinical benefit in advanced chronic myeloid leukemia and philadelphia chromosome positive acute lymphoblastic leukemia." *ASH Annual Meeeting Abstracts* , 114, 864.

[9] De Lavallade, H, Apperley, J. F, et al. (2008). Imatinib for newly diagnosed patients with chronic myeloid leukemia: incidence of sustained responses in an intention-to-treat analysis." *J Clin Oncol* , 26(20), 3358-63.

[10] Deininger, M. W. (2008). Milestones and monitoring in patients with CML treated with imatinib." *Hematology Am Soc Hematol Educ Program:* , 419-26.

[11] Delbaldo, C, Chatelut, E, et al. (2006). Pharmacokinetic-pharmacodynamic relationships of imatinib and its main metabolite in patients with advanced gastrointestinal stromal tumors." *Clin Cancer Res* 12(20 Pt 1): 6073-8.

[12] Druker, B. J. (2008). Translation of the Philadelphia chromosome into therapy for CML." *Blood* , 112(13), 4808-17.

[13] Fernandes, M. S, Reddy, M. M, et al. (2009). BCR-ABL promotes the frequency of mutagenic single-strand annealing DNA repair." *Blood* , 114(9), 1813-9.

[14] Giles, F. J, Kantarjian, H. M, et al. (1999). Multidrug resistance protein expression in chronic myeloid leukemia: associations and significance." *Cancer* , 86(5), 805-13.

[15] Giles, F. J, Rosti, G, et al. (2010). Nilotinib is superior to imatinib as first-line therapy of chronic myeloid leukemia: the ENESTnd study." *Expert Rev Hematol* , 3(6), 665-73.

[16] Green, H, Skoglund, K, et al. (2010). CYP3A activity influences imatinib response in patients with chronic myeloid leukemia: a pilot study on in vivo CYP3A activity." *Eur J Clin Pharmacol* , 66(4), 383-6.

[17] Hochhaus, A, Kantarjian, H. M, et al. (2007). Dasatinib induces notable hematologic and cytogenetic responses in chronic-phase chronic myeloid leukemia after failure of imatinib therapy." *Blood* , 109(6), 2303-9.

[18] Howard, S, Berdini, V, et al. (2009). Fragment-based discovery of the pyrazol-4-yl urea (AT9283), a multitargeted kinase inhibitor with potent aurora kinase activity." *J Med Chem* , 52(2), 379-88.

[19] Hughes, T, Saglio, G, et al. (2009). Impact of baseline BCR-ABL mutations on response to nilotinib in patients with chronic myeloid leukemia in chronic phase." *J Clin Oncol* , 27(25), 4204-10.

[20] Jabbour, E, Cortes, J. E, et al. (2007). Current and emerging treatment options in chronic myeloid leukemia." *Cancer* , 109(11), 2171-81.

[21] Jabbour, E, Jones, D, et al. (2009). Long-term outcome of patients with chronic myeloid leukemia treated with second-generation tyrosine kinase inhibitors after imatinib failure is predicted by the in vitro sensitivity of BCR-ABL kinase domain mutations." *Blood* , 114(10), 2037-43.

[22] Jabbour, E, Kantarjian, H. M, et al. (2007). Chromosomal abnormalities in Philadelphia chromosome negative metaphases appearing during imatinib mesylate therapy in patients with newly diagnosed chronic myeloid leukemia in chronic phase." *Blood* , 110(8), 2991-5.

[23] Jabbour, E, Kantarjian, H. M, et al. (2009). Imatinib mesylate dose escalation is associated with durable responses in patients with chronic myeloid leukemia after cytogenetic failure on standard-dose imatinib therapy." *Blood* , 113(10), 2154-60.

[24] Kantarjian, H. M, Cortes, J, et al. (2010). Optimizing therapy for patients with chronic myelogenous leukemia in chronic phase." *Cancer* , 116(6), 1419-30.

[25] Kantarjian, H. M, Giles, F, et al. (2007). Nilotinib (formerly AMN107), a highly selective BCR-ABL tyrosine kinase inhibitor, is effective in patients with Philadelphia chromosome-positive chronic myelogenous leukemia in chronic phase following imatinib resistance and intolerance." *Blood* , 110(10), 3540-6.

[26] Kantarjian, H. M, Giles, F. J, et al. (2010). Nilotinib is effective in patients with chronic myeloid leukemia in chronic phase after imatinib resistance or intolerance: 24-month follow-up results." *Blood* , 117(4), 1141-5.

[27] Kantarjian, H. M, Brien, S. O, et al. (2003). Results of decitabine (5-aza-2'deoxycytidine) therapy in 130 patients with chronic myelogenous leukemia." *Cancer* , 98(3), 522-8.

[28] Kantarjian, H. M, Brien, S. O, et al. (2003). Imatinib mesylate therapy improves survival in patients with newly diagnosed Philadelphia chromosome-positive chronic myelogenous leukemia in the chronic phase: comparison with historic data." *Cancer* , 98(12), 2636-42.

[29] Lucas, C. M, Wang, L, et al. (2008). A population study of imatinib in chronic myeloid leukaemia demonstrates lower efficacy than in clinical trials." *Leukemia* , 22(10), 1963-6.

[30] Melo, J. V, & Chuah, C. (2008). Novel agents in CML therapy: tyrosine kinase inhibitors and beyond." *Hematology Am Soc Hematol Educ Program:* , 427-35.

[31] Moore, A. S, Blagg, J, et al. (2010). Aurora kinase inhibitors: novel small molecules with promising activity in acute myeloid and Philadelphia-positive leukemias." *Leukemia* , 24(4), 671-8.

[32] Hare, O, Eide, T. , C. A, et al. (2007). Bcr-Abl kinase domain mutations and the unsettled problem of Bcr-AblT315I: looking into the future of controlling drug resistance in chronic myeloid leukemia." *Clin Lymphoma Myeloma* 7 Suppl 3: S, 120-30.

[33] Olivieri, A, & Manzione, L. (2007). Dasatinib: a new step in molecular target therapy." *Ann Oncol* 18 Suppl 6: vi, 42-6.

[34] Quintas-cardama, A, Kim, T. D, et al. (2010). Nilotinib." *Recent Results Cancer Res* , 184, 103-17.

[35] Radich, J. P. (2007). The Biology of CML blast crisis." *Hematology Am Soc Hematol Educ Program:* , 384-91.

[36] Rosti, G, Palandri, F, et al. (2009). Nilotinib for the frontline treatment of Ph(+) chronic myeloid leukemia." *Blood* , 114(24), 4933-8.

[37] Roychowdhury, S, & Talpaz, M. (2011). Managing resistance in chronic myeloid leukemia." *Blood Rev* , 25(6), 279-90.

[38] Shah, N. P, Nicoll, J. M, et al. (2002). Multiple BCR-ABL kinase domain mutations confer polyclonal resistance to the tyrosine kinase inhibitor imatinib (STI571) in chronic phase and blast crisis chronic myeloid leukemia." *Cancer Cell* , 2(2), 117-25.

[39] Soverini, S, Martinelli, G, et al. (2005). ABL mutations in late chronic phase chronic myeloid leukemia patients with up-front cytogenetic resistance to imatinib are associated with a greater likelihood of progression to blast crisis and shorter survival: a study by the GIMEMA Working Party on Chronic Myeloid Leukemia." *J Clin Oncol* , 23(18), 4100-9.

[40] Steelman, L. S, Pohnert, S. C, et al. (2004). JAK/STAT, Raf/MEK/ERK, PI3K/Akt and BCR-ABL in cell cycle progression and leukemogenesis." *Leukemia* , 18(2), 189-218.

[41] Stoklosa, T, Poplawski, T, et al. (2008). BCR/ABL inhibits mismatch repair to protect from apoptosis and induce point mutations." *Cancer Res* , 68(8), 2576-80.

[42] Tanaka, R, Squires, M. S, et al. (2010). Activity of the multitargeted kinase inhibitor, AT9283, in imatinib-resistant BCR-ABL-positive leukemic cells." *Blood* , 116(12), 2089-95.

[43] Weisberg, E, Catley, L, et al. (2007). Beneficial effects of combining nilotinib and imatinib in preclinical models of BCR-ABL+ leukemias." *Blood* , 109(5), 2112-20.